# Incurable and Intolerable

# Incurable and Intolerable

## Chronic Disease and Slow Death in Nineteenth-Century France

JASON SZABO

RUTGERS UNIVERSITY PRESS

NEW BRUNSWICK, NEW JERSEY, AND LONDON

LIBRARY OF CONGRESS CATALOGING-IN-PUBLICATION DATA

Szabo, Jason, 1965–
  Incurable and intolerable : chronic disease and slow death in nineteenth-century France / Jason Szabo.
    p. ; cm.
  Includes bibliographical references and index.
  ISBN 978–0–8135–4545–5 (hardcover : alk. paper)
  I. Chronic diseases—France—History—19th century.   2. Palliative treatment—France—History—19th century.   I. Title.
  [DNLM:   I. Chronic Disease—psychology—France.   2. History of Medicine—France.   3. History, 19th Century—France.  WZ 70 GF7 S996i 2009]
  RA644.8.F8S93 2009
  616'.044—dc22                                                          2008035431

A British Cataloging-in-Publication record for this book is available from the British Library.

Visit our Web site: http://rutgerspress.rutgers.edu

Manufactured in the United States of America

To the memory of my parents

# CONTENTS

# ACKNOWLEDGMENTS

Many years went into writing this book, and during this time I have enjoyed the support of a large number of individuals and institutions. First and foremost, I'd like to thank my mentor George Weisz, whose vast knowledge and probing criticisms were a source of inspiration. His many kindnesses helped me see this project to the end.

I also want to thank my family for their love and support. Dominique Leydet helped me in countless ways as this project took shape. My daughters, Béatrice and Claire, have been a constant source of joy and wonder. My research trips and writing deadlines were a perennial distraction, and I hope that they agree that the final product was worth the time and effort.

Numerous friends, colleagues, and associates have also been tremendously helpful. My colleagues at the Montreal General Hospital—particularly Dr. Chris Tsoukas—consistently supported my endeavors, even when requests for protected time were anything but convenient. Diane Daoust, Gail Pucci, and Debbie Cutler generously helped out with all forms of technical assistance. At various points, Donna Evleth, Robbie Cutler, Annie-Claude Thériault, Marianne Di Croce, and Theresa Howard assisted me in amassing and cataloguing the many source documents. The staff at McGill's Osler library—Pamela Miller, Christopher Lyons, Lily Szczygiel, and Mary Dixon—always cheerfully responded to my queries. Deanna Cowan, Ingrid Dixon, and the other reference librarians did a remarkable job tracking down an array of nineteenth-century books and articles. Without their devoted efforts, it would have been impossible for me to complete this research.

I also benefited from the financial assistance of numerous funding agencies and foundations. These included the Social Sciences and Humanities Research Council, Associated Medical Services, the Canadian Institutes of Health Research, and the Montreal General Hospital Foundation. Two individuals in particular, William Seidelman and Ron Collett, generously supported my work as a physician and as a historian.

Various friends and colleagues have read all or parts of this book. James Vatistas, Sebastian Normandin, Thomas Schlich, and Alberto Cambrosio were important sounding boards as the book was taking shape and read early versions of the manuscript. I also benefitted from suggestions from the members of the history of medicine working group at Harvard University. Beyond providing an example of impeccable historical scholarship, my post-doc supervisor, Charles Rosenberg, provided helpful suggestions on several particularly thorny sections. And in an exemplary display of collegiality, Harry Marks and David Barnes generously read the manuscript on two separate occasions. Their criticisms were at once insightful and constructive, and they deserve much credit for helping me take this book to the next level.

I would also like to express my gratitude and affection to my friend and partner Andrea Tone. An accomplished historian and first-rate writer, she carefully read the entire book at a critical moment in its genesis. Her editing suggestions, along with those of Elke Kluge, Ann Youmans, and particularly my editor at Rutgers, Doreen Valentine, made it much stronger than it would otherwise have been. Her encouragement, along with that of the wonderful editorial group at Rutgers University Press, made finishing this project more enjoyable than I ever imagined.

Finally, I would like to thank my parents, John and Jeannette, neither of whom lived to see this book completed. Without their love and support, I would never have taken on a project such as this, and I dedicate this book to their memory.

# Incurable and Intolerable

# Introduction

It is extremely difficult to tell someone that their illness is incurable and that they are going to die. I know only too well, because I have had to do it often. I have spent my professional life treating chronically ill patients, most of whom were infected with the human immunodeficiency virus (HIV). Before the advent of effective antiretroviral drugs, a diagnosis of AIDS was essentially a death sentence. With little to offer them, I watched hundreds of people go on to die a slow and agonizing death. Most of them were my age, or slightly older. None of them wanted to die. In trying to help them, I realized that AIDS was, in many ways, particularly troubling. It was seen by many, including some of my colleagues, as a disease of homosexuals. As such, many were uncomfortable in the face of it. But everyone at my teaching hospital struggled with something even more basic: the knowledge that, no matter how hard we tried, the patient would eventually die. As time went on, I realized that incurability exerted a powerful effect on all of us—patients, families, and caregivers alike.

That prognosis could so profoundly influence people's attitudes and behaviors toward dying and death is hardly unique to our time. While working as a medical historian on the controversies surrounding the French healing shrine Lourdes, I encountered innumerable references to a group of individuals known as "the incurables" (*les incurables*). By the turn of the twentieth century, tens of thousands of incurably ill people traveled to the Pyrenees each year in the hope of being miraculously cured. Curious, I decided to find out who these people were. I wanted to learn more about their lives and their experiences.

Much of what I discovered surprised me. I learned, for example, that the term *incurable* was generally applied to a series of chronic diseases and only rarely to acute illnesses. Some of these disorders, including scrofula (tuberculosis of the lymph glands), are now quite uncommon in Western countries. Others, such as darters (a series of devastating skin conditions caused by, among other things, syphilis and tuberculosis), have disappeared. Phthisis or pulmonary tuberculosis, while relatively common, is no longer considered incurable. Certain conditions such as cancer and heart disease are, of course, still deadly today. Yet the range of illnesses our predecessors considered incurable was clearly different from the disorders that we now perceive as irremediable, such as end-stage cancer and amyotrophic-lateral sclerosis (also known as Lou Gehrig's disease).

Throughout the nineteenth century, no incurable illness rivaled tuberculosis, the undisputed captain of death. Various chronic disorders were almost as formidable, however. Severe gout and other forms of rheumatism crippled those it didn't kill; the afflicted were invalids in an era before the advent of mechanized transport and the comforts of central heating. Organic heart disease and advanced syphilis were also known to be harbingers of death. Cancer, then as now, was most people's worst nightmare. Many lives consumed by illness, countless others profoundly affected. Unfortunately, over time, these stories have been largely forgotten.

In trying to convey these disorders' far-ranging effects, I decided to focus on the strategies—individual and collective, substantive and rhetorical—that nineteenth-century French society employed to understand them and to deal with their effects. This involved sifting through a range of nineteenth-century sources and archives, a process that led me to question our understanding of important aspects of nineteenth-century life. It is, for instance, widely believed that acute illnesses were the dominant, or at least the most emblematic, illness experience of this era. The now taken-for-granted story, promulgated by demographers, clinicians, and historians alike, asserts that sometime around the turn of the twentieth century, the Western world witnessed a dramatic epidemiological shift as acute infectious diseases such as smallpox gave way to chronic degenerative ones such as cancer.[1] Acute illnesses, in other words, were the harrowingly lethal disorders that plagued the masses before the advent of sanitation, germ theory, and, of course, antibiotics.

Without denying the historical importance of infectious diseases, both the magnitude and the timing of this alleged transition was less clear cut than most scholars have recognized. Throughout the nineteenth century, at least in France, contemporaries referred to chronic disease in alarmist terms. In a work first published in 1808, one of the country's leading physicians, François-Joseph-Victor Broussais, was adamant that "even more fearsome than terrible epidemics, which appear only under certain circumstances, which can be seen coming, are feared, and fought with all the resources of the healing art, the causes of chronic afflictions are constantly active, are not susceptible to being interrupted, and they rarely let go of their victims prior to having sacrificed them: so that if we recapitulate the different types of death over a given period, we find that they have deprived the nation of more men than all other diseases put together."[2] Another practitioner, laboring in a poor Parisian neighborhood in the 1830s, similarly insisted that lingering illnesses caused the lion's share of suffering and death among those in his care.[3] This was not simply an urban phenomenon: stunted growth and chronic ill health were commonplace in smaller towns and villages.[4]

Mortality statistics confirm the accuracy of these observations. In 1847 and 1848, the various chronic diseases included under the heading of "organic lesions" killed almost four times as many Parisians as all acute infectious diseases combined.[5] Even in the infamous cholera year of 1865, the number of deaths that can be ascribed to chronic "constitutional illnesses" rivaled those caused by acute infectious diseases, including cholera.[6] Cancer alone was responsible for almost 3 percent of the deaths that year, a figure that would have underestimated both its annual incidence and relative demographic weight.[7] Cancer was also symbolically laden, both within medicine and society at large. For contemporaries, it conjured up images of unspeakable physical misery.

Foreshadowing concerns that currently frame discussions of public health, early historical surveys of disease ecology highlighted the rising importance of chronic degenerative diseases. In an article published in one of the leading medical journals of the 1830s, the influential German physician J.F.K. Hecker insisted that there had been a dramatic change in Europeans' physical constitutions since ancient times; while their predecessors had predominantly been afflicted with a "gouty" diathesis, manifested by severe gout and kidney stones, far more devastating disorders had taken center stage over time. Between the second and seventeenth centuries, leprosy, syphilis, and scurvy had been the leading constitutional illnesses. Since the early seventeenth, however, Europe lived under the shadow of a scrofulous diathesis, explaining the shockingly high incidence of scrofula, tuberculosis, and other "lymphatic" diseases, including cancer.[8] Several decades later, the author of an ambitious health primer concluded that the family of chronic illnesses known as the diatheses (flaws of one's constitution) dominated human pathology.[9]

Although it involved the repackaging of a concept dating back to ancient Greece, the idea that certain high-profile chronic diseases were caused by specific diatheses became a central tenet of Western medicine during the first half of the nineteenth century.[10] At once a pathological process and a group of morbid entities, such seemingly unrelated conditions as gout, scrofula, syphilis, tuberculosis, eczema, and cancer were all considered diathesic. To contemporaries, they constituted a coherent clinical cluster whose murky inner workings and devastating effects were a constant source of concern. Despite everyone's best efforts, each of them regularly caused horrifying disfigurement, intense pain, and humiliating infirmities. In their most severe form, they led to progressive wasting and slow death, an experience that we now refer to as terminal illness.

To say that the historical impact of chronic illness is more profound than generally imagined is not to suggest that patterns of disease haven't changed over the course of the last two centuries.[11] Certain degenerative disorders of the middle-aged and elderly (for example, cancer and coronary artery disease) are more widespread today that they were in the past, and many infectious ones have either disappeared or become increasingly peripheral, at least in the West. Yet the fact remains that chronic disease had a far greater demographic and cultural impact in the nineteenth century than we have previously realized.

Various factors have contributed to their subtle, but significant, marginalization. On one level, their historical obscurity reflects a longstanding collective blind spot among scholars studying illness and death. Notwithstanding the apparent "discovery" of chronic disease during the last century, organized medicine (and an earlier generation of medical historians) preferred to focus upon its successes and triumphs.[12] While important innovations, such as insulin and antibiotics, have been showpieces for twentieth-century medical science, society's struggles with chronic illness and the chronically ill have remained largely in the shadows. Viewed as an annoyance or worse, individuals who harbored these illnesses have generally been seen as uninteresting and burdensome, a source of frustration, not gratification. It was only in the 1980s, mirroring a growing critique of physicians' insensitivity toward the chronically ill, that scholars began suggesting that a fascination with sociomedical progress had distorted even the most sophisticated historical narratives.[13]

Unlike most chronic diseases, epidemics have been magnets for historical study of the changing nature of scientific knowledge and the culture that produced it.[14] One reason that epidemics have attracted such attention is that they were exceedingly visible, collective dramas. Their sudden appearance and disappearance, the scope of their devastation, and their frequent disregard for social distinctions ensured that they have been, and will remain, seminal events in our collective history. These same characteristics have also made them highly politicized; they raise probing questions about the organization of society even as they pressure authorities to provide explanations and solutions. In many ways, our longstanding interest in acute outbreaks of illness calls to mind our perennial fascination with revolutions and wars.

The failure to emphasize the significance of differing patterns of mortality has further obscured our understanding of the past. Infant mortality, driven primarily by acute infectious diseases, was very high during the nineteenth century. Yet people who had reached the age of reason—traditionally defined as age seven—more often succumbed to a chronic incurable illness. If one sets aside the earliest and most dangerous years of life (as contemporaries generally did when discussing mortality patterns), one appreciates why they too viewed degenerative diseases as society's greatest killers.

Equally important, if perhaps more elusive, is the distorting lens of changes in medical knowledge. A particularly telling example of such distortion is the way in which tuberculosis came to be reconfigured after the discovery of the tubercle bacillus. Almost overnight, the disease came to be viewed as an infectious rather than a chronic, progressive one. Just as the modern understanding of bubonic plague has affected this disorder's fate as historical object, early histories of consumption betray a characteristic bias.[15] Until relatively recently, the triumph of the bacteriological paradigm over earlier "misguided" ideas about tuberculosis, and the way that scientific truth allowed for the development of curative treatments to replace quaint traditional ones, remained the dominant storyline.[16] Furthermore, a long-standing tendency to speak of tuberculosis in the same breath as a variety of acute, epidemic diseases makes it easy to forget that contemporaries viewed consumption—the leading single cause of death during the nineteenth century—as the close cousin of cancer, not measles.[17]

Incurables illnesses' dramatic effects on nineteenth-century patterns of behavior led me to question another deeply embedded assumption: the belief that our forebears had a much better rapport with suffering and death. The prevailing image of death from this period is of a dignified and peaceful passing, surrounded by devoted and caring loved ones. "Bad deaths," marked by loneliness and alienation, are viewed as a quintessentially late-modern phenomenon. The French historian Phillipe Ariès played a critical role in legitimizing this "Paradise Lost" narrative. In his influential study of Western attitudes toward mortality, Ariès insisted that traditional societies had a far more wholesome attitude toward death. Situation-specific rituals and norms ensured that the dying process was both edifying and natural. His second, related assumption was that good deaths became increasingly uncommon in the late nineteenth century, as doctors and hospitals increasingly took center stage. Rather than dying at home as they had for centuries, people increasingly died in the hospital in the care of strangers.[18] Technological and technocratic, death became taboo. The emergence of an ultramodern, cure-at-all-costs mentality in the twentieth century ensured that the dying were either ignored or lived out their days tied to a machine. Ariès's vision of history is so pervasive that even scholars who have sought to refine his work assume that physicians progressively took control over or "medicalized" death, to the detriment of all.

This tendency to romanticize "simpler times" is ubiquitous. Some, like the best-selling author Elizabeth Kübler-Ross, drew inspiration from childhood memories. Others went further back in time. The founder of the modern hospice movement, Dame Cicely Saunders, glorified the eponymous medieval institutions. In her mind, these refuges for sick and dying pilgrims exemplified good terminal care: devout Christians addressing the physical and spiritual needs of those on their final journey. In a telling gesture, the pioneering thanatologist Herman Feifel concluded the updated version (1977) of his highly influential *The Meaning of Death* with the statement: "man of the late Middle-Ages and early Renaissance participated in his own death. It is fitting that we in the late twentieth century recapture our sovereignty over death and, hence, life. In responding to our temporality, we shall find it easier to define values, priorities, and life goals, and move toward a more common sharing of our humanity—all too eroded in the present world."[19] Together, these and other authorities have cemented the belief that previous generations dealt with the physical, social, and emotional consequences of terminal illness in a way that merits both praise and emulation.

My own research leaves me skeptical of what I've come to see as a falsely idealized image of the past. Indeed, one of the major problems incurables faced throughout the nineteenth century was that they weren't medicalized enough, or at least not in ways compatible with their interests. To some extent, the problem was technological; the range of remedies available to cure and palliate chronic disease was limited. Medicine's technical limitations are only part of the story, however. Personal concerns and an array of sociopolitical factors encouraged the neglect of those whom science deemed beyond hope. The net result of these and other sociomedical forces was a degree of suffering and alienation that was more pathetic than praiseworthy.

In all fairness, we already have some idea of the impact of incurable illness during this period. Nineteenth-century American diaries and letters give a sense of the devastating personal consequences of consumption, a disease long associated with progressive debility and death.[20] American women's struggles with breast cancer were, if anything, even more baleful.[21] French consumptives, both before and after the discovery of the tubercle bacillus, of course fared no better than their American counterparts. Yet despite the horrors of illness, many sufferers struggled to find something redeeming about their experiences.[22] The history of the shrine at Lourdes makes this abundantly clear even as it provides a unique vantage point onto contemporary responses to severe physical and existential adversity.[23]

Building upon these precedents, this book aims to paint a picture of the emotional, medical, and institutional universe of the incurably ill. The stricken turned to many individuals and institutions in a desperate search for succor, leaving behind a compelling glimpse of their struggle. This was at once a highly intimate, emotionally charged, yet crowded social space. Consider, for example, the case of Mme. Louis, a young widow and mother of three. A shining example of upward social mobility, she nonetheless died penniless in 1843 after a valiant struggle with cancer. Echoes of the last year of her life come to us from a Parisian notable, Antoine Vée, who described how

> she was obliged to send away all her workers, and fought for six months courtesy of her own resources; all her savings being exhausted, her possessions either sold or hawked, she turned to us; she could have been received in a hospice, but that would have involved abandoning her children. . . . It is not without the most heartfelt of emotions that we learned that the day before she died, prey to the cruelest suffering, Mme Louis was still directing her cherished little ones, and tried to weave together a few [tresses] of straw, with her failing hands, to bring in a bit of money. How often is Paris not witness to painful scenes such as this?[24]

While Mme. Louis may or may not have known how fortunate she was by the standards of the day, her story was otherwise depressingly typical.[25]

Despite a plurality of voices, acquiring a clear picture of people's response to their predicament has proven more methodologically difficult, and ultimately more rewarding, than I had at first assumed. Finding allusions to incurability and the plight of incurables involved considerable detective work; for contemporaries, these were unappealing topics of discussion. The observations, feelings, discourses, and practices of those drawn into this netherworld are the evidentiary fragments that I relied upon to recreate this social world. Varying in length and content, they generally took one of three forms: discussions of the science of chronic progressive disease, observations about the experiences of the incurably ill, and fleeting-yet-heartfelt expressions of admiration, affection, discomfort, indifference, or guilt.

A series of letters describing patients' struggles to find relief and to come to terms with their experience proved particularly invaluable. One set of correspondences—upwards of six hundred letters written in the 1860s by members of a Catholic confraternity—provided important insights into the illness and death experiences of a broad cross-section of the population.[26] These and several other smaller collections were not only rich and at times highly personal but also provided an empirical anchor against which the observations and claims of others could be compared. Taken together, the wide-ranging discussions of chronic progressive disease offer a unique and poignant perspective on a country's scientific, social, and moral landscape.

Focusing on a concept (*incurability*) and a label (*incurable*) rather than a single disease draws attention to these disorders' most noteworthy feature: they were often progressively fatal and almost always associated with severe suffering. The torments of incurable illness are particularly rich in insights because of the difficulties and dilemmas they (ex)posed; they were exceedingly complex entities (scientifically, personally, socially) that left few untouched or indifferent.[27]

Ultimately, the experience of "being incurable" is best understood as the product of an intricate series of negotiations and interactions among various social actors—patients, families, physicians, alternative healers, religious and political authorities—each with his or her own agenda and challenges. Culturally specific and historically contingent factors, in turn, shaped how all concerned behaved in the face of chronic progressive disease.[28]

For physicians, the boundaries and meanings of incurability were inseparable from the all-important issue of medical prognostication. A series of competing theories sought to explain how, when, and why specific chronic diseases reached a point of no return. In retrospect, the most stable element in medicine's understanding of incurability was that it reflected a state of advanced, irreversible organ destruction or dysfunction; it was thus synonymous with certain specific diagnoses (for example, inoperable cancer, advanced tuberculosis, and degenerative neurological disorders). Despite broad areas of consensus, the science of incurability was consistently troubling and divisive. For various reasons, successive generations of French physicians disagreed over the prognosis and principal causes of the two most socially prominent incurable diseases, cancer and tuberculosis. Some optimistically asserted that they were easily cured; others saw them as all but inherently incurable, the product of an irreversible and inexorably fatal constitutional flaw. Amid all the noteworthy developments in late nineteenth-century medical science, the delineation of the true trajectory of these disorders, treated and untreated, remained contested.

Few of those involved were unaware of the scientific and social significance of these discussions. Given that medicine was a low-status profession that lacked credibility, explaining and justifying therapeutic impotence was a critically important exercise in damage control. Helplessness in the face of certain high-profile chronic diseases, in other words, was bad enough. Admitting ignorance as to their root causes would have been unthinkable. One perceptive practitioner put his finger on what was at stake, observing that "it is already compromising enough for the reputation of our science that there exists illnesses that it cannot cure, without being forced to acknowledge that we are unable to prevent them as well."[29] Being able credibly to explain their genesis allowed physicians to conserve one of their more coveted social and professional roles, providing advice to the "worried well."

For patients, the question "what is to become of me?" was inevitably tied up with another equally weighty concern—"why me?" As the century progressed, doctors increasingly concurred that some combination of nature and nurture generated a fatal flaw in the chronically ill. Particularly in the case of the diatheses, most efforts at deciphering chronic illnesses' hygienic, social, and moral messages cast aspersions on the integrity of the stricken.[30] Increasingly, the scientists and social commentators who joined the debate agreed that chronic progressive illnesses were special in the worst of ways. Environmental influences, so critical to the development of acute illnesses, could not by themselves account for chronic illnesses' complex phenomenology. Many, if not most, diatheses appeared to run in families. Their notorious resistance to what were seen as otherwise efficacious therapies also suggested that the patient's body, not the doctors' remedies, was the main problem. In 1875, a respected clinician whose pioneering observations on the vascular system have stood the test of time observed how

> if it is true that, in the greatest number of illnesses, we notice, to different degrees and in unequal measure, a remnant of a beneficial reaction, there are unfortunately some wherein it is impossible to identify any, and in which the disease imperturbably follows its fatal course from beginning until end. . . . Now, one may take note, where are these examples taken from? Do they arise from the sudden shocks of outside agents, that in a sense strike down the organism and allow it neither the time nor the option of reacting? No, I borrow them precisely from the realm of chronic diseases, in which all external impulsions escape us, illnesses that are created and conceived out of nothing [*de toutes pièces*] in the depths of nutritive life, illnesses in which the organism seems to draw from its own core all the elements of the pathological evolution, and to work, with a regularity that confounds us, toward its own annihilation.[31]

In societies preoccupied by violence, disorder, and vice, the dominant illness paradigm played to the interests of the upright and the affluent (provided they remained healthy); they could sleep easily knowing that virtue was generally rewarded in this life as well as the next. Similarly, by emphasizing that most people brought incurability upon themselves, an increasingly insecure group of elites could insist that a program of individual self-improvement (or selective breeding), rather than the overturn of industrial capitalism, held the key to a brighter, healthier future.

Enjoying a degree of social visibility rivaled only by cholera and smallpox, the deadliest diatheses similarly mirrored and reinforced prevailing cultural assumptions and norms. In other words, if epidemics sporadically carried off those predisposed by misery, vice, and poverty, then scrofula, cancer, and tuberculosis offered a constant reminder of the dangers of social transgression. Strikingly, even as older ideas about individual "essences" were superseded by bacteriological science, etiological discussions of tuberculosis remained deeply moralizing.[32] In the second half of the nineteenth century, well-worn concerns about the perils of biological and behavioral *laissez-faire* emerged as central elements in an increasingly codified and coherent ideology. In societies in which ideas of natural selection, degeneration, and contagion were common currency, incurables were increasingly seen as a biological fifth column, a leading threat to national vitality.

Admittedly, several prominent counternarratives of illness existed alongside these alarmist and accusatory ones. The best known and longest lasting of these was the Romantic myth of tuberculosis. Notwithstanding its triumphalism, there is reason to believe that this soothing narrative was more a rearguard action on the part of those with an interest, and the wherewithal, to "tell their own story." The existence of competing disease representations certainly raises the interesting issue of the links between poetics, self-perception, and illness experiences. They also beg the equally important question: why have specific terminal illnesses consistently enjoyed such unique evocative power?

Contemporaries' understanding of what was wrong with incurables had important, though not necessarily consistent, effects on their care. Physicians, in fact, exhibited complex and often contradictory attitudes toward the stricken. Acutely conscious of both the perils and the opportunities involved, doctors were often unenthusiastic helpmates. When they did take on the task, however, they always sought to set the terms of engagement.

Invariably, the preferred mise-en-scène was a carefully scripted affair in which patients were told as little as possible. Doctors employed many ruses to control the flow of diagnostic and prognostic information. Hopeful ambiguity, in many ways, was simply a question of prudence; medicine's limited diagnostic and prognostic accuracy, most contemporary physicians reasoned, made it preferable to "do everything" while hoping for the best. Besides, it was assumed to be counterproductive, even dangerous, to share dark secrets. In an unusually open marketplace, frankness and nihilism also appear to have been bad for business. A series of scientific assumptions and powerful social forces reduced the interpersonal dynamics between doctors and incurables to the axiom: "I won't ask, you won't tell, and the illness will speak for itself." Uncertainty, in this setting, was a lonely ray of hope in a gray sky.

One of the clearest outgrowths of such carefully cultivated ambiguity was rampant medical consumerism. As often as not, incurables turned to various healers and healing systems—simultaneously. New means of communication and transportation permitted the ever-widening dissemination of both people and information. In their many peregrinations, patients and families continued to cling to a set of intertwined beliefs. The first was that, despite appearances to the contrary, nature was essentially beneficent. The second, ironically, reflected an ongoing faith in human (or in some instances divine) agency. Many wanted to believe that finding a cure simply involved taking matters in one's own hands and making the right choice(s). Depending upon their personality, belief structure, stage of illness, and disposable income, patients engaged in a desperate search for the right doctor, the right medicine, the right vacation spot, the right mineral water, or, when things got really bad, a suitable saint or shrine.

At a stage when an illness's malign nature and distressing prognosis left few doubts, people struggled with the realization that their case was now hopeless. More than one rediscovered religion or redoubled their faith. Certain committed freethinkers, on the other hand, made a point of rejecting the Church and its rituals. Some particularly unfortunate individuals, horribly disfigured or broken by suffering, withdrew into mute despair or ended their own lives.[33]

As incurables' needs became more pressing, a striking discrepancy often emerged between physicians' discourse and behavior. Although few practitioners denied the importance of palliating suffering, many distanced themselves from incurables or withdrew altogether. Although by all accounts commonplace, such "abandonment" was always morally dubious in a society that viewed incurable illness as a trial of one's worth. Free to choose, many physicians took the path of least resistance. They had their reasons, some selfish, some perfectly understandable. More than anything, the specter of severe suffering over which they had little sway encouraged them to conclude that there was "nothing they could do."

Obviously, not all incurables ran equal risks of finding themselves neglected and ignored. From start to finish, the prospects of the poor were singularly grim. It was common knowledge that chronic disease disproportionately attacked those who could afford it least; their prognosis was correspondingly dismal. To add insult to injury, extreme poverty placed even the most basic comforts out of reach. The ensuing misery was one of the more depressing leitmotifs of the nineteenth century, shocking all those who took the time and effort to notice. This is not to say that those who could afford the best of everything had an easy time of it. Terminal cancer is painful even in silk sheets. Middle- and upper-class incurables would also have felt the effects of prevailing attitudes toward the proper and appropriate use of narcotics, an issue that, by the late nineteenth century, had emerged as a leading ethical dilemma in both France and the Anglo-Saxon world.

Hypodermic morphine emerged as a Janus-faced symbol of the promise and the peril of modern pharmacology. Broadly speaking, pressing socio-political concerns shaped responses to local and national drug problems. At an individual level, technology, social norms, and illness also interacted in fascinating ways. "Addiction" among the chronically ill played a critical role in the framing of so-called morphine mania. A growing fear of the drug, in turn, had important effects on physicians' behavior. The outcome of doctors' negotiations with those who could legitimately claim that they "had to have" their injection can only be understood within a broader normative frame-work, one informed by assumptions around what it meant to be a "good patient" who had died a "good death."

For all its religious overtones, this was not a single-constituency issue. There existed a strikingly broad consensus around what it meant to be a good incurable; lucidity, stoicism, and self-control were celebrated by bishop and freethinker alike. A conviction that certain cherished ideals should inform one's final illness performance partly explains why freethink-ing physicians and Catholic moralists were of a like mind when it came to morphine. Increasingly acknowledged as the experts on all questions of behavior, physicians confidently asserted that they alone could judge when a patient truly needed narcotics. A combination of high-minded ideals, fin-de-siècle anxieties, and the vagaries of human physiology together set the stage for the emergence of a striking consensus: only "unacceptable" suffer-ing justified recourse to the Pravaz syringe.

By century's end, morphine mania was arguably the most visible prob-lem associated with the care of the incurably ill. The most intractable was the strain that poverty-stricken incurables placed on contemporary chari-table institutions, particularly hospitals. Only too often, incurables were ready, even eager, to seek refuge far from home. The sources of this medical institution's drawing power were varied and complex; suffice it to say that patients and families often saw this as the lesser evil. In response to these demands, decision makers struggled to find a cost-effective system to deal with the problem of incurable illness. No one denied that these disorders had devastating physical and social consequences, or flatly rejected that, at least in principle, something had to be done. Yet in France, none of the country's institutions—the hospital system, the Catholic Church, or the state—proved up to the task.

Despite much pious self-examination, nineteenth-century decision makers generally focused their energies and attention elsewhere. In the immediate post-Revolutionary decades, hospital reform had been a primary concern. Inspired by the conviction that hospital beds should be the exclu-sive preserve of "patients," the social and medical elite decided that those who were merely destitute would henceforth have to turn elsewhere. With the benefit of hindsight, historians justly view this as a critical step in the hospital's progressive medicalization. Yet most have ignored one of the more striking paradoxes of contemporary administrative logic. For even as efforts were being made to keep the able-bodied out of these increasingly high-profile institutions, an elaborate system was also put in place to exclude some of the sickest people of all, those deemed hopeless.

This policy was based upon a series of interconnected arguments: incurables were depressing, scientifically uninspiring, and a waste of time and money. In the end, patients for whom there was "nothing left to be done" were subjected to a critically important category shift: they went from being a medical to a social problem. Equally significant, in all social policy discussions, incurables were inevitably lumped together with the elderly and the disabled. This ragtag community of hospice cases found themselves confined to a parallel universe in which the law of diminishing returns was ruthlessly applied; they competed for the meager crumbs that successive administrations spent on hospice relief during the nineteenth century.

An increasingly militant left-wing government eventually launched a comprehensive assault on the charitable status quo. Invoking certain Revolutionary ideals, radical republicans and socialists stressed that patients and hospice cases had a right to assistance; society, they increasingly asserted, also had a duty to provide for those incapable of earning their keep. A partial solution to the hospice problem was finally put in place in 1905 with the passage of a law guaranteeing the elderly, invalids, and incurables a modest pension for life.

Beyond bringing a fresh perspective to some well-worn issues—the cultural meaning and representation of illness, the history of charity, hospitals, and opiates—this work ventures into terra incognita. It embraces the messy world of nineteenth-century prognostics, motivated at least in part by a desire to understand the effects of this proprietary knowledge on the healing encounter. In taking up the art and science of palliative medicine, it helps us better understand a complex social system and nettlesome doctor-patient relationship. Finally, incurable illness illustrates the important role that, then as now, an idealized vision of a "good death" played in shaping attitudes and behaviors.

Although this study focuses primarily on nineteenth-century France, what it says about the human condition largely transcends questions of time and place. I have attempted to balance the issue of historic and cultural specificity with the recognition that certain attitudes, practices, and preoccupations cut across centuries, continents, and cultures. There are other histories of incurability waiting to be written whose details will vary as a function of local dynamics and changing circumstances. Yet many of the most important themes explored in this book—futility, uncertainty, shame, and spirituality, to name but a few—are as unavoidable as they are instructive. Nineteenth-century responses to severe adversity can and should inform our present-day efforts to deal constructively with chronic disease and terminal illness.

It should also be remembered that Paris was the Mecca of Western medicine for much of the modern period, and the teaching and research carried out there had lasting repercussions, particularly in the United States.[34] France's sophisticated theorists, quarrelsome practitioners, and scrupulous civil servants left behind a wealth of fascinating material on chronic progressive disease. The Parisian hospital system's highly revealing policies toward and experiences with incurables are also amply if elusively documented. Equally important, the awkward combination of traditionalism and dynamism typical of this period allows for an appreciation of the ways in which the illness experience was transformed by, yet transcended, technological, social, and political change. The country's deep social and ideological divisions underscore the less-than-predictable effects of contemporary identity politics. Finally, much of what we know about the history of Western attitudes toward death and dying was written by French historians using (primarily) French material. Their observations and claims are invaluable to the study of one of the principal antechambers of death.

While taking up a few of the issues that have been explored by historians working in the field of death studies, this book is less concerned with death and its rituals per se and seeks instead to decipher the immediate impact and broader cultural significance of a complex illness experience. In the process, it looks anew at the role of Catholicism in the care of the incurably ill. Religious faith was one of the few things that allowed people to overcome their aversion to suffering; dying and death also remained an appealing niche for an increasingly beleaguered institution. For the stricken and their families, the Church's rituals and doctrines were an important source of solace, primarily because they offered a measure of redemption commensurate to their suffering.

Focusing on the history of medicine, this work also adds its voice to a small but important current in cultural history that examines the fascinating interplay between religion, spirituality, politics, and illness.[35] In asking the question "how does a specific medical, sociopolitical, and religious environment affect people's response to chronic disease and terminal illness?" this book attempts to understand patients and caregivers on their own terms. Deciphering the complex rules, motives, and instincts that guided them will, I hope, help us better understand both our past and ourselves.

# 1

# "What Are His Chances, Doctor?"

## The Semantics of Incurability in the Nineteenth Century

When patients nowadays go to a physician, the questions uppermost in their minds are usually "What's going on?" and "Is it serious?" In responding to the latter, physicians have increasingly relied on prognostic templates that presuppose that each disease has a distinct natural history. These outcome models, in turn, decisively shape doctors' attitudes and management strategies. With self-limited or comparably benign diseases, the information exchange tends to be straightforward; physicians offer reassurance, encouragement, and suggestions for hastening recovery. When they suspect a progressive and incurable illness, physicians find "being in the know" extremely problematic.

While incurable illnesses have always had dramatic personal and social repercussions, our understanding of the label "incurable" has shifted over time. In the nineteenth century, a number of disorders and disabilities were granted this dubious distinction, but cancer and tuberculosis stood out. Their true prognosis was the subject of recurrent and often heated debate, as physicians argued about many aspects of these disorders' biology. The issue of whether they were, in fact, incurable was consistently the most troubling question of all.

Depending on how you asked the question, the answer varied. The form and content of French debates are noteworthy for several reasons. For much of the nineteenth century, France was the epicenter of empirical, scientific medicine. It was also a cauldron of social conflict and political change, pervaded by hopes and fears surrounding the notion of progress. For these reasons, perhaps, no other country illustrates the intricacies of medical prognostication quite as vividly. At the same time, the arguments exposed here offer unique insights into the contested process by which our Western, illness-specific, prognostic science emerged.

These exchanges also merit careful consideration in that a diagnosis of incurable had dramatic material consequences. It largely determined what was said and not said, done and not done, structuring both entitlements and prohibitions. These debates also illustrate the impact of various factors—objective and subjective, clinical and extraclinical, substantive and rhetorical—on medical reasoning. In the face of complex, even contradictory evidence, doctors' assumptions about the "nature of Nature" and skepticism regarding medicine's diagnostic and therapeutic limits determined their opinion of cancer and tuberculosis's incurability.[1] For most of this period, prominent practitioners were said to espouse extreme views, from starry-eyed optimism to dour pessimism. With the benefit of hindsight, we can see that the situation was much more complicated. For one, contemporary physicians distinguished between several different forms of incurability: natural, medical, and surgical. They also tended to use the word "cure" quite liberally. Together, these factors ensured that most doctors' prognostic pronouncements were nuanced rather than polarized, calling to mind their handling of other more visible controversies.[2]

## Defining Incurable

Though it was vitally important to patients and physicians, few elite doctors explicitly addressed the issue of incurability. In the only book-length analysis, an aspiring academic physician, Dr. A. Jaumes, wrote in 1848 that doctors' silence on this matter reflected their reluctance to talk about their failures.[3] Various sources make it possible to verify his observations, notwithstanding doctors' rhetorical reluctance. Nearly all learned studies of chronic disease(s) briefly examined when, how, and why patients came to be incurable. Because spas and thermal stations became beacons for the hopelessly ill,[4] hydrotherapists also left behind a wealth of information, including their opinions about who would or would not benefit from "taking the waters." Then there are the writings of alternative healers, licensed and unlicensed. In a genre that proliferated after 1830, these "irregulars" discussed the various incurable diseases over which their panaceas supposedly triumphed. Together, these works allow us to reconstruct contemporaries' use of the term incurable while exposing the framework that underpinned medical prognostication.[5]

In administrative circles, incurables were those whose affliction caused complete and permanent disability. It was common knowledge that various diseases and deformities were incapacitating and that therefore might merit special consideration. An 1830 text that outlined of the workings of the Parisian charitable system catalogued an exhaustive inventory of incurable conditions:

General tremors. Rheumatismal invalidity, gouty or secondary to luxation. Incurable paralysis, complete or incomplete. Urinary or faecal incontinence. Cardiac aneurysm or one involving the great vessels. Chronic or suffocating asthma. Encysted dropsy. Rickets, deformation of the chest, the pelvis, or the limbs. Incurable erosive dartres. Repulsive deformities or those that render a person incapable of working. Large hernias that are impossible to contain. Loss of a limb. Complete deafness. Deaf-mutism. Idiocy. Epilepsy. Incurable cancer. Complete and incurable blindness, or vision so diminished that the indigent is unable to work.[6]

Phthisis's absence from this list is particularly noteworthy. Several considerations presumably explain its omission. Medical opinion was divided over its prognosis, and many with early-stage disease were still able to work. Equally important, many people were concerned about the social and political repercussions of officially acknowledging its incurability. Public charity couldn't meet existing demands, let alone see to the needs of an army of incurable consumptives. An otherwise inclusive vision of chronic disease, attuned to their socio-occupational consequences, thus patently omitted the most ubiquitous "incurable" disorder.

Though a few acute illnesses such as rabies and meningitis were judged incurable, the term was typically reserved for chronic diseases causing severe distress or involving vital organs.[7] Not all chronic diseases were created or considered equal; those that produced visible anatomical lesions were understood to be particularly grave. The links between visibility—both in the clinic and at autopsy—and prognosis were central and decisive. In 1854, Napoleon III's personal physician, Dr. Louis Fleury, observed that the German inventor of a popular form of hydrotherapy, Vincenz Priessnitz, eventually spurned anyone suffering from "organic diseases" (that is, those with anatomical changes). Immediately after, Fleury cited a French pioneer for whom only pulmonary phthisis and cancer were absolute contraindications to hydrotherapy.[8] Two decades later, another noted hydrotherapist similarly stressed that, unlike most other chronic diseases, therapeutic waters could at most only prevent cancer and tuberculosis and not cure them once the disease had taken hold. Consistent with contemporary opinion, Dr. Joseph Beni-Barde explained that "the therapeutic effect is that much more considerable when the modified tissues deviate as little as possible from normal."[9]

In addition to cataloguing available treatments, Dr. Jaumes's commentary had a more ambitious goal: to describe and decode the complex behavior of chronic illness. Strikingly, his work began with a lofty statement of principle: no disease was inherently and inevitably incurable. Soon after,

however, he referred to a series of disorders that "show themselves to ordinarily be incurable" and that he termed "reputedly incurable."[10] Though this
latter moniker was much older, it became increasingly prominent between
1830 and 1880, when it was clearly part of the lay vernacular.[11] The source of
its appeal is obvious. It recognized common knowledge while avoiding rigid
and unpalatable dogmatism.

Jaumes's classification scheme subdivided incurable disorders on the
basis of their clinical trajectory. "Absolutely incurable" diseases were those
that were generally considered incurable at the time of diagnosis. They
included general paresis, true angina pectoris, cancer, phthisis, and pella-
gra along with less ominous disorders that became increasingly intractable
over time: strokes, asthma, hypochondria, hysteria, and inflammations
of vital organs such as the heart. The least incurable chronic diseases—
dropsy, rheumatism, and scrofula—were "relatively incurable." Their prognosis varied as a function of the patient's age, heredity, and the disease's
anatomical location.[12]

Incurability was thus at once malleable, inclusive, and relative. Stroke,
for example, was an acute and potentially reversible event. At some point,
however, the patient and his disorder were incurable. Yet the term also
conjured up images of lethality; Jaumes noted that "primitive, relative incurabilities [sic], like absolute incurabilities, are followed soon after by death."[13]
But not all chronic disorders were fatal, and the label incurable tended to be
reserved for illnesses we now call terminal.[14] For most of the century, the
same four or five disorders—cancer, epilepsy, general paralysis, tuberculosis,
and (sometimes) scrofula—were on doctors' and laypeople's list of incurable
scourges. Late in the century, these same disorders remained on everyone's
list.[15]

Most were part of a frightening family of disorders known as the diatheses. On the surface, this was a bewilderingly diverse—to the modern eye—
array of disorders that included gout/rheumatism, syphilis, darters/eczema,
scrofula, scurvy, tuberculosis, cancer, and rickets.[16] Contemporaries, however, perceived affinities: each was associated with a unique, highly specific,
morbid product (produit morbide) capable of attacking most organs in the
body. To varying degrees, they all caused disability, disfigurement, and
severe suffering. They were also singularly tenacious, "chronic illnesses to
the highest degree."[17] Worst of all, they were extremely treatment-resistant,
with prognoses ranging from poor to desolate. If one considers only the
deadliest ones, syphilis had the best prognosis and (hereditary) cancer the
worst.[18] Scrofula, while exceedingly serious, fell in between. Summing up
contemporary views, a mid-century authority on chronic disease noted that
"scrofula, by the fact alone that it is a diathesis, is a grave illness: no matter how mild its present manifestations, it demands to always be watched

very closely, because it always leaves the subject under the threat of more worrisome lesions. All the same, its prognosis cannot be compared to that of tuberculosis and cancer; and, among the diathesic afflictions, scrofula is certainly one where it is the easiest, if not to obtain a cure, to at least erase the manifestations."[19] Although heredity generally figured prominently, it was understood that the prognosis of reputedly incurable illnesses reflected both biological and social factors, including the severity and stage of illness as well as the patient's age and occupation.[20]

Contemporaries' fascination with the diatheses partly reflected demographics—they were all depressingly common among both rich and poor. The most serious of them caught people's attention because they were terrifying to behold. Death appeared both methodical and predictable. General paresis, epilepsy, and cancer were particularly fearsome as there were no credible cases of spontaneous recovery. They confronted everyone with an almost unthinkable idea: "Nature" had created diseases without providing a cure. The many similarities between cancer and phthisis also forced contemporaries to consider the distressing "what if" scenario forcefully articulated at the dawn of modern scientific medicine: what if phthisis's prognosis was actually as bleak as that of cancer?[21]

## Chronic Disease before 1840: Dueling Ideas and Disappointed Optimism

In the early nineteenth century, a group of Parisian doctors assiduously compiled case studies and performed postmortems in an effort to better understand disease. It was a dreary routine, which they themselves described as a "painful career."[22] In a country raw from the ravages of the Revolutionary and Napoleonic wars, they ministered to the sick poor, many of whom were mortally stricken with chronic progressive disease. Phthisis, the leading cause of death at the time, understandably caught their attention. Cancer, while less common, was typically brought up in the next breath. Two important figures in the history of medicine, Gaspard Bayle and René Laënnec, placed these disorders in a separate disease category because of their unnatural, "heteromorphic" lesions.[23] Partly on the basis of this precedent, cancer and phthisis remained conceptually distinct for almost a century.

Their importance to the development and triumph of the anatomico-pathological method must not be underestimated. These diseases shared two features that demonstrated this technique's power at unraveling the mysteries of illness. They had dramatic and relatively consistent natural histories; they also left physical lesions readily discernible at autopsy. These disorders made sense, pathologically speaking, legitimizing this approach to understanding the body.

Despite pathological anatomy's professional cachet, the scrupulous cataloguing of these disorders' physical ravages left many anatomists deeply unsettled. Laënnec, for example, wrote that

> before the features and development of tubercles were well known . . . physicians no more than the public had any doubts as to the possibility of curing the disorder with the proper treatment, especially when one had caught it *in time*, when the illness was still in *its first stage*. All physicians who are abreast of the recent progress in pathological anatomy today think, on the contrary, that tubercular disorders, like cancerous ones, are absolutely incurable, because nature only makes efforts that are contrary to this goal, and medicine makes only useless ones.[24]

For many, the advent of microscopic diagnosis in the 1840s irrefutably established the incurability of cancer, as doctors could now distinguish the benign tumors that had previously misled everyone.[25] Unfortunately, as medicine's diagnostic accuracy increased, proven cures of phthisis and cancer declined both dramatically and proportionally. Albeit counterintuitive today, scientific progress tended to sow despair rather than optimism until after mid-century.

By the late 1830s, prognostic discussions had a desperate tone. In a landmark essay from 1839, Dr. C. Rogée noted that most colleagues believed that phthisis was "more or less incurable." Even though this went against established wisdom, he hoped that newly emerging anatomical evidence of healed tubercles would change perceptions.[26] Marshalling available evidence, the English physician James Turnbull wrote a lengthy defense of consumption's curability a decade later (1850). He knew he had his work cut out since "the profession, as well as the public, have been so strongly impressed with the belief that the disease is necessarily fatal, that anyone who would have maintained the opposite would, until very recently, have been looked upon only in the light of a boasting pretender."[27] A few years later, a prominent French colleague explicitly blamed the anatomico-pathologists for fostering such pessimism.[28] Angered by the widespread conviction that they never cured phthisis, the author of an award-winning essay insisted in 1858 that "the words *never* and *always* should be banished from the language of medicine. Examples of a cure, for all their rarity, their excessive rarity, one in a thousand, one in ten thousand or more, exist all the same."[29]

The era's other leading incurable illness, cancer, was even more despair inducing. Augustin Grisolle was an experienced clinician and respected pathologist who went on to be president of the Academy of Medicine. In an observation repeated in the various editions of his highly regarded treatise on pathology, he observed that the disease's end result was always the same:

death. Successful outcomes were so rare, he insisted, that most practitioners would never see one during their lifetime.[30]

It bears mentioning that defeatism became the norm despite the fact that, from 1819 on, no one claimed that phthisis was naturally and inherently incurable. Even in the case of cancer, there were pockets of optimism, as evidenced by the brouhaha surrounding the Lyon Academy of Medicine's decision to award its annual prize in 1835 to Dr. Pierre Teallier. Teallier's book on uterine cancer was categorical: doctors had no idea what caused this inherently incurable disorder. Their advice about prevention, in other words, was both specious and presumptuous. Several members of the Academy rose in protest and successfully passed a motion distancing themselves from the author's opinions.[31] Similarly divisive discussions erupted twenty years later at Paris's Academy of Medicine, pitting defenders of cancer's surgical curability against an entrenched group of skeptics.

The dreary consensus that had emerged by the middle of the nineteenth century was actually the product of decades of heated disagreement. During much of this period, two competing discourses vied for adherents. By way of useful simplification, one could say that people gravitated toward one of two distinct ideologies, localism and constitutionalism. Localists believed in the local origin and relative lack of specificity of cancer and tuberculosis. Constitutionalists considered them unique and distinct from other diseases. "Diathesic" (*diasthésique*), they resulted from a mysterious pathological disposition that engendered and directed the growth and development of a specific morbid product, lesions that in turn caused death by wasting.

In retrospect, localists and constitutionalists were at loggerheads over three fundamental issues: first, were these disorders primarily caused by one's environment or by some innate disposition, a "flaw" inherent to the sick individual and inseparable from his biological identity? Second, when and why did these disorders become incurable? Finally, what were the limits of human agency in their prevention and cure? Debates about the nature of these diseases were thus inseparable from the issue of therapeutic styles and attitudes.

## The Anatomico-Pathological Vision of Incurability

In 1810, Gaspard Bayle published his magisterial *Recherches sur la phthisie pulmonaire*. Reflecting years of painstaking observation, it was part phenomenology, part pathological atlas, part natural history. Above all, he sought to dispel uncertainty about the diagnosis and prognosis of tuberculosis. The picture he painted was desolate; though rich in clinical material, Parisian hospitals boasted few successful outcomes. Firsthand experience and devastating autopsy findings led him to insist that, long before anyone feared the worst, the seeds of destruction had been sown. While admitting that it seemed incredible that "phthisis has already made dangerous advances before it has produced any notable symptoms, or has simply resulted in mild indispositions," he concluded that "it is difficult to resist the evidence and the multitude of facts that seem to prove that these lesions are ordinarily already incurable once one has recognized their existence."[32]

Cancer also caught Bayle's attention. He wrote a posthumously published monograph and coauthored the article "Cancer" in the summa of contemporary Western medical knowledge, the *Dictionnaire des sciences médicales* (1812–1822). While allowing that local irritation, physical and emotional suffering, and self-destructive behaviors left people vulnerable, an innate flaw was key; "there exists an inner disposition that suffices, in some cases, to lead to the development of cancer and without which all external causes, either local or general, cannot ever produce this illness."[33] This preceded another critically important observation, namely that "the diathesis can exist without any effect on one's health: it is a particular disposition of our tissues, whose nature is entirely unknown, and which most frequently fails to manifest itself by any tangible sign." By this the authors sought to distinguish the diathesis, or predisposition, from cachexia, a hallmark feature of end-stage illness.[34]

The notion of specific disease-causing dispositions increasingly dominated anatomico-pathologists' understanding of chronic illness.[35] Part of its appeal was that it allowed them to deemphasize the role of so-called *forces vitales*. These forces were the centerpiece of medical vitalism, a school of thought associated with the eighteenth-century German physician Frederic Stahl. For vitalists, bodily functions and mind-body relations were mediated by a series of invisible yet tangible forces whose proper functioning was essential to good health. Notwithstanding its venerable history and ongoing support in the medical faculty at Montpellier, vitalism proved increasingly unpopular in Parisian medical circles, partly because of its association with Catholicism.[36] The notion of flawed constitutions thus provided a palatable alternative to explain the genesis and development of tubercles and tumors, eczema and arthritis, scurvy and advanced syphilis. This shift, in turn, played an important role in the triumph of the anatomico-pathological method, a cornerstone of modern scientific medicine. The theory of the diatheses served as the critical link between a static catalogue of symptoms and autopsy findings, and a dynamic, physiological account of illness.

The biological particularities of each member of this group of diseases contributed to the elaboration of an overarching, composite picture. Gout, for instance, proved that constitutional vices produced tangible chemical abnormalities of the blood that caused unpredictable crises before turning inward and attacking vital organs. Syphilis, on the other hand, demonstrated that a foreign agent or "virus" could enter the body, corrupt the constitution, and destroy the human body from within. Rickets and scrofula, two leading chronic afflictions of childhood, demonstrated that diatheses were generally part of one's birthright.

Cancer and phthisis were the quintessential diatheses, however, dramatically illustrating the pervasiveness of the underlying physiological vice. Ubiquitous and socially prominent, phthisis also acted as a fixed point around which the other diatheses orbited. Scrofula was known to predispose to the disease; some theorists believed that the arthritic diathesis conferred protection. Cancer, however, stood out because apparent cures were usually only brief reprieves in a lost cause. Its natural history made a deep and lasting impression, as it suggested that the diatheses resisted even aggressive intervention. Two leading anatomico-pathologists, Bayle and Bruno Cayol, highlighted the effects of postoperative relapses on perceptions, noting how "one of the most remarkable effects of this diathesis, is the reproduction of the cancer after surgical removal. The wound heals completely, the patient recovers a most brilliant state of health, they sometimes even acquire a plumpness and a freshness that they never previously had, and nonetheless the cancer recurs after a greater or lesser period of time, either at the site of the scar itself, or in an entirely different part of the body."[37] Cancer's core message was dire: even radical surgery was simply palliative, as it did not address the patient's underlying flaw.

The clockwork lethality of the leading diatheses suggested that events were orchestrated, even predetermined, by a powerful malevolent force. There was a magical quality to them; they were intangible and elusive, yet capable of laying waste to the body. In one brief passage, a practitioner managed to put his finger on something that mystified everyone, namely that diatheses were illnesses *"emancipated from their causes."*[38] Because of their long latency, some likened them to a volcano waiting to erupt.[39] This paradigm served as the prelude, or pretext, for acknowledging medicine's impotence. Could one hope to change someone's biological essence? As one authority observed, "A diathesis never abandons the subject which it attacks, and upon whom it has impressed its inalterable seal."[40]

## A Competing Vision of Chronic Progressive Disease: Broussaisism

The anatomico-pathologists' views weren't uncritically embraced in the early decades of the century. Paris's leading Restoration-era physician, François Broussais, rejected their biological determinism. He was particularly troubled by their views on heredity, telling them to "stop, stop, or you fall into pure fatalism. Don't you see that you insult nature by supposing that it is capable of creating entire generations destined only to perish? Scorn therefore the voice of all the ages, and believe with us that there are no longer any diseases from heredity."[41] In his mind, diagnostic chaos was cause for celebration, not dismay. Toasting physicians' inability to distinguish between different pulmonary ailments, he insisted that "congestion" (*phlogose*) readily mimicked advanced tuberculosis before resolving spontaneously and completely.[42]

Broussais's prognostic views, albeit informed by his reading of the scientific evidence, also reflected his life experiences and politics.[43] He was convinced, for example, that he had been cured of consumption.[44] And if his predecessor Xavier Bichat's reading of the body was completely in step with the bureaucratic corporatism typical of early revolutionary ideals, Broussias's combativeness and iconoclasm earned him the title "Napoleon of medicine."[45] Descended from a staunchly egalitarian, anticlerical family, he joined the Revolutionary Army medical corps at the age of sixteen. News of his parents' gruesome murder by counterrevolutionary forces in the War of the Vendee that same year only fortified his republican convictions.[46] He quickly rose through the ranks, serving as military surgeon and advisor, before being awarded a teaching post at Paris's military hospital, Val de Grâce. For three decades, Broussais was an outspoken participant in the post-Revolution culture wars. Enormously popular with students, his lectures were standing-room-only events, reflecting his talents as an orator and the appealing simplicity of his therapeutic system. A consummate populist, he attacked the establishment and assiduously reached out to his core constituencies—students, military physicians, and the humble group of practitioners known as *officiers de santé*—for whom he symbolized resistance to the Restoration.[47]

Rejecting a fideism in which heredity was one of several intelligent forces structuring the universe, Broussais and other radicals insisted that mankind had no destiny other than the one it fashioned for itself. In their many acts of defiance, Revolutionaries highlighted the arbitrariness of human institutions and rituals, from the divinity of kings to the framing of time in reference to Jesus Christ. As events accelerated and violence spread, they sought to demonstrate that, since the trappings of existence were man-made, man was free to refashion his world.

Many of the leading anatomico-pathologists were, in fact, Royalist Catholics. None believed that an immaterial soul affected the workings of the body, though the emphasis they placed upon physical and moral order was certainly consistent with their conservative worldview. And without tarnishing his remarkable accomplishments, Laënnec's financial security and rise to power within Parisian medicine both depended upon the backing of powerful Catholic supporters.[48]

Quickly, however, the religious and political affinities of therapeutic pessimists became increasingly heterogeneous.[49] More than anything, they shared the conviction that medical science should remain above outside influences. Mistrustful of the human pressures of the clinic, purists insisted that only the cool logic of the natural sciences could reveal the laws governing human biology. Best known for his later work on cerebral localization and physical anthropology, the freethinking Paul Broca was also an accomplished surgeon-pathologist whose early work focused on phthisis and cancer. In something of a professional manifesto, he insisted that "when they [scientists] go back to their studies and laboratories, they must remain independent and never bow to party discipline. . . . An august goddess, Science thrones above humanity. . . . Only of her may it be said that she is made to command, not to obey."[50]

While recognizing the painful implications of their views, therapeutic pessimists stressed that scientific truth mattered more than social niceties. As one practitioner put it, "however despair-inducing the doctrine of the diathesis appears at first glance, one cannot reject it if it appears to be well founded, simply because our therapeutics still lack any direct means of destroying it. If this is the truth, one must proclaim it, because in the sciences all truths merit being told and must be told."[51] Responding to accusations of fatalism, Laënnec similarly insisted that "I believe, it is true, that there are many illnesses which we can neither prevent nor cure, at least in a certain and incontestable manner. The question is not, it seems to me, whether this is sad: the question is to know whether or not this is true."[52]

Broussais called such prognostic views a "monstrous fiction"; along with other like-minded contemporaries, he accused his opponents of withholding curative treatments and undermining patients' hopes for recovery.[53] He championed a simple therapeutic system grounded on a unitary theory of disease. Partly because of his wartime experiences, he maintained that cold, damp environments caused phthisis, not innate temperaments. He also sought to demystify cancer, insisting that it was caused by the same environmental factors responsible for other diseases.

Rejecting his rivals' embrace of disease specificity (reflecting their belief in the specificity of each diathesis), Broussais insisted that external irritation led to nonspecific inflammatory changes (*phlegmasies*) throughout the body. For various reasons, the stomach was usually the source of the problem. Other organs, particularly the lungs, could be subject to direct or sympathetic irritation, however. When extremely severe, inflammation was rapidly lethal; more often, it caused tissues to slowly degenerate, culminating in their transformation into malignant tumors or tubercles.

Broussais's image of the body was not that of a passive template upon which events played themselves out, but an entity that actively responded to unhealthy outside influences. Unfortunately, this defensive response often proved too intense or too protracted. His understanding of disease was thus grounded upon a paradox. Inflammation was both a normal reaction to outside irritants and the primary pathological mechanism underpinning human disease. In many ways, it resembled the experience of a besieged garrison that inadvertently set its own barracks on fire. Importantly, this pathological process was dynamic, contingent, and readily reversible. In a statement singled out by one eulogizer as his greatest contribution to medicine, Broussais insisted that medicine was poised to emancipate mankind, as "the vast majority of the poor souls that I found consumed by a chronic disease were simply the victims of an inflammation that had not been cured in its early acute phase."[54] Even seemingly desperate cases were potentially curable, if only because the disease-causing principle remained distinct from the patient's body until the end.

Broussais was an observant clinician, however, largely explaining why he too had a fatalistic streak. For a start, most people had little control over their environment and were unwilling to give up their bad habits. Equally important, tumors and tubercles eventually became treatment-resistant foci of further inflammation. He thus found himself admitting that "ordinarily, the cause that engenders a tubercle, produces thousands of them" before adding that "if tubercles are incurable, and it is not these that we must treat, at least in the majority of cases, it is the congestion [la phlogose] that precedes and produces them that one must strive to destroy."[55] Notoriously unpredictable, many cancers were also incurable. Only a vast experience, he warned his protégés, would allow them to know when a given case was truly hopeless.[56]

For him and his army of followers known as Broussaisists, it was neither biological necessity nor some mysterious twist of fate that made disease incurable but sociobehavioral factors. Patient blaming was a recurrent theme, vividly captured in one passage that stressed, "I am frequently called upon to treat terrible illnesses, which were allowed to pursue their course, or were worsened by the application of inappropriate therapies."[57] Charlatanism, not surprisingly, was a big problem.[58] Well-meaning families and friends, physicians regularly intoned, should call for a licensed MD immediately and refrain from giving medical advice of any kind.[59]

Those who turned to quacks had only themselves to blame. Yet Broussais and other elite physicians were highly critical of their colleagues, whom they also accused of committing terrible therapeutic errors. For several decades, Charles-Louis Dumas, professor of anatomy and pathology at the University of Montpellier, directed its clinic for the study of reputedly incurable illnesses.[60] In 1812, he published an exhaustive treatise on chronic diseases in which he presented an eclectic account of their genesis and evolution. In keeping with his vitalist convictions, he insisted that acute and chronic diseases were etiologically indistinguishable; doctors' mishandling of acute illnesses, along with heredity, explained why they went on to become chronic and refractory.[61] Dumas's message trickled down through the hierarchy; in 1807, one of his top students emphatically suggested that diagnostic incompetence and ill-chosen remedies destroyed patients' constitutions, transforming acute illnesses into chronic ones.[62]

The importance accorded to "artificial" (that is, human) factors extended to Broussais's analysis of poverty's effects on phthisis. Just as unhealthy environments were lethal over time, healthy ones could work miracles. This explained why phthisis could be cured "firstly, by aborting or resolving the tubercles, secondly, by allowing the progress of the illness to the point where nature has destroyed the degenerated matter and replaced it with a scar. The first type of cure, denied by Laënnec, is nonetheless possible. Every day the wealthy obtain it by going off to warm climes and there are even some who have had such attacks (of tubercles) a great many times and who have cured them, through the use of anti-phlogistics."[63] Although certainly no admirer, the Parisian medical luminary Gabriel Andral shared Broussais's views on poverty and disease. Entrusted to edit the fourth edition of Laënnec's landmark treatise, he inserted a footnote that emphasized, "in the hospitals the average length of phthisis is less than a year; in patients treated at home, and especially in those whom one can place in the most advantageous circumstances as to climate and alimentation, the duration of this illness is necessarily much longer and cannot even be calculated."[64]

If it was true up to a point, this disclaimer demands further scrutiny. A cynic would suggest that vagueness would have smoothed relations with a highly desirable clientele. By emphasizing, even exaggerating, the effects of social factors, doctors could justify the usual outcome—death—while condemning the poor to their own private incurability. They could then reassure affluent consumptives that they had another form of the disease, a decidedly more curable one.

Despite being tarred as a fatalist, Laënnec never actually claimed that phthisis inevitably ended in death. His writings, in fact, included statements that allowed him to be claimed by those on both sides of the curable/incurable debate.[65] While agreeing with his friend Gaspard Bayle that minimally symptomatic phthisis was generally incurable, he also believed that nature occasionally worked wonders when all hope seemed lost.[66] Citing clinical and anatomical evidence, he suggested that the cure of late-stage disease was possible, perhaps even common.[67] Such inconsistency is not the work of a muddled thinker loose with his words. Rather, it reflected the fact that several different forms of (in)curability awkwardly coexisted.

## Patterns of (In)Curability in Tuberculosis—Natural versus Medical

For all their differences, Laënnec and Broussais apparently had a grudging respect for each other. They also shared a common goal. Each helped legitimize a new science for understanding the body without losing sight of pathological anatomy's fundamental limitation. Unlike many other physicians, both men understood that dissection revealed nothing about the causes of disease, which necessarily acted upon the body physiologically.[68]

Their opposing visions of phthisis also overlapped in important ways. Laënnec recognized its natural curability while Broussais recognized that late-stage phthisis was generally fatal. Their biggest disagreement was over whether medicine could reliably and predictably influence the outcome. For Broussais, an early-stage consumptive was eminently curable; his "anti-phlogistics" (bleeding, leeches, and an austere diet) reliably prevailed.[69] He rejected the possibility of a biologically preordained outcome; one might turn back the clock no matter how superficially worrisome the symptoms. Hubris partly explains his ideas' extraordinary, if transient, appeal. Diagnostic uncertainty allowed him to reject his rival's modest therapeutic motto—"when in doubt, do something"—substituting instead the far more ambitious rallying cry, "when in doubt, assume and insist that you are curing the patient."

For Laënnec, phthisis was like a perpetual motion machine that, on occasion, inexplicably stopped. Nature, in other words, was capable of marshalling mysterious healing powers, albeit often only temporarily. Unfortunately, medicine was powerless to reproduce this feat. In his words, "the cure of pulmonary phthisis is not above the forces of nature; but we must admit at the same time that the medical arts do not possess any means to arrive with certitude to this goal. . . . One cannot fail to recognize an incurable illness when we see tried in turn against it almost all the most disparate remedies, medications with the most opposite effects; propose each day new remedies, exhume means that, previously too vaunted, had long stayed in a merited oblivion."[70] Elsewhere, he characterized the vast anti-tuberculosis pharmacopoeia as "sterile abundance."[71] Along with a widening circle of colleagues, he considered phthisis incurable because cures were unreliable, unpredictable, and unreproducible. They were natural, not man-made, wonders.

Not content merely to dismiss his opponent's claims, he accused Broussais of harming patients. Brandishing in-patient mortality statistics from Val de Grâce Hospital, he maintained that Broussais's patients fared worse than those of his colleagues. Public health records demonstrated that the widespread adoption of Broussais's "physiological" treatments had done more harm than good.[72] Coupled with their ward experiences, these attacks decisively shaped the attitudes of the next generation of practitioners. Speaking for a burgeoning constituency in 1833, one student concluded that "one recognizes with sorrow that the most carefully chosen remedies have always been useless, that they were frequently harmful, and that the efforts of the greatest masters have failed against this cruel illness."[73]

Laënnec's Parisian successor, Pierre Louis, kept up the assault in his monographs on phthisis (1825) and typhoid fever (1830). He is best known, however, for his 1835 study of blood letting in pneumonia. Aware of its growing influence in both the natural and social sciences, Louis single-mindedly applied the "numerical method" to medicine. The only way to judge a therapy's usefulness, he insisted, was to compare the average response rates between groups. His ideas were aggressively championed by the Société Médicale D'Émulation (established in 1832), which insisted that medicine was an empirical science whose practice should be guided not by subjective impressions and clinical experience but by rigorous evaluation. Only then could the profession objectively determine the best treatment for a given illness.

Although it secured Louis's posthumous fame, the numerical method counted more critics than enthusiasts during his lifetime.[74] Those with a sophisticated understanding of probability theory dismissed his case series as too small to bear the burden of proof.[75] Various detractors pointed out that clinical diagnosis was notoriously subjective, making intergroup comparison shaky at best. Critics also raised important epistemological concerns, particularly around the issue of causality. If useful at predicting outcomes, even the most accurate law of averages said little about the deeper nature of a given phenomenon.[76] At mid-century, leading physiologists such as Claude Bernard went a step further, suggesting that clinical science was a chimera; only laboratory-derived physiological insights provided a scientific basis for understanding illness and its treatment.[77]

Practicing physicians had other concerns, at once professional and deontological. Single-mindedly focusing upon disease risked dehumanizing medicine, while aggregate data ignored individual variability, subtleties that had traditionally directed doctors' clinical decisions. Critics contended that the numerical method was tantamount to healing by rote. It made a mockery of medical judgment and undermined physicians' already shaky authority. Rather than being subject to hard-and-fast rules, medicine was a healing art whose claim to expertise was grounded in accumulated personal experience and careful deliberation. Simply put, practicing according to the law of averages was incompatible with being an effective and compassionate healer, the only true source of professional legitimacy.[78]

In the end, the nineteenth-century medical elite came to view the numerical method as a heuristic aid rather than the basis of scientific medicine.[79] Louis's therapeutic skepticism, on the other hand, became quite entrenched. In the case of phthisis, the net result was growing despondency. A decade after Broussaisism's collapse, the second edition of Louis's work on the disorder from 1843 invoked phthisis's natural curability before noting, "If, in the present state of science, one cannot nourish the hope of curing phthisis, one can at least aspire to slow its evolution, with the help of well-planned care. But lest we cultivate any illusions as to the usefulness of the therapeutic agents used in the treatment of tubercles, one must remember that . . . after having been stationary for what can sometimes be a considerable period of time, it can then progress with great speed, without us being able to grasp the reason for such a profound change."[80] This represented the new dogma, marked by a collective discomfort with medicine's apparent powerlessness. When they suspected phthisis, physicians offered Band-Aid solutions while hoping that their efforts helped stave off the inevitable.

## Patterns of (In)Curability in Cancer— Natural, Medical, and Surgical?

If nearly as acrimonious, debates about cancer's prognosis differed in that essentially everyone acknowledged Nature's powerlessness.[81] This was troubling indeed for a profession whose therapies aspired to imitate its healing ways. "Nature be damned!" some insisted, unwilling to accept that medical science could do no better.

Always the optimist, Broussais believed that cancer's prognosis was excellent when the tumors were small and the patient well nourished.[82] Several leading surgeons—including Joseph Récamier, Jacques Lisfranc, and Frédéric Duparcque—agreed that precancerous or well-circumscribed growths were curable both medically (via internal and external remedies) and surgically (via surgical excision).

In 1844, a little-known practitioner named Stanislaus Tanchou published a book celebrating his successes and cataloguing the remedies that had proven effective during the preceding century, including hemlock, external compression, and carrot poultices.[83] Contemporary reception of this work was, to say the least, chilly. Alfred Velpeau, a member of the Academy of Medicine and probably the leading surgeon of his day, spoke disparagingly of the man and his ideas before pointing out, "I have seen enough of the women treated by Tanchou . . . to verify that the hopes of this practitioner were truly groundless: having no clear idea of what is currently understood by the term cancer, he confounded under this term all species of tumor or tumefaction of the breast, and the numerous observations, which moreover could not be more incomplete, that he borrowed from different authors, leave no doubts in this regard."[84] By the 1840s, the medical elite agreed that there was no effective medical treatment for the disease. Particular criticism was reserved for the most recent fad in breast cancer treatment—external compression—imported to France from England by Joseph Récamier.[85] Advocates were increasingly brushed aside, dismissed as having perpetuated the long-standing tradition of misdiagnosing diseases of the breast. Such confusion, a chorus of otherwise dissenting voices agreed, explained the brisk trade in panaceas. By mid-century, cancer was judged naturally and medically incurable. As with phthisis, peddling cancer cures had become a litmus test for charlatanism.

Far more controversial was whether cancer was curable via surgical excision. If the underlying diathesis was inherently incurable, Bayle and Cayol had nonetheless seen cases where surgery had apparently been curative.[86] This admission illustrates the extent to which the lines between "localism" and "constitutionalism" were blurrier with cancer than with tuberculosis. Although they admitted that the disease was caused by a specific constitutional disposition, therapeutic optimists insisted that it always began locally. Authorities such as Jean-Zuléma Amussat and Velpeau maintained that cancer only became "diathesic" (that is, destined to relapse) after a significant period of time. Such theoretical considerations were not an idle matter. They justified early, aggressive, and ostensibly curative surgery.

These surgeons long remained in the minority. Most practitioners accepted that surgery for late-stage cancer was potentially an effective palliative that sometimes prolonged people's lives. Early surgical removal was another matter altogether. Clinical and statistical evidence seemed persuasive: those lucky enough to survive the operation quickly relapsed. Radical cures, on the other hand, must simply be cases of mistaken identity. As the century progressed, most physicians came to believe that putative surgical cures, like medical ones, reflected errors in diagnosis.

Diverging views surrounding the diagnosis and prognosis of cancer prompted two heated debates at the French Academy of Medicine, in 1844 and again in 1854–55. Established by royal decree in 1820, this august body was entrusted to advise the government on matters of health policy. It also long remained one of the world's leading forums for discussing scientific theories and therapeutic claims.[87] The first of these blow-ups was instigated by one of the country's foremost anatomists, Jean Cruveilhier, who presented evidence suggesting that benign fibrous growths of the breast were common and generally misdiagnosed. He was particularly concerned by two regrettable consequences of such confusion. First, many women went through a cruel, even lethal ordeal for conditions that never "transformed themselves" into cancer. Second, many surgeons erroneously believed that early surgical intervention could cure cancer.[88] Though unwilling to declare it inherently incurable, Cruveilhier and others clearly believed that operations should only be performed late in the course of disease when the diagnosis was clear and unambiguous.[89]

Everyone acknowledged that breast cancer remained shrouded in mystery.[90] But Cruvielhier's arguments were taken to imply—quite correctly— that surgeons generally performed operations that were ultimately futile (if the tumors were malignant) or unnecessary.[91] Notwithstanding Cruveilhier's remonstrances, the ensuing discussion was incendiary.[92] As the *éminence grise* of French surgery, Philibert-Joseph Roux, noted, "as a result of the doctrine being put forward on benign tumors of the breast, almost all of surgery is called into question."[93] Elsewhere, he and others spoke of a widespread bias among physicians against nearly all forms of surgery.[94] In the ensuing debate, some members of the Academy worried about the effects that such backbiting would have on the public's already low opinion of doctors.[95] Roux also held Cruveilhier personally responsible for the death of those who chose to put off an operation until it was too late.[96]

Amid growing fascination with medical microscopy, competing opinions collided again in 1854 during the Academy's widely followed discussions on the microscope's usefulness in diagnosing cancer.[97] Internationally acclaimed for his technical prowess, Velpeau was now the leading spokesman for the early surgical removal of breast cancer. Invoking hundreds of operations and decades of hard work, he insisted that one could reliably diagnose cancer on clinical grounds. His highly tuned judgment allowed him to distinguish between three types of tumors: benign types that could be ignored, cancerous growths that were inoperable (that is, incurable) and better left alone, and early cancerous growths with all the features of operative curability. He ended his exposé by claiming that he had successfully cured several women who, microscope or no, had "true" cancer of the breast.

This animated debate pitted Velpeau's clinically centered defense of his surgical practice against a competing vision associated with the German-trained pathologist Hermann Lebert. Imbued with the latest Teutonic views about the specificity of the cancer cell, he and a growing number of young pathologists and surgeons defended the near-infallibility of the microscope at identifying cancer cells. In an interesting twist, a new technology confirmed the truth-value of an idea traceable to Hippocrates, that of cancer's inherent incurability. The microscopists were categorical: radical cures of cancer, even Velpeau's, were simply not cancer.

In the end, Velpeau carried the day on most of the technicalities raised during these discussions.[98] The critical issue of cancer's (in)curability remained unresolved, however. Looking back, this isn't surprising. Each side had an airtight case grounded in careful empiricism, a credible theory, and a foolproof defense of last resort.[99] Proponents of its curability argued that a single case sufficed to overturn their opponents' law-of-nature position. After presenting examples from the recent past, Velpeau told the Academy, "Among the patients cured for at least five years, it is said that I have only cited the case of three. What does it matter?! Were there only one, if it is authentic and perfectly established, this suffices for the opinion that I defend; but there are more than three, the most remote of which goes back more than five years."[100] Skeptics, on the other hand, disingenuously pointed out that his cure rate matched the frequency with which he had admitted to misdiagnosing breast lumps years earlier.[101] And what of the countless curable tumors that reliably relapsed after surgical removal, just as their theory predicted?

Divergent experiences partly explain these differences in opinion. Already in 1844, Velpeau alluded to the distance separating physicians and surgeons. The former generally cared for those in whom surgery had failed. Surgeons, on the other hand, preferred to dwell upon their successes.[102] Indeed such "competing objectivities" have been invoked to explain why different medical subcultures can see the same illness differently.[103] Yet the divisions ran even deeper, as the belligerents couldn't agree even on the epistemological ground rules. For purists, the exceptional case established the rule of curability, *tout court*. Velpeau's opponents, while recognizing that some tumors could be successfully removed, insisted that everyone with true cancer would eventually succumb.

The relative immobility of this position speaks to a more general feature of academic medicine, however. Simply put, it was professionally humiliating to be wrong about such an important issue. Velpeau, who probably had the most to lose, noted that if he was right "we would make them turn their back on three or four years of research, that would no doubt be a great loss for them; but they ask me, without scruples, to sacrifice the results of thirty years of hard labor."[104] Yet despite Velpeau's best efforts, he didn't transform contemporary cancer care. For one, his credibility was undermined by his inability to keep track of patients beyond four or five years. The surveillance mechanisms that have come to play such an important role in the study of the disease simply did not exist. Furthermore, several respected colleagues like Pierre Gerdy and Paul Broca argued that, if surgery was often beneficial, the cancerous diathesis was irremediable. Most important, however, patients themselves preferred to bide their time.[105] In the face of concerted resistance, Velpeau threw up his hands, observing that "operations have always and continue to provoke such dread, that practitioners have never abandoned the idea of curing breast cancers without them," hoping that surgical anesthesia would change people's behaviors.[106]

For quite some time, such optimism was apparently misguided. Surgeons, it is true, could point to small but encouraging case series. An 1871 article in a leading medical encyclopedia, for example, insisted that the risks and benefits of surgery were favorable enough to justify operating immediately in most cases.[107] Apparently, the majority of physicians and patients disagreed, preferring to put off an operation until it was absolutely "necessary."[108]

Alternative healers also espoused a decidedly antisurgical bias, and many promised cures that avoided the knife. In an interesting twist, a trained MD who practiced on the fringes of Parisian medicine for thirty-five years turned the usual pattern of accusation on its head. While acknowledging that his panacea didn't cure the disease, Dr. Denis de Saint-Pierre warned patients to "evade in any case the murderous scalpel of the doctor who would operate on you; such operations have only cured those who never had cancer."[109] Such opinions long influenced patients' treatment decisions. In 1881, a member of the elite Surgical Society of Paris reminded his colleagues that "while the impostors who claim to cure cancer without surgery, destroy it with caustics for many months and allow the morbid matter to penetrate more deeply, and when the patients finally come to ask us to operate on them, the lesion can no longer be widely removed at a stroke as we might have done had there not been so many months lost."[110] Throughout the century, surgeons found themselves in a bind that knew no easy solution: should they promise quick fixes like their competitors and look askance when patients succumbed? Or defend a realistic, yet far less seductive view: though generally incurable, cancer could be held in check if promptly removed.

## The Science of Prognostication

Between 1820 and 1860, practitioners could draw upon several forms of scientific evidence—clinical, pathological, and theoretical—to decide whether chronic diseases were (in)curable. In the case of cancer, there was a characteristic pattern to practitioners' attitudes. After a period of relative optimism, a steady diet of relapses led most to take a dim view of both its prognosis and surgery's usefulness.[111] Convinced that operations should almost be banned because they only added to patients' suffering, one surgeon admitted in 1846, "I did not always have such a definite opinion on this practical issue. At the beginning of my medical career, I followed the well-worn path; I operated on cases of cancer."[112] Another practitioner insisted that doctors' therapeutic practices were "an affair of age, habit, and temperament." Young, enterprising practitioners tended to operate indiscriminately; in Dr. Benoit's words, they were "exclusively surgical in the most rigorous and worst sense of the word." Hardened veterans, on the other hand, often erred in the opposite direction, inappropriately resigning themselves to inaction.[113]

A similar dynamic existed around phthisis. Young physicians often started out bright-eyed and optimistic, only to become hardened nihilists. The respected Montpellier professor Jean-Baptiste Fonssagrives was among the most vocal critics of a socialization in which "physicians, flush with youth and enthusiasm, avid to cure and sustain that sacred fire of life that is confined to their care, delude themselves mightily on the power of their

ministry and the value of the arms that they carry with them. Convinced
that, in principle, there exists no incurable illness, they end up, as a result
of a series of failures and setbacks, to doubt the usefulness of their interventions, and tend more and more toward skeptical expectancy. This is an
exaggeration of another sort."[114] Like much of the medical elite, he thought
that young doctors needed to be realistic, patient, and skeptical, particularly
with respect to the latest wonder drug.

In frustration and despair, disappointed idealists often turned on those
who had "misled" them.[115] Broussais, for instance, ended up a whipping boy
for an entire generation of physicians.[116] Criticisms continued to surface
long after his death, though they had more to do with celebrating progress
than settling scores. In 1875, one earnest physician emphasized "how many
patients, in effect, did doctors kill, especially under the influence of Broussais's ideas. . . . Is it possible to conceive that we could ever have bled phthisics?"[117] Although practitioners still didn't cure many people with the disease,
they could at least celebrate the fact that they didn't do that anymore!

Broussais's dethroning was only one instance of collective (dis)enchant-
ment; his anti-phlogistics were neither the first nor the last panacea to fail
the test of time. Among the more famous examples was the inhaled iodine
debacle, a mid-century therapy heralded as a miracle cure by a member
of the Academy of Medicine, Pierre Adolphe Piorry. After several glowing
reports led to its widespread adoption, it was relegated to the shadowy world
of alternative medicine. For as a fellow Academician noted decades later,
the reality he witnessed when temporarily replacing Piorry on the wards
was starkly different. Struck by the pestilential atmosphere, Hermann Pidoux laconically noted that the patients were miserable and begged him to
stop the treatment. He acquiesced a week later, convinced that the remedy
did more harm than good.[118] Such exaggeration, it appears, was more the
rule than the exception. Though quantitative analyses are lacking, much of
the experimentation surrounding reputedly incurable illness was initiated
because of doubts about other people's therapeutic claims.[119]

Things eventually got so bad that Fonssagrives wanted his colleagues
to unambiguously declare tuberculosis "incurable." Insisting that the profession's desperate, misguided search for a cure had undermined its credibility and integrity, he stressed how "the history of therapeutics is full of
the thoughtless apotheoses whose fastidious repetition is one of the causes
for the skepticism within and outside of medicine."[120] This foible was widespread enough to have been immortalized in an eighteenth-century apho-
rism that was still cited a century later.[121] This bit of popular wisdom noted
how a woman asked a medical luminary his opinion on a remedy very much
in vogue. Michel Philip Bouvart's response was "hurry up and take some
while it's still curing people!"[122]

## Variations on the Theme of Incurable

If Bayle's claim that the biological behavior of cancer and tuberculosis were indistinguishable failed to outlive him, these two disorders remained closely linked in everyone's mind. New ideas about tuberculosis, for example, were reflexively applied to cancer.[123] Cancer's grim phenomenology, on the other hand, long haunted discussions around the world's leading "reputedly incurable" illness.

Pioneering anatomists' evocation of the diseases' many similarities eventually drew the ire of high-profile revisionists. In his award-winning book on phthisis from 1873, Hermann Pidoux emphasized the differences between them, writing, "When I hear Laënnec profess the spontaneous or natural cure of tuberculosis during its second and third stages, after having declared that in its first stage it is just as incurable as cancer and all other organic productions; then to affirm its absolute medical incurability, I believe that I must be dreaming."[124] Ironically, Pidoux admitted that these two disorders differed from other serious chronic diseases; cancer occupied the highest and tuberculosis the lowest ends of his scale of organic illnesses.[125] He was adamant, however, that people not allow cancer's incurability to obscure the truth about tuberculosis. In his mind, any disease that resolved spontaneously was, by definition, medically curable.

His exertions also confirm that medical incurability, an inability to reliably and predictably halt disease, was of overriding significance.[126] Clinicians had several types of evidence at their disposal, yet it was their personal experiences with therapeutic failure that consistently proved most compelling. Anatomical evidence in favor of tuberculosis's natural curability, for example, was long viewed with skepticism because such observations were therapeutically irrelevant.[127]

More than anything, the vision of cancer and tuberculosis that reigned at mid-century was strikingly awkward. Tuberculosis was theoretically (that is, naturally) curable but medically incurable. Cancer was all but inevitably incurable: naturally, medically, and surgically. In a setting where medicine's usefulness was seriously compromised, the euphemism "reputedly incurable" clearly offered everyone a comfort of sorts.[128] Yet with tuberculosis, this label came under increasing scrutiny before eventually being rejected. As part of a campaign to transform perceptions, authorities drew attention to the body's success at controlling tubercles. In almost the same breath, they began to claim that if "sick" bodies were capable of defeating the enemy, medical science could too. Increasingly of one mind, they began to deny that every consumptive had to accept that the die was irrevocably cast.

# 2

## Reinventing Hope in the Late Nineteenth Century

Despite their dismal track record treating cancer, physicians in the 1860s were again questioning whether the disease was inherently and inevitably incurable.[1] Reluctant to admit defeat, they embraced the spirit of a colleague's earnest reminder that "when old age and death alone will remain untreatable, then medicine will have attained [its] goal."[2] Three decades later, despite growing worries about humanity's progressive physical degeneration, physicians were increasingly optimistic. Much of the medical elite embraced an outwardly paradoxical worldview: modern medicine was winning the battle against humanity's greatest scourges even as France (and the rest of Europe) was believed to be regressing biologically.[3]

When it came to the two deadliest diatheses, there was a broad tendency to put the best spin on existing accomplishments. This ethos, discernible first with tuberculosis and only slowly and incompletely around cancer, was aggressively promoted by important opinion leaders. It also eventually received the explicit doctrinal, if not financial, support of the state. Beyond the message's emotional appeal, efforts to convince ordinary people of the relative benignity of early tuberculosis and cancer were linked to the emerging public health crusade and the need for medical policing. In other words, in order to convince people to come forward and accept the dramatic consequences of these diagnoses, it was necessary to hold up the promise of a cure.[4] The process by which the medical profession first managed to convince itself that the diseases were readily curable will be outlined here.

The emergence of this buoyant prognostic narrative reflected the combined effects of several phenomena. The first involved rewriting the natural history of these disorders via the selective use of scientific insights. Doctors also championed the use of new therapeutic markers whose net effect was to further blur the distinction between "curable" and "incurable" strongly in favor of the former. Additionally, their enthusiastic promotion of certain high-visibility innovations encouraged the idea that human agency had a major effect on the course of these disorders. Finally, the profession put forward an account of therapeutic failure that was a paean to medical progress, discounting the still commonplace outcome of these disorders: death. In the end, the link between prognostic perceptions and scientific progress was convoluted at this critical turning point in history. This was mostly because curability in the setting of chronic disease was not tantamount to their permanent eradication by a specific, targeted pharmaceutical remedy or surgical intervention.

## The Physiological Basis of Incurability

In retrospect, neither Broussais nor his adversaries could completely account for the biological and social complexity of chronic illness. Mid-century theorists incorporated insights from both the anatomico-pathologists and the Broussaisists; that being said, the diathesis emerged as one of Western medicine's conceptual pillars.[5] In the process, its meaning was radically transformed. In the 1870s, one practitioner noted that quibbles aside, everyone accepted that "the word diathesis, from the Greek, means disposition. It is in this sense that it was employed by the ancients, notably by Galen and his school. Since, the meaning of this word has completely changed, and today one generally employs it to designate not a simple predisposition, but an illness that exists already."[6]

In an otherwise uninspiring 1888 lecture at the Paris medical school, an authority on chronic disease provided a cogent summary of contemporary medical constitutionalism. Max Durand-Fardel summarized the explanatory schema physicians had relied on for over a half-century, noting how

> among the diversities in the physiological states, one could take note of certain types, which are the *temperaments*. The classical temperaments are based on the mode of this or that vital function or this or that group of organs. [These] can become accentuated so that the equilibrium that maintains the complex elements of the organism in harmony comes to be broken: from there are born *constitutional states*, which are not yet illness, but which are no longer perfect health. Here one can recognize certain more or less determined types that stamp on the economy the mark of this or that system . . . the lymphatic, nervous, arthritic, bilious, anaemic, hemorrhoidal constitutions. It is not yet illness and yet is no longer perfect health: it is a way of being that impresses on accidental illnesses a particular physiognomy.[7]

In certain individuals, these constitutional irregularities crossed the line between the normal and the pathological, marking them off as diathesis-carriers. Initially understood as a state of heightened susceptibility, diatheses came to be seen as a treacherous physiological no-man's land.

This evolution was not fortuitous. On the one hand, Broussais's spectacular fall from grace fuelled skepticism about inflammation's role in human illness. Equally important, constitutionalism allowed medicine to integrate new knowledge into an age-old view of the body's workings.[8] In the 1840s, one practitioner stressed the importance of this rehabilitation, insisting that humoralist ideas were not only sanctioned by tradition and experience but "elicit new research that is liable to vindicate and enlarge the field of scientific medicine." Dr. Trinquier was confident that "the moment is not far off when a new humoralism, fortified by all the discoveries of the anatomical and chemical sciences, will reign where, still recently, the word was reproved and subjected to bitter criticism."[9] In fact, Western medicine did embrace neo-humoralism because it could account for both individual susceptibility and the effects of external factors (diet, climate, and so on) on health and well-being.

Beyond creating a critical bridge between things past and present, this conceptual shift also represented a tentative first step in the transformation of Western biomedicine's understanding of illness: a move from "specificity" (every disease is unique and specific to the sick person) to "universalism" (there exist discrete disease states, resulting from physiological changes that are constant and universal).[10] Despite the ongoing relevance of individual idiosyncrasy, nineteenth-century constitutionalism encouraged a habit of mind in which diseases were framed as biologically consistent, ontologically discrete entities. Decades before experimental physiology reified this idea, the existence of specific diathesic principles underpinned a new paradigm: different individuals suffered from the same disease. As part of their efforts to put forward a credible account of these disorders' physiology, constitutionalists increasingly focused on three salient aspects of human existence: habit, heredity, and misery.

In struggling to give substance to their theories, they explored analogies between chronic disease and other biological processes. These disorders' obstinacy and cascading nature led them to the idea of a morbid physiological habit. This notion proved critical, as it established a link between the original vice and the disease's symptoms and lesions. In 1875, the respected clinician Maurice Raynaud stressed the logic of assuming that "diseases resulting from some internal cause are of the chronic type," noting that "one conceives, without being easily able to give the reason, that a healthy organism, surprised, in a sense, by an outside aggression, makes an effort to rid itself of it, and succeeds in a variable amount of time. Either he is cured, or he dies; but the battle cannot last for long. One can conceive, on the other hand, that an organism sufficiently vitiated in the core of its substance to evolve on its own according to a pattern more or less distinct from normal, continues as it began, having no reason to change direction."[11] Chronic diseases were the price paid by bodies that, incapable of knowing any better, became locked into an immutable pathological rut.

For many, such ingrained compulsions called to mind the obsessive monomanias of the insane. Expressing a widespread view, Raynaud insisted that the diatheses were the product of a "morbid habit at its highest power," in his words, an "addiction."[12] Not coincidentally, these views emerged amid growing interest in this phenomenon. Indeed, the term *alcoholism* was coined during the same period.[13] Like the defective will of the drunkard, the bodies of the chronically ill were plagued by physiological obsessions resistant to the most carefully planned therapeutic regimens. In summarizing the root causes of incurability, Jaumes stressed how "addiction adds something more to the incurability of the illnesses that are already incurable by and of themselves," before adding that, in chronic afflictions, heredity combined with habit was a potent cause of incurability.[14]

Jaumes's comments hint at the extent to which medical constitutionalism was both founded upon and instrumental to the growing hegemony of hereditarian determinism. After the 1830s, the measured skepticism of the first generation of anatomico-pathologists increasingly gave way to certainty.[15] People didn't merely resemble their parents; they also inherited their constitutional flaws.[16] Countless people came into the world, in other words, preordained to develop cancer, phthisis, or scrofula. It was this sad fact, most believed, that explained why Broussais's foolproof remedies had failed. Speaking for a rapidly growing constituency, a disillusioned student observed in 1833, "It is not possible, at least in practical medicine, to deny the hereditary nature of certain maladies, among them scrofula and tuberculosis."[17] Though many found it disheartening, by the 1870s it was universally accepted that the diatheses were eminently hereditary.[18] Depressingly intractable social and political troubles partly explain hereditarianism's appeal to anxious European and American elites.[19] The science also appeared airtight. Heredity alone could explain why certain bodies seemed "programmed" to self-destruct.

In cases where entire families succumbed to the same chronic disease (common enough with phthisis), its fateful role seemed obvious. Yet contemporary understanding of heredity's workings was flexible enough to account for illness in families seemingly free of all "taint." Drawing upon the theories of the famed naturalist Jean-Baptiste Lamarck, it was increasingly accepted that acquired characteristics could be transmitted from parents to offspring. This, along with the belief that an atavistic or buried family trait could skip a generation, allowed theorists to account for divergent patterns of biological experience. Like many similarly ambitious explanatory paradigms, mid-century hereditarianism was essentially unfalsifiable.

Completing contemporaries' understanding of the genesis of chronic disease was the view that such patients suffered from "physiological misery," understood as a profound disturbance of the nutritional and lymphatic systems. This notion was articulated in 1861 by Apollinaire Bourchardat, a respected professor of hygiene who went on to be named president of the Academy of Medicine. "Misery" became increasingly central to contemporary understanding of chronic disease.[20] An interest in nutrition—both as a cause of disease and as a potential treatment—was reasonable given the diatheses' association with poverty and wasting. Yet misery and heredity also explained why the rich, living lives of relative ease in the healthiest environments, often succumbed to the same chronic diseases as the poor. Misery, it was increasingly asserted, came in two equally pernicious forms—internal and external. In detailing the genesis of phthisis, the widely cited clinician Hermann Pidoux insisted that everything made sense if one remembered that inadequate food, unhealthy environments, and inhuman toil were not the only reason that people developed the disease. The vices to which only the rich were privy, notably gluttony and idleness, were equally destructive. Notwithstanding his sensitivity to the plight of the working class, Pidoux was no proto-socialist; he roundly condemned their excesses and debauchery.[21] He was, however, particularly critical of wealthy, aristocratic consumptives. Like much of the bourgeoisie, he viewed illness as a sign of their physical and moral inferiority.

Habit, heredity, and misery together allowed constitutionalists to construct a physiologically credible explanation that encompassed the varied and complex behavior of chronic progressive disease. Its malleability allowed theorists to vary its contours to suit their tastes and inclinations. It also furnished an interpretation that seamlessly annealed the precepts of physical and moral physiology. Invoking discrete diatheses would also have helped physicians in their daily dealings with patients; it provided a cause for an unhappy state of affairs while justifying their impotence. Equally critical, these notions were ill-defined enough to allow physicians to reenvisage a more hopeful therapeutic ethos.

## The First Stirrings of Optimism, 1860–1880

For all its flaws, clinical science long remained the arbiter of the (in)curability of cancer and tuberculosis.[22] The dark mood that prevailed at mid-century seemed reasonable enough: tens of thousands of people died from these diseases every year, including those who could afford the best of everything. The continuing proliferation of miracle cures provided further evidence that nothing worked very well. Given French medicine's notorious skepticism, it is not surprising that many experienced clinicians still hadn't embraced "the doctrine of curability" in the early 1860s.[23] Given this entrenched incredulity, it is all the more noteworthy that, within a generation, prognostic pessimism was increasingly dismissed as ill-founded.

The critical first step in this process involved repackaging the tuberculous diathesis as potentially treatable, and by the 1860s it was no longer automatically equated with incurability and death.[24] A growing number of physicians and patients believed that a suitable climate or hydrotherapy could work marvels on even the unhealthiest constitution. To a degree, this optimism mirrored and was fuelled by social forces. Spa owners and spa physicians, often one and the same, aggressively advertised their waters' healing properties, to say nothing of the amenities (casinos, concert halls, parks, and the like) that graced their establishments.[25] Economic growth also created a burgeoning and buoyant middle class. In an era of scientific and technological progress, even the impossible seemed possible. It was only natural that such warm feelings spilled over into medicine, leading one doctor to proclaim in 1858 that "we do not believe in the notion of the impossible: the utopia of the day before is the truth of tomorrow; today, only systematic incredulity remains absurd."[26]

During these same years, an important conceptual shift encouraged physicians to think big. In rehabilitating the view that inflammation played a critical role in the genesis of cancer and tuberculosis, Rudolph Virchow revived the hope that they were dynamic, remediable disorders. He also successfully demystified the tumor cell and the tubercle. On the basis of painstaking pathological research, he demonstrated that their cellular components, if admittedly bizarre, were normal cells transformed by a concrete and identifiable force, which he theorized to be inflammation. Post-Virchow, no one defended Laënnec's notion of "heteromorphic" elements, with their nebulous and sinister overtones. Virchow thus stripped discussions surrounding these disorders of their most metaphysical element: the diathesic transformation of the body.[27]

Hopeful rhetoric was also a welcome balm to a profession struggling with futility and despair.[28] No matter how well-founded one's skepticism, hope continued to flourish. Decades before belief in tuberculosis' curability became common currency and a century before the development of effective antibiotics, even an arch pessimist admitted that pipe dreams sustained both patient and physician.[29] Despite all the evidence to the contrary, no one liked to think that medicine was powerless against the disease. Doctors, in other words, were ready to lose a battle well-fought. What they couldn't accept was that it was lost from the outset.[30]

Over time, willing credulity increasingly colored practitioners' attitudes toward available therapies. Though none seemed to work well independently, surely they were effective if combined intelligently. In an 1874 apologetic, one Parisian notable admitted that doctors traditionally had exaggerated the effectiveness of their therapeutic discoveries. He believed that each had found its place, however, before insisting that doctors should acknowledge their "therapeutic faith" in the range of available remedies.[31] Dissatisfied with the morose views of their immediate predecessors, he and a growing number of physicians chose to tell a different story about tuberculosis. Viewed from a distance, the second half of the nineteenth century stands as a watershed moment in the history of chronic disease. Though the treatments on offer came almost directly from the traditional *materia medica*, perceptions of the prognosis of tuberculosis (and to a degree cancer) had taken a 180-degree turn by the 1890s.

The bacteriological revolution was one source of inspiration. Though Koch's 1882 discovery of the tubercle bacillus didn't have immediate therapeutic implications, it dramatically affected perceptions. It added to the astonishment and excitement around modern medicine, an enthusiasm earnestly cultivated by practitioners of all stripes.[32] It also shifted attention away from the patient's body. The fact that tuberculosis was caused by a foreign pathogen made it reasonable to assume that the bodies of at least some of its victims were inherently healthy. This line of reasoning culminated in the Parisian professor Joseph Grancher's assertion that the pathological changes found at autopsy reflected physiological abundance, not misery.[33] In addition to being one of France's leading pediatricians, Grancher was popular with students and well-connected politically. His optimistic beliefs eventually found an inspiring, if controversial outlet. L'Oeuvre de Grancher, founded in 1903, took poor children from tuberculous households and arranged for them to be raised in the healthy country air.

If clearly an important catalyst, Koch's discovery cannot alone account for this changed mind-set. Rather, the main impetus came from a group of elite physicians who encouraged everyone to ignore the usual, banal patient experience (they still died!) and concentrate instead on more uplifting evidence of progress. By using the word *cure* creatively and focusing upon their healthiest patients, they could claim that the deadliest diatheses were in fact readily curable. Through the selective use of knowledge and evidence, a new and improved gospel of hope was delivered to an increasingly receptive audience.

## Case Study Number 1—The Curability of Tuberculosis 1860–1900

A few years before his death in 1869, a leading mid-century physician, Adolphe Grisolle, expressed doubts about accumulating anatomical evidence that, in the minds of some, corresponded to healed tuberculosis. Concerned by the shocking discrepancy between clinical experience and some anatomists' claims, he warned that "one should not consider all individuals with scarred tubercles at autopsy as having been cured of phthisis; by this count nine-tenths of the human race would be phthisics and pulmonary tuber-culisation would be, among the grave afflictions, the most curable of all."[34] Grisolle put his finger on something that was still true in the 1860s: autopsy evidence remained the only compelling source of hope.

Admittedly, optimists could point to exceptional cases, cured after exhibiting all the signs and symptoms of tuberculosis. Though always controversial, such anecdotes were enough to convince some.[35] Over time, a pedagogical exercise based on vague recollections took the form of a concerted effort to collect and disseminate such reports.[36] Eventually, an informal international collaboration to publicize them emerged, part of an effort to win the battle of perceptions. In 1890, Georges Daremberg insisted that "the physician who directs the treatment of consumptives must be profoundly persuaded that pulmonary phthisis is curable," noting that "Laënnec already believed in its curability; today clinicians the world over have verified this assertion. . . . I too have followed several consumptives for ten years who, completely cured, have taken up their occupations again, have married and had healthy children. I can even say that the consumptive (cured for ten years) that I know best is me. Thus let me loudly proclaim that the cure of consumptives is possible, since I have succeeded so well in my job as a patient."[37] Diagnosed with phthisis in his twenties, Daremberg nonetheless went on to be an accomplished clinician and respected medical journalist. His articles appeared in high-profile medical periodicals such as *Progrès medical* as well as the leading organ of the French intelligentsia, the *Journal des débats*. He also published several books on tuberculosis before succumbing to the disease in 1907, aged fifty-seven.

Beyond convincing the lucky beneficiary, "doctor stories" were par-ticularly compelling for many physicians.[38] In a few high-profile instances, famous clinicians even requested postmortem validation of their diagnos-tic suspicions.[39] Yet even such exceptional cases were unable to bear the full burden of proof. As one skeptic noted, "We believe that the value of the few cases of cures that can be cited has been exaggerated." They cer-tainly couldn't compare to the countless thousands who perished accord-ing to what many took to be the law of nature.[40] Even optimists indirectly acknowledged that, taken alone, the cures constituted flimsy evidence. One of the better-known optimists was Sigismund Jaccoud, professor of clinical medicine at the Paris medical school and perpetual secretary of the Academy of Medicine. In a series of lectures in 1881, he could find no better way to describe such events than "providential."[41]

Unfortunately, Providence was neither a reliable helpmate nor scien-tifically credible. Many medical observers, in fact, leveled harsh criticism against credulous colleagues who placed too much faith in these narratives.[42]

Without denying that some cases ended happily, Montpellier professor J. B. Fonssagrives cautioned that "the usual thread of the prognosis of phthisis is non-cure . . . the reputedly cured consumptive is ninety-nine times out of a hundred a patient who has become an invalid."[43] By 1881, Fonssagrives struggled to convince his colleagues that recent therapeutic hubris had done more harm than good. Tuberculosis, strictly speaking, was still incurable. While his concerns were many, one that frustrated him most was doctors' ambiguous and misleading use of the word "cure."

## What Does It Really Mean to Cure?

In 1864, a would-be optimist pointed out that diatheses, even when left untended, could remain quiescent for months or years. It was important to keep this in mind because with many miracle cures, "the story often goes back only a few months, or one or two years at most."[44] In retrospect, the putative cure of phthisis referred to several possible outcomes, ranging from a momentary improvement in symptoms to a permanent resolution of all signs and symptoms of disease. These categories were obviously not mutually exclusive and the duration of each outcome varied.[45] One of Jaccoud's *Clinical Lessons* usefully illustrated this phenomenon, for he noted,

> I had the satisfaction of seeing the patients leave the hospital after three or four months of treatment, their constitutions regenerated, allowing them to take up their occupations and their daily lives without fatigue; the lesions were very often the same as at the moment of entry, but the organism was now capable of resisting their extension and consumptive influence; and a year, eighteen months, two years passed before these individuals were obliged to leave their jobs to come back and seek succor; in two cases, this delay, which is the measure of the relative cure, was even three years.[46]

Jaccoud repeatedly used the term "relative cure" in his lectures.[47] He wasn't alone; a fellow member of the Academy, Hermann Pidoux, called such reprieves "quasi-cures."[48] By the 1890s, people actively debated whether the use of such terms was appropriate.[49] Immersing himself in the controversy in 1892, Daremberg proposed to do away with all modifiers, proposing that the term cure be reserved for a tubercular who "during ten years, has taken up their occupations without having had an episode of coughing up of blood, a bout of fever attributable to a burst of activity of the tuberculosis, a single sputum with bacilli."[50]

Often, however, "cure" was an elastic term that referred to anything other than rapid progression to death. Sometimes the word was used so loosely that it led to accusations of professional misconduct.[51] Yet even if one allows for the corrosive effects of self-interest, the question remains: why didn't doctors simply say tuberculosis was treatable? The issue was partly semantic, a linguistic legacy of the recent past that left everyone with no other idiom for describing the effects of their treatments. Yet it probably reflected something more basic: a desire to play up one's accomplishments amid uncertainty and self-doubt. In their struggle to believe in themselves, doctors referred back to their highest calling—the predictable, methodical, and permanent eradication of disease. Pidoux certainly preferred to frame his efforts this way, insisting that "the question is not to know whether or not these cures are as solid as those [we have seen with] pneumonia, and whether or not the subject is susceptible to a relapse. I say that he is cured, as one can be in the case of a chronic illness. Medicine is thus not impotent against Phthisis."[52]

## The Creation of a New Form of Tuberculosis—"Imminent" Disease

Barely twenty years after Grisolle rejected suggestions that tuberculosis was the most curable chronic disease, Joseph Grancher proclaimed to Paris's medical students that he knew "of no chronic disease upon which therapeutics has more of a hold."[53] In under a half-century, tuberculosis went from being among the most incurable chronic diseases to arguably the least. How was this possible?

The sanatorium movement's emphasis on rest and aggressive nutritional support probably did help some patients. Yet France had no public sanatoria until well into the twentieth century. Improvements in overall health, an offshoot of rising living standards, may also have made tuberculosis less consistently lethal. Yet changing perceptions, rather than declining mortality rates, seem to have been decisive. By late century, those who got identified as tuberculosis victims increasingly included people with early, even preclinical, disease. Just as the word cure was increasingly fluid, a diagnosis of tuberculosis became far more ecumenical, embracing cases that Laënnec and other pioneering anatomico-pathologists, in their quest for diagnostic accuracy, had tried to exclude. Aware of the temptation that such practices posed, Pierre Louis had specifically warned of the "many errors into which we would be drawn, if we sought to establish [the diagnosis] at the beginning of the affliction." Given that early-stage phthisis often improved spontaneously only to relapse a short time later, Louis also saw little merit in curing such cases.[54]

Between the mid-1830s and the 1870s, elite physicians rarely made boastful claims about their ability to reliably cure well-established tuberculosis. Everyone was eager to offer advice to affluent individuals who believed that they had a tuberculous taint, however. Catering to the worried well appears to have been one of the more desirable aspects of medical practice.[55] Growing numbers presumably agreed with Pidoux that such cases were the most important because they were the most curable. He was among the first to insist that diathesis-carriers exhibiting subtle symptoms and minor physical signs had curable tuberculosis.[56] Here, too, he was an avatar, though the importance eventually accorded such claims probably exceeded his expectations.

Fewer than ten years later, Jaccoud spoke of "imminent tuberculosis" while insisting that "without a doubt the practical utility of these presumptive elements is very often annihilated because the physician intervenes too late, that is to say at an epoch when it is not a question of a possible illness, but of a confirmed one." He used this as a pretext to proclaim that "medical intervention is often too tardy, the negligence comes either from the patient or the family, or the physician, ill aware of the value of presumptive signs of tuberculosis, believes himself authorized to do nothing, from the moment that he detects the absence of existing lesions; no matter the cause, what is certain is that in a large number of cases, the premonitory period is not used, or is so tardily, that the so-called prophylaxis is actually confounded with the treatment of confirmed illness." Elsewhere, he used the term "virtual illness" to describe high-risk individuals who were not yet symptomatic.[57]

In 1890, Grancher provided a forceful account of a heretofore ignored phase of the disease. Believing it to be a truer reflection of events inside the body, he argued that there were four stages to tuberculosis not three, as clinicians since the time of Hippocrates had believed. While acknowledging that the physical signs were subtle and almost nonexistent during the germinal stage, their detection was crucial because "*a precocious diagnosis, made at the stage of germination, is that much more useful, because at this time, therapy is all powerful at stopping the evolution of the tuberculous process.*"[58] He then provided an expansive case definition: anyone with pleurisy or anemia and subtle lung findings had "germinal tuberculosis." Anyone convalescing from another serious illness was a "candidate for tuberculosis." Fortunately, they were all curable. He also insisted that these patients' unimpressive physical signs matched autopsy findings observed during the previous hundred years.[59] Subtle findings signaled early tuberculosis, which thousands and thousands of autopsies had purportedly demonstrated was readily curable.

Grancher recognized that his ideas might be too radical for some. He wasn't sure his colleagues would accept that germinal tuberculosis existed, admitting that "it may take considerable time to bring along their convictions on these two points: that a precocious diagnosis is possible and that therapy at this point is often very effective."[60] Perhaps deep down he knew he needn't worry, for his was a message destined to please. Beyond challenging their diagnostic acumen, the successful detection of germinal tuberculosis allowed doctors to do what they most wanted: "cure" patients.

Grancher's ideas quickly carried the day. Within a few years, he and other opinion leaders were forcefully encouraging ordinary citizens to engage in active self-diagnosis. In the introduction to a 1900 work that popularized the new gospel, a noted authority on tuberculosis asserted, "It is to the mother, it is to the head of the family that you address yourself, to them that you show how tuberculosis of the lungs is the most common of chronic diseases. After which you prove that it is surely the most curable of the prolonged ills that decimate humanity. . . . You say, in effect, to the patient who reads you: 'you will be cured if you firmly wish.'"[61] The book's author, Dr. Élisée Ribard, aimed to teach mothers to recognize childhood tuberculosis long before it became obvious. Single episodes of haemoptysis, colds that lasted more than three weeks, protracted bouts of bronchitis, even a severe and prolonged sense of weakness, he warned, constituted the first manifestations.

He also highlighted the important distinction that doctors were now making between a tubercular and a consumptive, informing them that "today, telling a patient that he is tubercular is no longer pronouncing his death, but really giving him encouragement. . . . Be on your guard, you must at all costs rid yourself of this enemy; it has already produced tubercles that are impairing your breathing; soon it will make poisons, will spread them in your body; and from tubercular you will become consumptive/ *now one almost always dies from consumption.*"[62] The shifting meaning of "tuberculosis" and "tubercular" was the cornerstone of the revised doctrine of curability. Perhaps unwittingly, Grancher demonstrated how paramount this new disease was to this nascent ideology of therapeutic hope. The outcome of old-style tuberculosis was the same as it had always been; when patients had reached the disease's first stage, they were almost invariably incurable.[63] Decades before the advent of effective antibiotic therapy, semantic shifts drove the perception that medicine was poised to conquer the disease.

Physicians came to believe, and convinced many others, that relatively vague, even innocuous symptoms signaled tuberculosis, albeit an eminently curable form. Although this optimistic vision was widely embraced, lingering doubts remained. In 1905, Daremberg observed that "when you have cured him [the patient with early symptoms and minimal signs], you will certainly meet charitable souls, even among your colleagues, who will not restrain themselves from repeating that you have cured someone who was not sick."[64] Such concerns were used to great effect by Thomas Mann. One of the deep, unresolved tensions in his early twentieth-century masterpiece *The Magic Mountain* is whether its hero, Hans Castorp, is sick or whether the sanatorium doctor invented his illness with the help of a powerful new technology, the x-ray.[65] This all-important innovation allowed doctors and authorities to peer more effectively into people's bodies in search of latent disease.

## Case Study Number 2—The Cure of
## Uterine Cancer, or the Triumph over Fear

An 1883 thesis on uterine cancer candidly admitted that "in spite of our efforts, surgeons' hardy ones or the patiently sustained ones of physicians, we are but little more advanced than the contemporaries of Hippocrates."[66] By all accounts, this form of cancer was particularly awful. Predominantly afflicting young women, its suffering left everyone grappling with feelings of alienation, helplessness, and pity. Yet amid the gloom, a string of important discoveries fueled hopes that treatment of all forms of cancer was entering a new era. In 1892, an *éminence grise* of French surgery proclaimed that "the essential thing is to not despair and cross our arms, when we think about what we have done in the last twenty years for scourges as fearsome as pyemia, septicemia, erysipelas, puerperal fever, rabies, foot and mouth, tetanus, tuberculosis, etc. . . . if cancer remains the only disease whose essence remains unknown, it is that we have taken the wrong approach to understanding its development and to resolving all the unknowns that at the moment surround most aspects of its history."[67] While some fruitlessly searched for a "cancer bacteria," debate raged over whether it was a hereditary diathesis or an infectious disease. Opinion remained divided, yet even hard-core "constitutionalists" increasingly accepted that cancer began locally and only subsequently infected the rest of the body.

Less clear was whether precocious, radical surgery definitively rid the body of the disease. Amid this uncertainty, surgeons everywhere set off in search of the gynecological Holy Grail: the undisputed cure of a case of uterine cancer. Buoyed by refinements in anesthesia and antisepsis, optimists were increasingly adamant that it was possible to cure the disease. All that was missing was proof.

These events unfolded at a time when the emerging field of operative gynecology was at a critical crossroads. In the case of ovariotomy (that is, the removal of one or both ovaries), developments had been dramatic. Dismissed as unconscionably dangerous in the 1850s, by the mid 1880s it was regarded as a relatively safe and increasingly legitimate intervention. And although still controversial—particularly in France where it was slow in catching on—the procedure played a critical role in establishing the field of abdominal surgery.[68] The belief that a woman's overall physiological and psychological well-being mirrored her reproductive health helped rationalize a dramatic increase in operative interventions, both in Europe and North America. By the early twentieth century, American doctors had performed an estimated 150,000 ovariotomies, partly under the guise of protecting women's emotional stability and mental health.[69] In light of this, one understands why one physician noted in 1891 that "many men who started as gynecologists are now our most brilliant surgeons."[70]

In many ways, uterine cancer represented the ideal test case for modern surgery's curative potential. It was anatomically singular, at the interface between inside and outside the body. Surgeons everywhere assumed that success here would provide a critical proof of the concept, opening the body to ever-more radical procedures. Yet for over two decades, it could neither be guaranteed nor proven that surgery was up to the task. It was, in fact, only in 1904 that a pioneering German surgeon presented a case, cured for more than twenty-six years, which others judged to have "establish[ed] the operative curability of uterine cancer."[71]

With a mortality rate around 70 percent when the treatment first became widespread, the only thing clear about total hysterectomies was that this operation was deadly. Published descriptions, along with one singularly bad experience, led the most accomplished French ovariotomist to "abandon them with pleasure to surgeons whose ardor for flashy surgical novelties has not been put to the test." This admission was followed by a warning, imploring practitioners to be extremely cautious "because it is impossible to cite any cases of cure from the numerous hysterectomies carried out for true cancer." Those who survived the operation, Professor Koberlé insisted, succumbed faster than those treated conservatively.[72] Another equally prominent surgeon suggested that palliative approaches were less dangerous and equally effective, as evidenced by the prolonged survival of those who declined surgery. Rare instances of survival several years post-op, Dr. Després insisted, reflected errors in diagnosis. Even the diagnostic gold standard—microscopic confirmation—was incapable of settling the matter, because "too often we have the microscope say what we want it to."[73]

That same year (1887), an American colleague used an address at the Ninth International Medical Conference in Washington as an occasion to condemn the practice of total hysterectomy. While conceding that the operation may have been a justifiable experiment in earlier times, Dr. Reeves Jackson suggested that it was time everyone recognized that "the operation, instead of being more beneficial than preceding and comparable methods, has been proven to be actually injurious. It has not prolonged life; on the contrary, it has shortened and sacrificed it. It has only lessened suffering in those who died. It has not only given worse results that any other method of treatment, but worse than those of the disease left to itself. . . . [How long] should the destructive work go on? Shall there be any limit?"[74] Contemporary statistics uphold his rebuke. From 1878 to 1904, the published mortality rate of vaginal and abdominal hysterectomy was approximately one in three. In 1891, mortality rates were as high as 30 percent; by decade's end they remained a staggering one in five.[75] These figures may, in fact, have underestimated the risks, as surgeons apparently failed to report bad outcomes.[76] Clearly discouraged, a proponent of aggressive surgery for uterine cancer eventually admitted in 1891 that "no matter what the procedure employed, it is always a palliative procedure as with everything that addresses cancer."[77]

Yet some surgeons in France and abroad persisted; to use an expression applied to late twentieth-century transplant surgery, they had the "courage to fail."[78] Aptly characterized as radical, they were a beleaguered yet vocal minority on both sides of the Atlantic.[79] Prodded by their many critics, several stood up to justify their actions. Among the most voluble was Louis-Gustave Richelot. In 1885, he told the influential Surgical Society of Paris that "we have the right to hope for, in a small number of cases, a radical cure of cancer; all surgeons, in all years, seemed to believe in it, acted as though they believed in it; this search for the cure is the best means for finding the procedures that come closest to this or gives our patients the longest survival."[80] The ensuing decades-long controversy exhibited striking similarities to debates around tuberculosis. Key discussants created innovative and ingenuous ways of defining "cure" while focusing attention on those in the earliest preclinical stages.

Collectively, proponents of hysterectomy generally made a critically important value judgment: a single good outcome justified everything else. One thus understands a young student's calculation that "even if we had only one chance in a hundred, the death sentence being without appeal in the case of nonintervention, vaginal hysterectomy must be preferred to all other methods, because all others have failure as their final outcome."[81] One member of the Academy of Medicine was deeply concerned by the "moral hazard" associated with this line of reasoning. He intimated that, in their single-minded pursuit of a cure, radical surgeons were motivated more by a desire to demonstrate their operative dexterity than by their patients' best interests.[82] In some cases, the risk was real, not imagined. Accusations of venality, publicity seeking, and inadequate consent abounded and, it would appear, were not wholly unmerited.[83]

In an effort to deflect criticism, hysterectomy's proponents insisted that high operative mortality rates simply reflected inexperience. Invoking the learning curve, a particularly important factor in the case of surgery, served two essential functions. It justified failure while framing operative death as a technical rather than a moral issue—a regrettable, though necessary, price of progress. Projecting into the future was particularly important in the bleak early years. Richelot, for instance, argued in 1885 that "to summarize,

Gentlemen, I do not believe that I am deluding myself in saying that the reduction of the time required for the most difficult part of the vaginal hysterectomy will constitute a veritable progress, as it will shorten the duration of the operation, diminish the violence of the maneuvers and surely prevent hemorrhages. . . . Antisepsis will do the rest and the operation thus corrected will give, I hope, fine successes."[84] Careful to highlight incremental improvements in operative mortality, radical surgeons sought refuge in cancer's complexity. Undaunted by unflattering statistical evidence, Richelot insisted that "the facts that concern the physician are too delicate and composed of elements too diverse for such fictive method to ever become clinical truths, and analysis must always correct the brutality of the numbers."[85] He was convinced that statistics hadn't had the last word, if only because surgeons had generally operated on the sickest patients.

Despite refinements in operative techniques, surgeons continued to have trouble finding women with early-stage disease willing to undergo an operation. Therein lays a critically important difference between these social dynamics and those around other heroic interventions. Late twentieth-century transplant surgeons faced many of the same issues (uncertainty, high surgical mortality rates, low "success" rates, calls for a moratorium) and used similar rhetorical techniques when discussing their failures (the scientific merit of their efforts, the need to look past the present and into the future). Yet in this latter case it was dying patients rather than relatively healthy ones who were risking their lives.[86] Nineteenth-century gynecologists thus fought an uphill battle; yet while waiting for someone to come forward with definitive proof, they slowly began to emphasize how hysterectomy was associated with several types of "cure."

The prominence eventually accorded "operative cures" was an early manifestation of a broader trend. Surgical narratives in the 1880s adopted the practice of pronouncing as cured anyone who didn't die immediately. One illuminating example of a now general phenomenon appeared in a series presented to the Parisian Surgical Society in 1892. It chronicled the case of a thirty-seven-year-old woman "rapidly cured" although "dead in May 1890, seven months after the operation"; followed by that of D. Z. "operative cure without incident . . . Pelvic and genito(thigh) pain: must have succumbed in a hospice where the patient was admitted."[87] The choice of "cure" over, say, "survival" was not innocent; it suggested that physicians were beginning to accomplish the Herculean task of saving those previously dismissed as hopeless.

During a critical time in the debates, advocates proposed an even more radical shift in the therapeutic goalposts. Aware that almost everyone relapsed in the first twenty-four months, Richelot noted that "in some statistics, one calls cured patients who have gone past two years."[88] Four years later, a medical student parroted his professor's verbal acrobatics, noting how "speaking of complete cure [in uterine cancer] we rally completely to the opinion of M. Pozzi who wishes to substitute the term 'durable cure.' Given that we can never speak of a definitive cure in the case of cancer . . . as he says so well, 'a temporary cure is still a cure.'"[89] Conceptual and linguistic gymnastics played an equally important role in the case of breast cancer; in defending radical mastectomy, the high-profile American surgeon William Halstead accorded pride of place to the prevention of local recurrences rather than so-called ultimate cures.[90]

Some went even further in blurring semantic boundaries, insisting that interventions that provided a semblance of a cure, however temporary, were preferable to those that only assuaged symptoms. Eventually, such reprieves emerged as the main justification for putting patients' lives at risk. Dismissing certain forms of statistical evidence put forward by his opponents, Richelot argued in 1891 that "what one must know, to judge the operation, is the number of months or years that it adds to life, if one can determine it; of most interest is the time that passes prior to the appearance of the relapse."[91] Within two months, he had refined this line of reasoning, reiterating that the average survival of all patients was both irrelevant and misleading; the thing that mattered most was how long it took for the tumor to recur.[92] Richelot did not specify whether he invented this therapeutic yardstick or imported it from outside of France. What is clear is that he was the first French surgeon to promote radical surgery exclusively on the basis of a precept that would become central to doctors' understanding of prognosis within oncology: disease-free survival.

## Why Are They Still Here? Incurable Illness in an Era of Exuberance

Physicians had to be linguistically nimble whenever they discussed incurability, acknowledging medicine's limits without undermining its authority. Not surprisingly, bad outcomes required more discursive dexterity as diseases became reputedly curable. In the case of cancer, experts increasingly blamed unenlightened colleagues and misguided patients. At the Second International Conference on Cancer (1910), one of France's leading surgeons characterized ignorant or sloppy physicians as a deadly menace. Worse, countless patients delayed seeking reputable advice, availed the services of incompetent healers, or simply refused treatment.[93]

Given the disease's legendary tenacity, it was understandable that most cancer patients lost the battle. With tuberculosis, the profession faced a true conundrum. If it was the most curable chronic disease, why did so many people with it die? Over time, therapeutic optimists managed to explain away this paradox. The Parisian professor Noël Gueneau de Mussy's *Clinical*

*Lessons* on phthisis set the standard. He began his lecture by asserting that "almost all the depictions of this illness that have been traced in recent years were based upon observations made in the hospital, that is to say in conditions that precipitate the evolution of the illness, and render its outcome almost inevitably lethal. Misery and debauchery, the double fruit of ignorance, become the auxiliaries of this murderous diathesis, and render its attack more irreparable."[94] This brief passage provided the blueprint for subsequent discussions. Slowly but surely, the biological determinism of the anatomico-pathologists gave way to social and behavioral determinism.

The archetypal working-class consumptive's health, everyone knew, had been destroyed by a combination of misery, overwork, and vice. Compounding the problem, such patients sought help too late and inevitably received suboptimal care. Was it any wonder that they were incurable?[95] In the evolution of doctors' prognostic perceptions, commonplace clinical experience was increasingly deemed conceptually irrelevant. Social factors, not biology, explained the medical misfortunes of the poor and indigent.

Yet what was one to make of the many rich sufferers who also withered away and died? Physicians put forward several explanations. Hereditary forms of the disease, they averred, were understandably lethal and refractory.[96] As with working-class patients, doctors also increasingly blamed wealthy tuberculars whenever things went awry; they became incurable because they did too many wrong things and not enough right ones. For some, immorality and excess led to irreparable internal misery. More often, however, subtler forms of personal negligence were invoked to explain the mixed track record of the "new" and highly effective therapeutic regimens.

Citing German statistics that showed that only 6 percent of sanatoria patients died during their first admission, several French leaders insisted that this regimen also prevented and cured relapses.[97] The problem was one of discipline: too few patients submitted to therapies that were long, tiresome, and demanding. The pitfalls were legion. As Daremberg noted, such therapy "must be scrupulously supervised, especially when some improvement begins to be felt. At this point, the patient believes himself cured and can by his imprudence lose in a few weeks the fruit of several years of sage and enlightened care."[98] Though the road was long and arduous, the patient was ultimately responsible for his or her recovery.

If prognostic views had become increasingly optimistic over time, one thing endured: individual physicians' insistence that they were not at fault when a patient's disease proved incurable. A disillusioned medical student spoke for all when he remarked that "unfortunately, in the society in which we live we are too often forced to be content with [preventive] treatments which would be far more useful if everyone could follow the precepts of the [medical] arts. This power, in effect, does not always exist: too little fortune, freedom; here the passions; but all that is outside of the physician, he sees the ill but cannot remedy it."[99] Amid the differences of opinion, discussions around (in)curability consistently referred back to causes specific to nature and the environment, to medical virtuosity and to the sick themselves. The relative importance accorded each varied over time. Together, however, they constituted the conceptual foundation for coming to terms with a singularly disturbing sociobiological experience.

## Conclusion—Out with the Old, In with the New?

Throughout history, the meaning and definition of incurability have been unstable and contingent, subject to the vagaries of scientific progress and disease ecology. In the twentieth century, certain breakthroughs have led to dramatic and high-profile shifts. Sometimes, as with diabetes and AIDS, one should speak of transformation rather than cure.[100] With other high-profile disorders, however (bubonic plague, neurosyphilis), the situation is less ambiguous: specific therapies can eradicate the responsible microorganism. In the case of nineteenth-century France, the shift from "reputedly incurable" to reputedly curable was gradual and contested, reflecting an animated, century-long exchange.

It is worth emphasizing that in all Western nations, contemporaries recognized that there existed two biologically distinct disease entities called cancer and phthisis/tuberculosis. Despite improvements in nutritional status, their prognosis also remained grave and relatively stable. It is unlikely that case fatality rates were so dramatically affected by early twentieth-century therapies as to make the disease eminently curable in a presentist sense. Even if most doctors embraced the semantic shift in an era of thunderous scientific optimism, some influential practitioners and members of the general public were clearly unconvinced.[101] Ironically, in 1905 a leading optimist insisted that tuberculosis among the poor was actually more incurable than in Laënnec's day.[102]

Reflecting contemporaries' porous understanding of therapeutic efficacy, prognostic science was largely a matter of perceptions and choices.[103] It varied, in other words, according to the particular subject whose (in)curability was being considered. Further, physicians who insisted that all manner of treatment benefit represented a form of cure made it even more difficult to distinguish "curable" from "incurable."

One should not equate linguistic manipulation with a lack of sophistication, however. Explanations of medicine's powerlessness were often scientifically savvy and attuned to the big picture. They share, in fact, many affinities with recent analyses of the political and economic forces driving tuberculosis's ongoing incurability in many parts of the world.[104] Assessing treatment benefit in chronic disease remains problematic even today, despite the availability of powerful diagnostic, technological, and statistical tools. If we worry aloud now about the scientific validity of randomized control trials in this setting, nineteenth-century practitioners had no choice but to do what they could with far less.

It is also important to emphasize that, for both personal and social reasons, prognostic indeterminacy long suited many people's interests. In many ways, it was only with the passage of a French pension law on July 14, 1905, that objectively diagnosing incurability became a matter of pressing public interest. With the flick of a pen, a specific sociomedical identity—occupationally disabled because of incurable illness—became a political reality with financial implications for the entire citizenry.

Interestingly, it was assumed that the law's application would be unproblematic. Just as one could use a birth certificate to measure "old age," its framers assumed that determining whether someone was "incurable" was straightforward. Doctors' input was thought unnecessary; incurability was assumed to be so obvious that the community could judge the matter. Yet amid growing concern that too many compensation-demanding incurables were abusing the system, a ministerial decree (August 3, 1909) accorded doctors an important gatekeeping function. Henceforth, only medically certified invalids and incurables could receive compensation.[105] Tellingly, this provoked a brief turf war between hospital and community-based physicians, who were accused of lacking the necessary impartiality to fulfill this important duty.[106]

Driven by fears that the process was too subjective and physicians overly indulgent, efforts were made to impose a uniform assessment method. In 1911, Dr. E. Ravon published a scoring system that assigned a numerical value to various disabilities and diseases. Only a disability rating of 50 percent or more entitled the sick person to a pension. The list was remarkably thorough, though like the vocabulary of curability itself it left ample room for interpretation and negotiation. Not surprisingly, cancer and tuberculosis figured prominently. Everyone with a malignant tumor automatically qualified. Partly because of concerns about bankrupting the state, it remained unclear whether tuberculosis was covered by this law or not. Ravon insisted that those in the disease's second stage needed to be judged on a case-by-case basis; those who could still put in a day's work were expected to. Only patients in the third stage, with weeks or months to live, automatically qualified.[107] Beyond its attention to detail, this classification system exemplified a process that became increasingly pronounced during the twentieth century: the objectification, bureaucratization, and standardization of misery.

It also points to something more fundamental and human about incurability: it is at once obvious yet highly subjective. The century-long controversies explored here demonstrate that the more complex and laden the question (socially, economically, politically), the more difficult it is to get at "the truth." Prognostic science was particularly freighted as it raised deep-seated questions about the nature of Nature and the meaning(s) of illness. Plagued by a sense of personal and professional vulnerability, doctors readily took credit for easy successes. As we shall now see, bad outcomes invariably elicited a search for scapegoats.

# 3

---

## "I Told You So"

### The Rhyme and Reason of Chronic Disease

During the nineteenth century, the science of chronic disease was intimately tied up with questions surrounding the meaning of life. If Sir Thomas Sydneham's centuries-old suggestion that mankind brought such sicknesses upon itself still represented the dominant conceit, Sir James Paget put his finger on something equally decisive.[1] In struggling to explain terminal illness, naturalism gave way to metaphysics. Addressing the Royal College of Surgeons in 1853, Paget acknowledged that malignant tumors and tubercles were singularly disturbing because "we trace no fulfilment of design for the well being of the body: they seem all purposeless or hurtful." Only Divine Will, inscrutable yet impeccably just, could explain this distressing state of affairs; for as he noted, "If our thoughts concerning purpose were bounded by this life, or were only lighted by a ray of an intellectual hope, we could not discover the signs of beneficence in violences against nature, or in early deaths. . . . But, in these seeming oppositions, faith can trace the Divine purposes, consistent and continuous, stretching far beyond the horizon of this life . . . untimely deaths should make us timely wise."[2] A profound aversion to the thought that "there is no point to all this" drove speculation about the moral logic of chronic disease, especially the deadliest diatheses. Successive generations of European and American pedagogues generally shared the belief that terminal illness was the penalty inflicted upon a misspent life.[3] One advantage of slow death, however, was that it offered the chance for personal and spiritual redemption.

Nineteenth-century explanatory narratives rejected the possibility that the diatheses were random events. Like insanity, they were read as a sign of individual weakness and social breakdown. Partly for this reason, an aura of disrepute consistently tarnished them. Along with alcoholism, the most ubiquitous and frightening constitutional illnesses—cancer, tuberculosis, syphilis, and scrofula—were linked to notions of individual and collective degeneration.[4] Albeit more pronounced by century's end, the association of these disorders with physical, intellectual, and social decline was a long-standing leitmotif. In both old world and new, it was assumed that all forms of deviance exacted a heavy toll. Incurable illness provided tangible proof of this deadly association and thereby played a critical role in reinforcing contemporary moral and behavioral norms.

## The Many Meanings of Chronic Disease

In struggling to understand a world rife with illness, contemporaries were guided by the assumption that they had experienced a biological fall from grace. In 1807, a young physician insisted that chronic diseases were much neglected by the ancients. This was due to their supposed rarity in days past: depraved habits, unnatural diets, and luxurious ways were modern vices, after all.[5] While agreeing that the number of those afflicted was increasing, one Restoration-era priest blamed the Enlightenment and French Revolution for this distressing state of affairs. At the inauguration of a hospice for incurables, Father Léraillé insisted that "the cause of our irremediable infirmities [resides] in our discords or the shameful libertinage which from the upper classes descended into the obscurest ranks, producing monstrous excesses."[6] Yet the didactics of chronic disease were never one-sided. If many American health reformers similarly implicated a long series of moral transgressions, other theorists turned such logic on its head.[7] Anticipating claims subsequently embraced by certain eugenicists, a French expert insisted in 1867 that "Christian civilization, by showing that the value of human life resides more in his intellectual power that in physical strength, by conserving and in elevating, contrary to the customs and practices of antiquity, people with sickly constitutions, has potently contributed to the development of chronic illnesses, and has, so to speak, furnished the raw material."[8] Throughout the century, writers from across the ideological spectrum exhibited a perennial concern about the deleterious effects of civilization.

Among the clichés in Hubert Lauvergne's 1842 ethnography of death and dying was that civilization was "fertile *ad infinitum* in poisons to the physical nature of man"; it denatured constitutions and planted the seeds of various organic illnesses.[9] He was not alone in his views. Linking modern life, nervous ailments, and insanity has been a strikingly tenacious cross-cultural paradigm.[10] Yet "Progress" had even deadlier consequences than nervous exhaustion. Citing cancer's rarity among the natives of Guyana, the father of modern dermatology, Baron Jean Alibert, insisted in 1833 that there was a direct correlation between a society's cultural refinement and its cancer risk.[11] Others used Parisian mortality data to prove the existence of these links.[12] Despite occasional flashes of skepticism, this belief was widespread and enduring.[13] Members of Paul Broca's Anthropological Society, for example, showed a perennial interest in the relationship between race, civilization, and cancer, insisting that ethnomedical studies proved that primitive peoples were relatively immune.[14] This belief that modernity causes cancer has obviously persisted into the twentieth century, notably among those of a "holist" bent.[15]

Tuberculosis was the other leading marker of social and physical decay. In 1879, one Franco-German authority suggested that as simple life gave way to luxury and excess, "tuberculosis progressed even among the [American] colonists living in the towns and countryside."[16] Yet as with neurasthenia, experience with consumption led people to blame specific aspects of the modern socioeconomic order. Increasingly, it was urbanization, with its stresses, strains, and miseries that was implicated. Painting a somber picture of the effects of urban poverty, François Broussais rued the proletariat's embrace of various "artificial stimulations." While acknowledging that "everywhere man is avid for stimulation and wants to feel alive," strong coffee and strong liquor were far more injurious than the salubrious pursuits of country life.[17]

Broussais's lament echoed a fear that figured prominently in the emerging public health movement: the city's fatal attraction for ruddy peasants, drawn by the siren song of wealth and luxury. Only too often, tuberculosis was all that they had to show for their troubles. Variants on this morality tale, already discernible in the 1830s, became increasingly strident over time.[18] The worrisome association between tuberculosis and urban migration and societal decay represented an elaborate trope that figured prominently in most late-century discussions of the disease.[19] Because of this, sanitary reform and urban renewal became rallying cries among American and English public health advocates. In France, a romantic attachment to the land and paranoia about demographic decline made much of the rhetoric more explicitly antiurban.

Concerns about broad cultural trends and population health provided the backdrop against which physicians assessed patients' individual vulnerability to illness. Beyond being a source of professional pride, predicting who would fall sick was a deadly serious matter. For if TB occasionally appeared in those who seemed biologically sound, far more common were those "whose nature rendered them propitious to the appearance of the disorder, *tuberculosis patients by original sin.*"[20] Certain patterns of physical development were deemed cause for concern. A narrow chest, spindly limbs, high cheek bones, pallor, and flushing elicited an avalanche of hygienic advice. Most worrisome of all, however, was the lymphatic constitution, the touchstone of chronic disease. One student described the afflicted as "beings offering only flaccidity and softness in the tissues, only weakness and slowness in their functions, delicacy in their organization, pallor in their entire habitus; they are all asthenia." If most assumed that the effeminate and languid were at great risk, this truism came with a worrisome caveat: "one must also include in this class of men those who, under a fine appearance, often disguise the greatest weakness and inertia."[21]

Often enough, reading the biological tea leaves proved fractious and unnerving. Many parents of lymphatic children were actually proud of their child's appearance; as one physician observed, "They do not suspect that below this fine, rosy, transparent, delicate skin, is hidden a vice, terrible as the poison within certain flowers that decorate our flower beds."[22] This imagery illustrates an important burden that was associated with certain chronic diseases; the appearance of a diathesis invariably raised suspicions, putting the stricken at the center of a discomfiting dialectic: Why me? Why him? Physiological explanations increasingly fractured along national and linguistic lines. Strikingly, however, the importance accorded to consumptives' constitution, if anything, gained momentum in the era after germ theory changed everything.[23]

The precise relationship between tuberculosis and the other diatheses remained contested; different theorists spoke of affinities, antagonisms, and transformations. Most authorities were convinced that there was a link between scrofula, tuberculosis, and cancer, however. The leading causes of hereditary phthisis, Noël Guneau de Mussy explained to the University of Paris medical class in 1858, were vice, poor hygiene, parental age, and health status. Cancerous parents, for instance, frequently engendered tuberculous children.[24] Such convictions, in turn, reinforced perceptions that the diatheses were distinct, self-perpetuating disorders caused by bad blood.[25]

Hygienic discussions at once identified those whom biology had seemingly condemned while holding up the promise of individual and collective redemption. For it was assumed that sound advice and right living would enable people to enjoy the fruits of modernity with impunity. All but the most foreboding theorists presumed that physical constitutions, like ecosystems, could be preserved and partially restored. If each had its own rich and variegated history, social movements such as phrenology and temperance were bound by a transcendent faith in the power to transform the world one life at a time. Activists of every stripe were confident that eugenic marriages, prenatal hygiene, and careful child rearing would reliably produce a nation of "healthy, moral, and intelligent children."[26] Yet getting a good start was only the beginning. Maintaining good health involved a lifelong struggle against temptation.[27]

Nineteenth-century jeremiads had a strikingly formulaic quality to them. Stomach cancer, it was intoned, was caused by thwarted ambition, bitter emotions, and alcohol abuse.[28] Gout was the product of gluttony.[29]

Repeat offenders, most liked to believe, could expect an early grave. Reflecting contemporary wisdom, Herman Pidoux warned that consumption would remain rampant until society "corrected the loose morals, the habits of luxury and indolence, the excesses of the table, the torments of ambition and all the stings of life that never cease to overexcite and exhaust the rich classes, to first foment gout with all its tortures, and later phthisis with its languor and mortality."[30] The stories of dissolute bourgeois men who died alone and consumptive vividly illustrated the depths to which the socially superior could descend.[31]

Whenever talk turned to tainted constitutions, syphilis and other sexually transmitted diseases invariably came up. Late-century physicians and social reformers, for example, highlighted its horrors as part of an effort to reform public morals. Venereal disease and prostitution were framed as interrelated social menaces, threatening individual bodies and depleting the nation's vitality.[32] Syphilis, like alcohol, also framed late-century discussions of tuberculosis.[33] Without questioning the stridency and organizational aplomb of Victorian moral crusaders and their successors, the idea that the fin-de-siècle "syphilis phobia" was unprecedented historically should be viewed skeptically, however.[34] The disorder had long figured prominently in discussions of chronic disease.

For many, syphilis was the first link in the pathological chain. In a widely cited treatise on hereditary disease published in 1808, one of the doyens of French medicine, Antoine Portal, argued that most chronic conditions were caused by the scrofulous vice, best treated with anti-syphilis mercurials.[35] Others were less diplomatic in their considerations of causality. The physician credited with founding modern dermatology, Baron Jean Alibert, claimed that "nobody doubts that most of the scrofulous individuals of Paris are disguised syphilitics" and listed its principal causes as venereal excess, class hatred, and arrested moral development.[36] As time went on, the medical elite took a more nuanced position; venereal disease was a predisposing rather than requisite cause of the other chronic diseases. Many practitioners continued to insist that most organic illness was caused by syphilis or the toxic effects of mercury, however.[37] One successful mid-century charlatan, for example, insisted that his panacea acted against the root cause of chronicity. Claiming that darters, syphilis, and scrofula "are fomented by an inner virus of an identical nature," he maintained that this virus "determines and complicates 19/20[ths] of the other Chronic Diseases."[38] His views were obviously self-serving and simplistic. One suspects, however, that they mirrored the common understanding of morbid physiology, notions that, in turn, allowed the patent medicine market to thrive.

These were not simply working-class views; aberrancy and ill health were closely linked in everyone's mind. Like countless others, René Laënnec assumed that syphilis and masturbation, alone or in tandem, caused phthisis, insanity, and wasting.[39] Even in the United States, where such subjects were comparably taboo, it was assumed that the sins of the father weighed heavily; as historian Charles Rosenberg has observed, "Children conceived by a sexually exhausted father and sexually abused mother would, according to such [hereditarian] formulas, suffer from one of those diathetical conditions that guaranteed a brief and miserable life."[40] The cycle of immorality didn't stop here, however, as consumptives were also assumed to have voracious sexual appetites. Repeated inquiry led the ever-skeptical Pierre Louis to dismiss the idea; just like other chronically ill patients, consumptives' physical ills decreased their sexual drive. Without speculating why this former view was so pervasive, most patients apparently found the idea ridiculous.[41] Despite such remonstrance, learned discussions of consumptives' prowess remained commonplace a half-century later.[42]

Many also drew connections between sexual misconduct and uterine cancer.[43] Interestingly, when facts suggested otherwise, the facts were simply set aside. Discounting statistical evidence indicating that prostitutes were not particularly prone to uterine cancer, a leading surgeon countered that most were simply too young to have developed the disease. Obliged to account for its appearance among the virginal, he invoked deviance of a different sort; he crassly suggested that nuns, doomed to celibacy, were unable "to resist the temptations of onanism" and masturbated themselves to an early grave.[44] Beyond indulging in a hackneyed male sexual fantasy about convent life, these comments belied a widely shared assumption, that abnormal or immoderate sexuality was injurious.

Admittedly, everyone acknowledged that factors beyond one's control caused illness. Dramatic personal upheaval and changing social circumstances were known to be physically ruinous. Physicians and moralists also spoke sympathetically of dutiful spouses, usually wives, whose singleminded devotion fatally undermined their health. Yet when authorities summed up their insights, the dictates of medical moralism generally eclipsed all else. Jaumes's study of incurability revealingly concluded that "incurable illnesses, for the most part, come from the hygienic errors which we commit and especially faults which accumulate from generation to generation."[45] A mid-century advice book was even more judgmental. Mankind was naturally healthy, it optimistically averred. Chronic illness was the punishment meted out for flaunting the laws of morality and of hygiene.[46] Most discussions of chronic disease thus included a warning and an indictment, which together constituted the moral ecology of disease. Over time, the struggle between optimists and pessimists grew more one-sided as the scientific establishment increasingly spoke of the progressive degeneration of the human species.

## Chronic Progressive Diseases and the New Intentionality of Nature

Though no nation was spared, France experienced more than its share of upheavals during the nineteenth century, as simmering unrest erupted sporadically in violent protest and civil war. If everyone but the Royalists looked to the future rather than the past, the country's mid-century experiment with mass democracy left many profoundly disheartened. Some have suggested that the resulting disillusionment, coupled with experience treating cretinism, decisively affected Benedict-Auguste Morel's ideas about "degeneration."[47] This asylum director from the working-class city of Rouen gained international recognition for his theory of human evolution, which posited that contemporary France, and all mankind for that matter, was caught in a downward evolutionary spiral.

In formulating his ideas, Morel drew on a variety of disciplines, including anthropology, physiology, and natural history. He was also influenced by deeply felt metaphysical and spiritual convictions. His Viennese Catholic upbringing had been austere and devout, experiences that eventually spawned a strongly rebellious streak. Given his own struggles with poverty, one understands why he was drawn to Philipe Buchez's vision of Christian socialism with its emphasis on egalitarianism and social action. In the end, Morel formulated a compelling synthesis in which Christian teleology and creationism were forged to scientific concerns with heredity, the environment, and national decline.[48]

Preoccupied by what he and others believed was an alarming increase in the incidence of insanity, Morel pointed to the physical and moral squalor produced by rapid industrialization. Combined with alcohol abuse, these urban environments produced individuals who were physically and mentally stunted. Through the implacable workings of heredity, their condition worsened across generations, culminating in idiocy and sterility. Given his professional training, Morel not surprisingly focused on degeneration's neuropsychiatric manifestations: alcoholism, hysteria, epilepsy, and idiocy. Yet he and others considered certain chronic diseases to be their somatic equivalent.[49]

The notion of degeneration is generally viewed as a late-century phenomenon, an outgrowth of fin-de-siècle anxieties and prejudices. Discussions of deviance, criminality, and insanity increasingly focused on biological rather than social factors. Faced with growing numbers of chronic and intractable cases of insanity, psychiatrists' early-century optimism progressively gave way to somber hereditarianism, and by century's end, experts on both sides of the Atlantic concluded that many, perhaps most, criminals and lunatics were born incurable.[50] Concerns for France's future only darkened after the Franco-Prussian War and the violent paroxysms of the Commune (1870–71).

The progressive reworking of Morel's ideas played a critical role in articulating these fears, providing a scientific idiom for making sense of a wide range of antisocial behaviors.[51]

Yet for somatic emblems of degeneration (which included scrofula, cancer, tuberculosis, and syphilis), late-century views differed more in intensity than in kind. In this case, hygienic confidence had always been half-hearted. Decades before Morel committed his ideas to paper, others had expressed concern that humanity was regressing biologically. A carefully reasoned study of hereditary diseases from 1817 painted an unapologetically somber picture. Unwholesome urban environments and dysgenic marriage practices were paving the road to ruin, prompting the warning that "such insouciance, or rather iniquity, is one of the principal causes of the degeneration of the human species that we see in the large cities and the depopulation that is the necessary consequence."[52] Even a fervent opponent of hereditarianism, François Broussais, acknowledged in 1834 that misery, poor hygiene, and vice ensured that poor constitutions "become habitual; tubercular productions, lymphatic degenerations of all kinds, form soon after; death strikes the young prior to the age of marriage; if they make it to that point, their children will not reach adulthood, they will not pass the stages of dentition, or they will be carried off by scrofula or eruptive phlegmasias; thus families are extinguished after a small number of generations."[53] Over time, sociopolitical, intellectual, and ideological trends increased the receptiveness of industrialized societies to this somber view of modernity. As with most late-century hygienic campaigns, efforts at combating degeneration were an indicator of Malthusianism's declining influence. In the first half of the century, the upper class saw no compelling reason to address the laboring classes' woeful physical and moral state.[54] For various reasons, however, the belief that chronic ill-health and premature death were, as Malthus suggested, the natural order of things progressively yielded to the fear that a decaying breeding stock would undermine the French nation in its struggle to survive.[55]

The fear of (de)evolution arose as Darwinism was destabilizing traditional ideas and assumptions, and its basic precepts decisively shaped attitudes towards chronic disease. For a start, the wastefulness of natural selection shattered earlier images of Nature's beneficence. Equally important, Darwinism posed a threat to Church teachings and Christian teleology. The resulting crisis of confidence encouraged the pursuit of secular forms of transcendence, both cultural and biological. Philosophers as different as Hippolyte Taine and Friedrich Nietzsche celebrated the critical importance of genius in the transmission of culture even as social Darwinists such as Herbert Spencer defended the dominance of specific classes, races, and nations. This chauvinistic theory of history, in turn, legitimated colonialism, militarism, and the more virulent strains of nativism.

In many ways, Darwinism's impact in France was modest compared to its hold on the Anglo-Saxon world. The country's leading scientists and learned societies barely acknowledged his writings. This "conspiracy of silence" greatly dismayed Charles Darwin, whose candidacy as a corresponding member in the French Academy of Science was rejected eight times between 1870 and 1878.[56] Partly this reflected France's indigenous and largely hostile evolutionary tradition. It also mirrored French savants' disinterest in the mechanics of species transformation; the country's intellectuals instead focused their attention on human prehistory and the divisive issue of spontaneous generation. Empirical to a fault, they found Darwin's ideas overly speculative. In their minds, the evidence didn't support his bold assertions.[57]

Although it didn't take the scientific community by storm, *The Origin of Species* certainly didn't go unnoticed. The notoriety mostly reflected the circumstances surrounding its introduction to the French reading public. Unable to find a scientist willing to translate the work, Darwin settled on a little-known *femmes de letters*, Clémence Royer. Her opinionated footnotes were problematic enough. Worse, her fifty-page introduction was an antireligious polemic that included claims—particularly about the origins of life—that Darwin had refused to entertain. Greatly dismayed, he eventually arranged for a competing translation. The damage was done, however, and Royer's comments played into the hands of those who judged the work seditious and atheistic.

Reassured by the entrenched scientific opposition, the Catholic hierarchy kept a low profile until Darwin turned his attention to the origins of man. In 1877, the devoutly Catholic Constantin James published *Du Darwinisme ou l'homme singe*.[58] This incendiary text included a laudatory letter by Pius IX attacking Darwinism as both absurd and morally corrupt. Yet in subsequent decades, important rifts appeared in Catholic opinion. Swayed by its growing scientific legitimacy, certain Catholic scientists and theologians endorsed Darwinism's basic tenets. Many authorities remained committed to the fixity of species, however, and leading Catholic journals more or less rejected all forms of evolution until well into the twentieth century.[59]

If its social and scientific trajectory varied considerably from country to country, Darwinism had one consistent effect: it validated hereditarian thinking and stimulated interest in biological and social meliorism. The most infamous of the resulting reform movements was eugenics, a term coined in 1883 by Englishman Francis Galton. Between 1890 and 1930, eugenics movements were founded in over thirty countries, adapting the transcendental "Galtonian gospel" to local conditions.[60] Interestingly, Clémence Royer anticipated one of the movement's important strands, known as negative eugenics. Near the end of her preface to *Origin of Species*, she called for the elimination of "the weak, the infirm, the incurable, the wicked themselves and all the disgraces of nature . . . which they perpetuate and multiply indefinitely."[61] In France, her preaching fortunately fell on barren soil. The country's eugenicists focused their attention on improving socioeconomic conditions rather than limiting the reproduction of undesirables. Liberal hostility to state intervention, long-standing fears about depopulation, and Church opposition helped the country avoid the state-sanctioned abuses that were perpetrated in the United States and particularly in Germany.[62]

In France and elsewhere, however, this intellectual ferment paved the way for a compelling new understanding of chronic progressive disease: it was nature's way of eliminating losers. Just as insanity and idiocy brought neuropsychiatric degeneration to a close, cancer and tuberculosis eliminated the physically degenerate. In 1859, two years after Benedict Morel published his famous observations, a leading member of the Paris medical faculty told the students that "when one envisages the frequency of tuberculization and studies the causes," it was obvious that "even as substances that cannot be assimilated are chased out of the organism, radically spoiled organisms are eliminated from the bosom of the living collective."[63]

Intentionality emerged as an integral part of the metaphysics of terminal illness. Hermann Pidoux, for instance, described cancer and tuberculosis as the "ultimate" chronic illnesses, disorders that "finish people off."[64] He and other authorities increasingly took the position that these disorders served an important housekeeping function.[65] The country's leading expert in the emerging field of cardiology, Michael Peter, boasted of the social benefits that came with Nature's self regulation; when one or both parents were defective, he told the medical class, "the descendant, infinitely degenerate, unfit for the struggle for life, finishes himself and his line off by tuberculising himself."[66] Terminal illnesses thus emerged as the booby prize of natural selection, a development that contributed to their being layered with racial and class biases.

In 1888, a leading medical encyclopedia included a comprehensive table that summarized long-standing ideas and anxieties regarding humanity's fall from physiological grace. Several somatic disorders contributed to human degeneration, including syphilis, scrofula, tuberculosis, leprosy, rickets, and cancer.[67] The importance of these diatheses to Morel's theory—and hereditarianism more generally—should not be underestimated. Along with insanity, alcoholism, and idiocy, both venereal and wasting diseases provided tangible proof that some people were morally and biologically unfit. Terminal illness also served as a microcosmic template for population degeneration. In this, chronic progressive illnesses played a critical role as both signifier and signified. They were at once a potent cause of species' decay and emblematic of the process.[68]

Having long existed as parallel narratives, the conceptual histories of psychiatric and somatic diseases become interwoven at mid-century, seamlessly connecting ideology and biology. After the 1860s, their destinies became increasingly enmeshed and the process of physical/mental/moral degeneration almost inseparable.[69] A few internationally acclaimed psychiatrists such as Paul Moreau de Tours and Benjamin Ball posited a direct link, suggesting that physical disorders like tuberculosis and scrofula could mysteriously metamorphose into mental illness and vice versa.[70] However fleetingly, the concept "degeneration" captured the spirit of an age and briefly broke down the barriers between the most devastating disorders of psyche and soma. In societies preoccupied with order—biological, social, and political—chronic progressive illness and insanity were disturbing reminders of mankind's self-destructive potential.[71]

These disorders have also been lightning rods for discrediting mythologies and representations.[72] Predictably, syphilis has consistently been demonized, and even the vocabulary used to describe it has contributed to the censure.[73] Yet talk of inner vices, hereditary taints, and paternal syphilis consistently pervaded discussions of cancer and tuberculosis as well.[74] When evidence suggested that heredity played a modest role, critics countered that most patients lied about their families.[75] Logic that today seems circular was accepted in a setting marked by distrust of others and firm convictions about how the world worked.

One can appreciate that being labeled a degenerate or a degenerate-to-be was a humiliating experience, and people understandably tried to shield themselves and their families. The opprobrium around certain diatheses was evident in an 1879 discussion at the Academy of Medicine. The blue-ribbon panel mandated to examine the reliability of Parisian death certificates identified several important pitfalls. Most practitioners were unwilling to list syphilis and suicide as causes of death, while "some will not declare that their clients died from cancerous or tuberculous afflictions, or other hereditarily transmitted diatheses, out of fear of being prejudicial to the interests of the client's children."[76] The authors' use of legal phraseology was not accidental. Marriage was generally part business, one in which the label "damaged goods" seriously undermined one's prospects. In the early twentieth century, tuberculosis's stigma was so pronounced that Georges Daremberg maintained that most wealthy families

do not dare bring their consumptive children to consult with a physician for tuberculosis patients, or if they do, ask him to say he doesn't know them. The families would never admit that the father or mother or sister of a young girl died from tuberculosis; all relations are severed with the physician who treated the deceased. If they run into them, they feign to not recognize them. You see how little one can rely on the sincerity of families, when you seek sanitary information with a view to marriage. The most honorable, the most religious, hide the truth without scruples.[77]

The fear and stigma surrounding the disease continued to haunt the recovered tubercular; many apparently sought to conceal their past the way a "recovered alcoholic" or "recovered drug addict" might do today.[78]

There's little doubt that Koch's discovery of the tubercle bacillus and changing sociopolitical circumstances had significant effects on patients' experiences. The stridency of the accusatory discourses, channeled via a more effective public health infrastructure, also had an impact on perceptions. Along with late-century concerns about degeneration, these factors led to the profound stigmatization of those afflicted with syphilis or consumption.[79] Despite this, it is important to not overemphasize the decisiveness of the historical break. If changing perceptions increased patients' sense of shame, this was an issue not of kind but of degree. Late-century shifts involved the stripping away of a paper-thin veneer rather than the whole-scale construction of a radically novel attitude. Fully understanding the history of stigmatization requires that we consider the sights, smells, and miseries of terminal illness, the anti-aesthetics of suffering, if you will.

# 4

## Death, Decay, and the Genesis of Shame

This refuge is for you, Oh unhappy child
Whose tainted blood torments,
Though innocent, you are left to weep
A mother's misfortune or a parent's errant ways! . . .
You, upon whom the world, instead of delights
Heaped scorn or even its abuse
Because of a vice that inheres in your drooping frame.

—*Adélaïde Perrin et les jeunes filles incurables* (1875)

Ritual and narrative have long been sources of solace in the struggle with adversity. In the Christian tradition, illness represented the price of original sin, a symbol of the transitoriness of earthly existence, and a foretaste of hell's torments. Most importantly, however, disease was a vehicle of spiritual awakening and growth and a divine reminder that earthly life should be spent preparing for the hereafter. Such chastisement was particularly important for the wealthy; it was a precious corrective for the deadliest of sins, vanity.[1] To this day, spiritual reflections on sickness remain an important strand of devotional literature. Yet beginning in the mid-eighteenth century, a secular imagery of virtue amid hardship began to emerge. In his novel *Nouvelle Héloïse* (1769), Jean-Jacques Rousseau presented a new and sentimental image of death and dying. At its climax, the stricken heroine slips serenely away, surrounded by her loving family and undisturbed at the prospect of divine judgment.[2] In the century that followed, consumption epitomized this new ethos; even now, the mortally stricken poet is emblematic of the "Romantic age." During its nineteenth-century heyday, the disease was equated, metaphorically at least, with a nobility of spirit that left one vulnerable to disease. Physical dissolution, in turn, offered even courtesans the chance to attain personal and spiritual perfection.

Building on the oft-cited observation of the noted American essayist Susan Sontag, some have suggested that consumption was not a stigmatized disorder of the "other" like syphilis or cancer until the late nineteenth century.[3] The literary and social elite supposedly embraced and internalized their predicament; consumption, so cast, was "a source of cultural value" and "a focus for a certain kind of fashionable narcissism and self-dramatisation."[4] In the case of France, we'll see that that this flight into fiction was more self-protective than self-celebratory, a phenomenon that shares features of something that modern stigma theorists term a "separate system of honor."[5] My aim in revisiting this much-discussed issue is to explore the relationship between representation and the range of lived experiences and to examine the internal logic of stigmatization, particularly the symbiosis that exists between chronicity, incurability, and suffering. Wasting diseases, in particular, have inspired searching questions and incriminating discourses. This largely reflects their unique phenomenology; the living dead stirred up such apprehension that people simply couldn't ignore them.

## Consumption in the Romantic Era:
## Sublime Defeat or Banal Suffering?

It is difficult to delineate the exact chronological boundaries of European Romanticism. Originating in Germany, it spawned a series of indigenous national movements, each with its own dynamic and specificities.[6] Furthermore, one also finds quintessentially "romantic" elements in works outside this period. In many ways, it is easier to speak of its apogee, between 1780 and 1840. Given its lasting effects on Western culture, however, even marking its decline is problematic, all the more so because Romanticism was many things to many people: a literary guild, an ethos, a sensitivity, a way of seeing/knowing/being in the world, and a manifesto (both artistic and personal).[7] Its heterogeneity and numerous internal contradictions only increase the label's indistinctness. In short, there's an omnipresent danger of either seeing Romanticism everywhere or of circumscribing it too narrowly. Despite this, one can readily identify the methods, sensibilities, and concerns that characterized Romantic art and analyze the historical context in which these works were produced. Romanticism can thus be partly understood by examining the specific cultural products and the particular circumstances—material, political, social, and intellectual—that inspired their creation.

This sixty-year period witnessed the emergence of a new breed of artist whose identity was deeply and inextricably enmeshed with his work. Certain themes—like the exuberance and careless destructiveness of nature—were integral to the Romantic ethos. Equally characteristic was the growing fascination with distant times, exotic places, liminal states, and the hidden genius of simple folk and "noble savages." All these areas of interest were marked by a striking exaltation and spontaneity. The period's best works were also stylistically and experientially probing. In the pursuit of an ideal, Romantic art, particularly poetry, explored humanity's other self: primal, hidden, dangerous, and sublime. Unlike the Classicism that preceded it, high art was no longer content to hold up a mirror to nature. Through the rich use of symbol, imagery, and myth, the artist offered a glimpse of a deeper truth or unrealizable ideal. The Romantics aspired to (re)create a sense of harmony with nature, with humanity, and with the divine, a quest all the more poignant because it was assumed to be unattainable.

Events inside and outside Germany played a central role in the movement's genesis. Romanticism was partly a backlash against the French Enlightenment, with its dispassionate rationality and pursuit of geometric certainties. Romantic artists and philosophers also sought to get beyond the tranquil contemplation of nature. Believed by some to mark the high point of Romantic philosophy, the German philosopher Johann Gottlieb Fichte insisted that even his discipline was ultimately about doing rather than knowing. He was both a passionate witness to world events and a fervent German patriot; enormously influential in his own day and beyond, Fichte viewed knowledge as "simply an instrument provided by nature for the purpose of an effective life, of action." Many artists and intellectuals were of the same mind, valorizing creations that dared to be heroic.[8]

In the realm of both art and politics, the French Revolution and its aftermath—the Terror, the rise and fall of Napoleon—were transformative. At once sources of hope and dismay, these events inspired successive generations of Romantic artists. The lessons they drew varied. Among the most destabilizing was that there was no foreordained order to things. They also demonstrated that the forces of unreason could exert as powerful an influence on the course of history as any science of good government.

That a brave new world didn't rise out of Europe's ashes was another source of frustration and inspiration. Obsessed with order and stability, the Restoration was dismissed as stultifying and narrow-minded. Amid a range of opinions about the nature of the ideal society, it was universally assumed that there had to be more to life than social climbing and soul-destroying ennui. A few famous individuals such as Alphonse de Lamartine and Victor Hugo turned to politics. Most withdrew into themselves; as one literary historian has observed, "The poetic response to the age's severe political and social dislocations was to reach for solutions in the realm of ideas."[9] In a very real sense, the same was true of illness, grief, and loss.

Consumption was an important literary vehicle and a potent Romantic symbol. Like insanity, it was associated with genius and excessive sensitivity. It thus embodied a cruel paradox: a beautiful person enveloped by a horrible disease. In the representation of experience, aesthetics and biology were gently interwoven. Phthisis's premonitory signs—mild weight loss, glossy whiteness, and rosy cheeks—were also marks of beauty. Spitting up blood, emotionally distressing yet physically painless, announced the beginning of the end. Yet even during the descent into oblivion, these personages remained larger than life. A fitting end, marked by a final act of love and renunciation, completed the tableau. Death was the ultimate aesthetic gesture, fulsome and fulfilling. From beginning to end, Romantic-style suffering was ethereal and uplifting.

The emotionally taut imagery that pervaded portraiture, literature, and contemporary narratives is so compelling that some scholars have suggested it provides a window onto actual experiences. There is some merit to this. Even the more rarefied elements of the Romantic narrative weren't completely divorced from reality. Consumption was rich in pathos, partly because remissions both troubled and inspired. It was a disease, one diarist noted, "which more than any other tortures the heart with hopes and fears."[10] Some sufferers, it appears, consciously patterned their behavior to match literary representations.[11] Consumption lent itself to emotionalism partly because it left some people's sense of dignity relatively intact. It was a long-standing cliché that consumptives were naturally insouciant; as one expert noted in 1879, "even when things are totally desperate, phthisis veils life's ills and the horrors of death."[12] Their *belle indifférence* in the face of impending death was generally credited to youthful naiveté and nebulous changes in the brain.[13] That being said, cultural practices and conceits helped sustain this aura of unreality. Romantic-era art and contemporary palliative practices both sought to deny the harsh reality of physical decay and premature death.

Equanimity tended to be in short supply when people's physical condition deteriorated, however. One mid-century expert noted how "at the beginning, consumptives are carefree, because they suffer little or not at all, and yet how frightened they become when they experience a crisis of breathlessness or spit up blood. Their mood understandably improves as their physical state improves; but all it requires is for their cough to get worse, that fever, night sweats appear, and they begin to worry again."[14] Even among those committed to self-fashioning, bodily decay left little room for the sublime. On the basis of the diaries of four famous consumptives (Anton Chekhov, Franz Kafka, Katherine Mansfield, and Marie Bashkirtseff), sociologists Claudine Herzlich and Janine Pierret insist that each case was marked by an inverted mythology. "In the beginning these writers felt as if their illness had removed them from ordinary life and engaged them in an abstract confrontation with passion and with death, a confrontation in which the body was barely implicated," they observed. With time, however, "each of them discovered the weight of the most material limitations—symptoms, the invasion of the self by illness, the difficulty of maintaining relations with others, exclusion from the world. In this manner all of them gradually discovered that they were sick."[15]

Sick bodies unfortunately tended to tyrannize both mind and spirit. In 1806, respected surgeon and essayist Marc Antoine Petit observed that "the first egotist must have been a man who was suffering: pain multiplies the *human ego* a hundred-fold."[16] In 1898, in an era marked by widespread interest in the emerging field of psychology, another physician invoked the "frenzied individualism" and the "ferocious narcissism" of the chronically ill before bemoaning the fact that "yesterday he made a show of his specu-lative mind, or related anecdotes, or confided his projects; today he can only speak of his illness, complete with fastidious harpings."[17] Rather than encouraging spiritual refinement, chronic ill health tended to engender self-absorbed complainers.[18]

Yet in an era when marks of distinction were critically important, the elite desperately clung to an idealized vision of themselves, even those who were terminally ill. That the beau monde, at the turn of the nineteenth century, increasingly preferred to die in seclusion is telling in this regard. Read by some as a sign of worldly sophistication, it also helped preserve a sanitized image of the self.[19] Even when death was a public affair, great care was taken to impart the desired impression. The composer Frederic Chopin provided one such example. His passing was preserved for posterity in grand Romantic style. The private diary of the noted author George Sand paints a very different picture of the brilliant artist, however. At one point, she com-plained of her lover's inability to "vanquish the worries of his imagination." Elsewhere she called him a "detestable patient" who behaved as though "his spirit had been skinned alive."[20] More than anything, idealized representa-tions were culturally consonant abstractions that embroidered virtue on an ugly necessity.

Iconic European consumptives were also not early-century Everymen; most sufferers were not affluent or gifted artists. For the old, the crippled, and the poor, dignity and self-worth were in very short supply. A leading Romantic *femmes de lettres*, Madame de Staël, had few illusions, observing that "certain physiognomies escape degradation by virtue of the splendor of their spirit, but the human form, in its decadence, often takes on the most vulgar expression, which barely allows for feelings of pity."[21] That certain stigmata of consumption were aestheticized also does not mean that the disease was free of stigma. In the early nineteenth century, scrofula was a shameful disease that people sought to conceal. Yet it, too, was associated with intellectual precocity and artistic genius. The stricken also displayed the animated features and waxy beauty central to the esthetics of tuberculosis.[22]

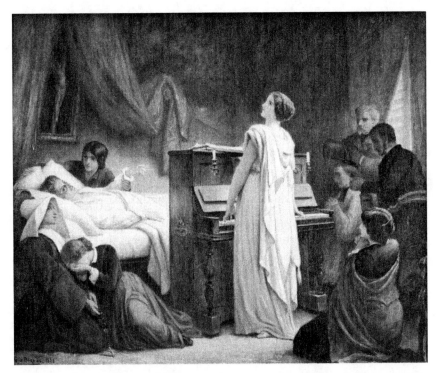

FIGURE 4.1. A picture postcard based on Felix Joseph Barrias (France, 1822–1907), *The Death of Chopin*. Chopin's longtime friend and admirer, the Countess Delphine Potocka, apparently sang for him as he lay dying. The original hangs in the Polish National Museum. Reproduced with permission from the National Museum of Cracow.

Most important of all, life for most sufferers consisted of more than writing poetry or active self-fashioning. Even the social elite understood success in material terms—raising healthy and successful children, living a long life, accumulating wealth or honors. It was in the orbit of daily life, in other words, that one looked for answers to questions such as What have I accomplished? What have I become? What am I bequeathing to posterity? By nearly all measures of success, consumption was anything but poetic.

Among the most troubling constants of chronic illness was that it made a mockery of all pretensions.[23] In 1885, a homeopath observed, "In sickness, all men are equal, and the misery of the rich is just as great as that of the poor . . . does one suffer less in a palace than in a hovel? For me, a patient is more pitiful than the poor, because the poor still posses the greatest of all goods . . . Health!"[24] Convinced that gentility and tuberculosis were incompatible, a member of French high society insisted, "I know of nothing more hideously fetid than the bedroom of a rich consumptive;

it is a scrupulously closed space, where air, along with hope, are forbidden entry; weather stripping on the doors, weather stripping on the windows; thick drapes enveloping the bed, where the poor consumptive stews in his sweatiness and in air twenty times re-breathed, twenty times soiled by contact with ulcerated lungs."[25] People's sense of self tended to be as devalued as their living spaces. Although southern Europe was a popular destination for affluent consumptives, its inhabitants were convinced that the disorder was contagious. During a health-seeking journey, George Sand bitterly complained that in Spain, "whoever is consumptive is pestiferous, leprous, and scabious."[26] Wealth, in other words, didn't insulate people from harsh treatment at the hands of others. At the same time, consumption also undermined gendered distinctions. Because of its association with prostitution, working-class female consumptives were increasingly tarred with the masculine vice of promiscuity. Chronically ill men, on the other hand, found themselves feminized: condemned to live like bourgeois women, idle and dependent.[27]

Yet for those who could permit themselves the luxury, "internalizing" tuberculosis was infinitely more appealing than invoking other explanatory paradigms that centered upon contagion, heredity, and vice.[28] For most people, the possibility of hereditary transmission was particularly upsetting. Patients with a distressing skin condition known as darters, one expert noted, preferred to believe they'd caught it from someone else because "no individual wishes to accept that a shameful disease should inhere in his own economy."[29] Tellingly, the people most intent on romanticizing the disease were singularly vulnerable on the issue of heredity. Wealthy consumptives presumably had fewer excuses for falling ill, be it malnutrition, substandard housing, or back-breaking work.[30] Romanticism provided the elite with an elaborate and compelling counternarrative: consumption was not a shameful, contagious, and hereditary disease but the tragic fate of high-minded idealists.

Such rationalization was presumably a source of comfort to some. In a very real sense, Romanticism, like Christianity, was singularly preoccupied with transcendence and redemption. The prize, however, was not eternal life but one's personal or artistic legacy. Using a largely secular idiom, it championed a long-standing and poignant ideal: an artful life and a good death were a bulwark against oblivion. In a world where religious certainties had been gravely undermined, idealism was a pleasing alternative to the harshness and cynicism that Honoré de Balzac so magnificently caricatured in his cycle of novels, La Comédie humaine. Mixing accurate accounts of historical events with detailed descriptions of Parisians' daily struggles, Balzac compellingly conveyed the lives of a city and its people. The result, on many levels, wasn't pretty; many of his most memorable fictional characters were harsh, grasping social climbers. They were also relentlessly ironic and judgmental, like the great novelist himself.

In the end, poets and literati had many reasons for choosing to portray consumption as sublime. It nonetheless remained a physical and emotional trial, as evidenced by the voluminous medical literature. Here a radically different vision of the disease emerges, one rife with "gruesome images of decay, putrefaction and stinking effluvia, no less repulsive than cancer."[31] Physicians' testimonials, I'd suggest, represent a privileged vantage point that lifted the artistic veil and revealed the terrible burdens imposed by consumption and other chronic, progressive illnesses.[32]

### Better Left Unsaid: Consumption in the Romantic Era

Prior to the twentieth century, North American and northern European societies didn't attempt to systematically segregate consumptives.[33] Fear and prejudice were translated into other forms of disapproval, however. Self-interest, conspiracy, and shame pervaded the question of marriage, and prospective spouses were screened for contagious and hereditary diseases. On this score, tuberculosis was clearly stigmatizing. An overview of marital hygiene from the leading compendium of medical knowledge, *La Dictionnaire des sciences médicales* (1819), stated that scrofula, widespread and comparably benign, didn't preclude marriage. The same was not true of "nervous" diseases (imbecility, dementia, and epilepsy), uterine cancer, and phthisis.[34]

In a setting marked by mutual suspicion, families were known to conceal health-related information.[35] The problem was so widespread that the reappearance of undeclared, preexisting consumption was considered grounds for annulment in France.[36] At the very least, a tuberculous "taint" dimmed one's marriage prospects on both sides of the Atlantic. It is telling that many early-century medical treatises warned the poor against marrying social superiors who were obviously ill. Though it is impossible to know how widespread this phenomenon was, for every family tempted to marry up the social ladder there was necessarily another ready to marry down.

Two twentieth-century phenomena further illustrate the hazards of accepting the romanticization of consumption at face value. Fashion designers in the 1990s, most notoriously Calvin Klein, were accused of glamorizing drug abuse by using models whose "look" called to mind heroin addiction.[37] AIDS has also spawned a rich iconography, much of which self-consciously exploits Romantic themes and symbolically laden forms.[38] Even a nineteenth-century classic, *La Bohème*, was recently reset with a dying AIDS patient replacing the consumptive heroine.[39] One would be hard-pressed to claim that AIDS or drug abuse is valorized as a cultural or physical ideal. Nor do these narratives shield sufferers from recrimination, exclusion, and shame. At most, refashioning shameful medical conditions helps blunt the slings and arrows that are part of the sufferer's lot.

In short, the fact that bright, socially connected people consciously crafted an ethereally inviting image of consumption does not mean that it wasn't also a source of shame and stigma. Anyone tempted to take such poetics literally forgets that Romantic art was never about reality. Illusion and displacement were one of its central preoccupations and most effective literary conventions. Most Romantic artists were animated by deeply felt ideological commitments and a keen sense of pathos; in the mind of one literary critic, this partly explains why Romantic poetry's "greatest moments of artistic success are almost always those associated with loss, failure and defeat."[40] At a day-to-day level, chronic ill health was clearly more baleful than beautiful. To better appreciate these disorders' impact, it is worth briefly considering some insights on the related issues of deviance and stigma.

## The Stigma of Incurable Suffering

In 1963, sociologist Howard Becker published a groundbreaking study that insisted that deviance could only be understood by examining the social worlds, motivations, and interactions of those on either side of the label "deviant."[41] Among his most powerful claims was that this was not a universal, immutable category but one imbued with socially determined, value-laden assumptions. Focusing on the discredited members of society ignored the motivations and biases of those who passed judgment.

That same year, sociologist Erving Goffman published his now-classic study of stigmatization. Merging previous work on identity formation and the social world of asylums, he argued that a stigma was the product of a dynamic process involving predicaments, relationships, and strategies.[42] Because of negative stereotypes or a perceived performance gap between themselves and normals, stigmatized groups were devalued by the rest of society. Ashamed and diminished, they struggled to find ways to attenuate or conceal their perceived inadequacies via an active process he called "passing."[43] Goffman also maintained that normalcy and stigma are fluid concepts and that most people face an affront to their identity at some point in life.[44] Notwithstanding this important corrective that suggested that stigmas were ubiquitous, the "failings" he focused upon—severe disabilities, racial background, insanity, and homosexuality—were all highly stigmatizing in the 1960s.

Over time, insights from a school of thought known as labeling theory were applied to more forms of deviance, including physical illness. In a landmark study of the medical profession from 1970, Elliot Friedson denied that somatic illnesses were objective, biologically anchored, processes. He believed that they were largely socially constructed, by which he meant that diagnosis and treatment essentially took something that had no stable ontological status and "made it what it was." Equally important, Friedson suggested that society's response to illness varied according to both its imputed seriousness and perceived legitimacy, which ranged from illegitimate (that is, stigmatized) to unequivocally legitimate.[45]

Social scientists have emphasized the intertwining effects of biological and social factors upon people's disease trajectories.[46] Considerable attention has also been paid to the challenges faced by the chronically ill at different points of their "careers." Terms such as biographical disruption and identity crisis have been used to capture these disorders' far-reaching and deeply felt effects.[47] Many authors have also explored how patients adapt to chronic illness. By nature dynamic and unstable, adaptation invariably involves reconciling one's pre- and post-illness identities as well as forging a future amidst uncertainty, suffering, and loss.

Together, this body of scholarship had provided important insights into the process by which people do or do not find themselves devalued. With most chronic illnesses, one can speak of enacted stigma (something humiliating actually happens) or of felt stigma (activities are voluntarily curtailed out of a fear that something might happen).[48] Most chronically ill and disabled people also struggle with a delicate dilemma: wanting to have their predicament empathically acknowledged versus the desire to conceal their limitations.[49] Complicating matters further, the physically deviant do not represent a monolithic block; personal, financial, and social factors affect self-perception.[50] Power relations are also critical to the selective singling out of certain defectives; as one scholar recently reiterated, "Stigma is entirely dependent on social, economic, and political power—it takes power to stigmatize."[51] Importantly, it also takes power to resist.

Historically, the stigmatization of certain categories of patients has occurred through successive steps. First, illness subsumes identity; one is considered a patient rather than a person. Second, this new identity becomes a source of distress and shame. Many of the disorders that have traditionally been singled out, like plague and cholera, are both terrifying and disruptive.[52] Over time, "epidemic" and "scapegoat" have become virtually synonymous; victim-blaming, discrimination, and vilification have sustained distinctions between an able-bodied self and a sick (and often foreign) other.[53]

Shame and censure have also loomed large in the setting of chronic disease.[54] Given their effects on self-worth, all possess a certain stigmatizing potential. Various nineteenth-century commentators remarked that protracted suffering prompted feelings of inadequacy, even self-loathing.[55]

Misery, shame, and concealment went hand in hand, leading one mid-century onlooker to speak of "the wounded pride of the wounded life."[56] In an influential study of suicide, the respected psychiatrist Brierre de Bois-mont observed that physical pain and "social death" led many incurables to end their lives. In one of several illustrative suicide notes, a downwardly mobile artisan described his life as a "sorry existence." Humiliated by his inability to work, his perceived abandonment by master and coworkers was more than he could bear.[57] On this score, women's domestic responsibilities proved a mixed blessing. Though it imposed extra hardships, keeping house and home together apparently left them less prone to feeling useless than male breadwinners.[58]

The financial consequences of chronic disease were another source of humiliation and guilt.[59] An incurably ill artisan who had watched his world progressively disintegrate left the following words for his family and posterity: "My dear daughter, for six months your strength has been used up, you've silently pawned your possessions; soon we'll know the horrors of hunger. It is better that the person who is good for nothing departs; you have just gone out to make another sacrifice; upon your return, you'll no longer have me as a burden."[60] If the affluent did not risk going hungry, they faced other troubling affronts. Failing health frequently led to a loss of self-respect and social status, leaving them fearful and emotionally vulnerable. Making matters worse, rapacious relatives not infrequently began to circle when it appeared that a chronic illness would end in death.[61]

Harsh material conditions magnified people's suffering and the incrimi-natory power of illness. This was particularly manifest in the first half of the century, a period of rapid urban growth and widespread misery. It was a time when the affluent looked down on their inferiors with a mixture of dismay and disgust.[62] In a society organized around distinctions of rank, class, and wealth, incurables consistently counted among life's losers. Perhaps unaware of how denigrating the image was, Hermann Pidoux insisted that, to under-stand consumption, one needed to remember that "the more the organism is debased, the more illness is ascendant; the more it degenerates, the more it engenders. It lives from it: it is formed of its alterations and its garbage."[63]

Institutional policies towards incurables left little doubt that they were persona non grata. Already deeply self-conscious of their infirmities, they shouldered the extra burden of knowing that society had washed its hands of them. Though only one affront among many, this form of neglect stoked class hatred. The poor often enjoyed a cruel satisfaction at the thought of their social superiors falling ill; as one health primer noted, "Gout and its atrocious crises are the least punishments for this envied and reputedly happy life. Cancer, tuberculosis, apoplexia, serious neuroses, kidney and heart diseases daily leave [bourgeois] families in mourning and avenge the misery of the poor soul who dies in the hospital."[64] Rather than prompting a show of solidarity or solicitude, chronic illness tended to be experienced as a humiliating form of defeat.

This predicament put even intimate relations to the test. All too often, healthy people responded by closing ranks and avoiding the stricken. Relations between these two "enemy camps" were often strained, one ironic observer noted, if only because

> the well person sometimes lets slip his sense of joy that he's not the patient . . . he boasts of his luck, his hygiene, his biological factors, he feels the worth of his health; he speaks of his skill at maintaining it; it is his masterpiece which he embellishes day by day; and he severely judges the clumsy person who let his body sink into imbecilic suffering; he looks for quarrels. Let us flee this patient; he is ugly; he is dirty; he moans without shame; it suffices to come close to feel disenchanted with life: he is an upsetting reminder of the worst side of the human condition; he is the image of misery and distress.[65]

Only love, charity, or self-interest could effectively counterbalance such feelings. To be fair, many contemporaries displayed remarkable degrees of devotion. In 1829, a widowed milkmaid was awarded one of several annual Prizes for Virtue (Prix de vertu) by the Académie Française. Her award recognized twenty years of devoted care to an epileptic and handicapped child whose parents had abandoned her as an infant.[66] Yet despite such acts of heroism, there remained an almost unbridgeable gap, particularly when an affliction was both incurable and "repulsive."[67]

Prevailing attitudes at once mirrored and reinforced patients' sense of suffering and loss. One of the critical subtexts to incurability was summed up by the questions "what's wrong with you?" and "why don't you just get better?" In the 1830s, a Parisian charlatan discussed diathesis sufferers' desperate and unsuccessful attempts to purge their tainted blood. These disorders poisoned the physical and moral existence of both rich and poor; many sufferers' futures were so bleak that they were all but lost to society.[68] The opprobrium surrounding incurability was regularly translated into morally laden analogies. In a high-profile debate at the Academy of Medicine, one elite physician accounted for cancer's grim prognosis as follows: "individuals soiled [entachés] by a diathesis, comparable to hardened sinners, fall back, on the least provocation, into the same illness, I would say almost into the same pathological sin from which we had cured them more or less often."[69] The conviction that incurability was caused by some personal failing, in turn, weighed heavily upon the stricken. Stripped of social distinctions they'd enjoyed when in good health, innumerable chronically ill patients were dogged by a guilty conscience and the sense that they were physically imprisoned.[70]

More than anything else, heredity lent itself to feelings of inadequacy and blame. Via a nebulous though taken-for-granted process, socioeconomic, biological, and moral failings were supposedly transmitted to one's children.[71] For contemporaries, heredity allowed them to make sense of past, present, and future while anchoring their understanding of the notion of risk. Equally important, prevailing beliefs were predicated upon and enshrined a system of natural justice whose basic assumption was that virtue was rewarded and transgressions punished. Simultaneously morally laden and moralizing, hereditarian ideas were seamlessly embedded in prevailing social thought.[72]

In aristocratic societies, the appearance of a familial illness was a dramatic event that left one wondering whether the "deadly germ" was isolated or pervasive. It also meant that the peace and happiness of many a family depended upon their physician's sense of discretion. Many families sought to conceal information only to have the "indiscretion of illness" thwart their plans.[73] Like a stain with indelible ink, the development of a hereditary disorder such as consumption was a critically consequential and lasting social signifier. Beyond opening up an emotional can of worms, it risked changing the "clan identity" forever. Patients and their families risked being labeled disease carriers, poised to transmit their blemish to the yet unborn.

Throughout the nineteenth century, certain diatheses were subject to particular forms of censure. Though it never became state policy, two experts called for legal sanctions prohibiting marriage between individuals who each had a consumptive in the family.[74] Others maintained that a familial taint precluded certain otherwise natural and desirable activities. Reflecting the belief that hereditary diseases could be transmitted in multiple ways, in 1864 a mid-century physician reiterated the long-standing view that "a woman *can* and *must* breastfeed her child, when she is in good health, and has, among her ancestors or immediate relations, no scrofulous, tuberculous, or cancerous parents."[75]

Before considering why some disorders were consistently singled out, it is important to recall a few salient characteristics of the stigmatization process. The most important is that all chronic diseases can be associated with indignity and shame; stigmatization is not and was not an all-or-nothing phenomenon but a continuum marked by increasingly dramatic effects on identity and self-worth.[76] At the same time, various forms of psychological and social adaptation helped mitigate their impact. In the end, however, whether one's illness evolved well or badly was critically important. The most deadly and incurable diseases were also those that most profoundly soiled one's identity.[77]

## Terminal Illness and the Specter of Contagion

Some illnesses have been constructed in ways that raise few questions about the physical and moral integrity of the stricken. In struggling to account for society's relatively forgiving representation of heart disease, Susan Sontag has persuasively suggested that we have come to see it as reassuringly mechanical, readily accepted in terms of normal wear and tear.[78] Furthermore, many serious heart and kidney ailments are more palatable because they are episodic, at the borderline between acute and chronic. In the period before antibiotics, they tended to be more treatable and somewhat less onerous than either cancer or tuberculosis; depletive medicines (diuretics and others), digitalis, and nitroglycerine offered patients a respite from their travails, albeit often only transiently. Death often came suddenly, an ending whose brevity helped circumvent a protracted and disobliging scrutiny of the person's identity. The issue of ebbs and flows and of broken parts dominated discussions of their phenomenology; they were quite explicitly *not* diseases of consumption, wherein one withered away and died.

The deadliest diatheses, on the other hand, haunted the nineteenth century because of their troublingly predictable denouement, slow and lingering death. The terms *diathesis* and *cachexia* (the severe wasting seen with terminal illness) were so closely linked that people used them interchangeably until mid-century.[79] Even after disease and symptom were no longer synonymous, they remained integrally yoked in the minds of both physicians and the lay public.[80] Several features of scrofula, tuberculosis, and cancer were particularly disquieting. Their methodical lethality suggested that they were governed by a malevolent force; they also caused severe suffering and disability, exposing the human condition at its worst and most vulnerable. Finally, they led to physical deterioration so pronounced that the stricken seemed more dead than alive. Faced with unspeakable misery, contemporaries' fears and anxieties were consistently channeled into hand-wringing about biological and moral contagion.[81]

Many existing histories suggest that tuberculosis was deemed contagious only late in the century. The issue was not so clear-cut in the minds of contemporaries. Even the separation of Europe—before the triumph of bacteriology—into contagionist (south) and anti-contagionist (north) medical camps requires qualification. In France at least, popular prejudice consistently allowed for the possibility of person-to-person transmission.[82] The medical elite were also less than categorical. The Parisian notable Gabriel Andral acknowledged in 1837 that while the risk of personal contagion had been exaggerated by some, it was unreasonable to dismiss such concerns outright. Phthisis shared obvious affinities with other infectious diseases, to say nothing of the "miasmas" that patients' lungs and skin exuded. He concluded that those in daily contact with consumptives needed to take certain precautions, particularly when the illness reached its final stages.[83] In subsequent decades, such studied ambiguity was the norm.[84] Even a leading anti-contagionist cited the dangers posed by exhalations produced by the bodies of dying consumptives.[85] Similar concerns also surrounded cancer. Considered contagious until the late eighteenth century, a series of unsuccessful inoculation experiments had seemingly proven that it could not be directly transmitted.[86] Lingering doubts remained, however, and a certain reserve was recommended to those who cared for the stricken.[87] That such fears were pervasive is hardly surprising, given long-standing beliefs about the dangers of foul odors and a growing fixation with olfactory experience.[88]

Along with everything else, the diatheses produced unforgettable sights and smells. In the case of scrofula, the odor was comparably benign, likened by one expert to freshly butchered meat.[89] Tuberculosis was another matter; a leading spa physician spoke of "the nauseating odor *sui generis* that soils the warm and condensed atmosphere of these revolting rooms. . . . One can often detect it all the way into neighboring rooms occupied by healthy families or patients not suffering from phthisis."[90] Certain cancers were even more repulsive to behold and to smell. One student described the bodily discharge of uterine cancer as so "eminently fetid, [that] they usually sustain around the patient a loathsome atmosphere in which the repulsive odor sends away her entourage and turns the poor thing into an object of repulsion."[91] The fact that the stricken gave off dangerous effluvia for months served to further stoke contagionist concerns.

Long before the emergence of late-century hygienic crusades, then, miasma and caregiver fatigue were understood to pose a threat to the well-being of others. From a public health perspective, hereditary transmission complicated the issue of contagion, for both infectious and hereditary disorders involved the passage of something undesirable from one body to another.[92] Even the language used to describe familial diseases was pregnant with contagionist metaphors. One had to carefully choose a spouse, one physician warned, as "an unfortunate alliance, a guilty lack of concern for the health of a delicate child, is enough to introduce the evil into a household and to bring, in little time, the ruin of a long series of robust generations."[93]

Robert Koch's identification of the tubercle bacillus in 1882 exacerbated an already difficult situation. Proof of person-to-person transmission provoked an epidemic of "pthisiphobia," and the status of tubercular became what deviance theorists call a "master status." It eclipsed, in other words, all other biosocial attributes and permanently marked the stricken in the eyes of others.[94] Koch's revolutionary discovery compounded a long-standing process whereby consumptives were progressively devalued. The requisite ingredients for their devaluation preceded his discovery; the triumph of hereditarianism and the identification of a specific microorganism deprived elites of recourse to other less stigmatizing narratives. Consumption, to use Erving Goffman's conceptualization, went from being simply discreditable (which gave the upper classes enough leeway to tell stories to and about themselves) to fully discrediting. As poetics went by the wayside, a dirty microorganism and a horrible illness were literally all that they had left with which to work.

Equating filth and illness was hardly new, even with tuberculosis. Yet during the late nineteenth century, tuberculosis was increasingly cast as a lower-class and racially determined disease, the product of vile habits, bad blood, and hygienic ignorance. Mobilized by fear, various countries embraced the hygienic gospel with a vengeance as middle-class reformers launched crusades against dangerous behaviors and dangerous practices such as spitting. Certain "dangerous" people, notably black American domestic workers, were subjected to particularly severe censure and surveillance.[95] For both their own good and the health of society, the indigent poor and foreign born were shown how to clean up their lives.[96]

Motivated by concerns that specific lodgings acted as sinks of contagion, French authorities established municipal *Casiers Sanitaires* in the 1880s and 1890s. For several decades, mortality data were analyzed in an effort to identify "tuberculosis houses." Like-minded French and British authorities launched a similar hunt to identify "cancer houses."[97] Often spearheaded by Progressives eager to improve living conditions, these studies failed to explicitly state whether the root problem was the building or its people. Over time, a growing emphasis on obligatory decontamination implicated the latter. The dominant message was that dying consumptives and cancer patients left behind dangerous residues that might pose a long-term risk to future inhabitants.

Catalyzed by uncertainty and fear, the prevailing hard science was palpably alarmist. Late-century discussions of hereditary taints are particularly revealing. On one level, the resurgent interest in the role of the "host soil" in infection illustrated the difficulty people had setting aside centuries of received wisdom. It also reflected a growing recognition that interactions between host and microbe were complex, confronting theorists everywhere with the issue of differing susceptibility.[98] Yet it also echoed a long-standing and pervasive prejudice: cancer and tuberculosis patients were defective, dangerous, or both. In an era of impersonal microbes, the fact that certain people fell sick could have been ascribed to bad luck. Instead, injunctions continued to have an old-fashioned, morally vindictive ring, as when one expert insisted that "tuberculosis patients are afflicted with a parasitic condition; but besides this, they are tributaries of the stains which their ancestors bequeathed them."[99] Among other things, the pervasiveness and staying power of this belief reflected the importance of "moral contagion," the emotional effects that diathesis carriers had on those around them.[100]

## Moral Contagion and the Anti-aesthetics of Suffering

If the danger was as much psychological as physical, contemporaries' pre-occupation with moral contagion decisively shaped cultural attitudes. In essence, diathesis suffers were like Gorgons, a danger best avoided by diverting one's gaze. The antipathy was particularly intense towards those with disquieting physical deformities. It was widely known that the prospects of those who did not succumb to a highly destructive skin ulcer known as lupus were dim.[101] The effects were particularly dramatic when the disease attacked the face; most patients became "an object of disgust and even of horror," and one of the few opportunities left open to them was to serve other patients in a hospice or almshouse.[102] When the mutilation was severe and social ties tenuous, the result was exclusion and neglect. Near the end of the biographical novel *The Life of a Simple Man* (1904), the narrator "Old Tiennon" recounted how an elderly acquaintance with cancer of the face

> suffered without respite and he spent long nights without sleep. And he suffered also in mind, for he felt that he was an object of loathing to all. He was not allowed to sit at the table: they poured his soup on his bread in a special bowl, which remained unwashed for weeks; they no longer allowed his grandchildren to come near him; the servant refused to wash the cloths which he wrapped round his face; and he heard his daughter-in-law say one day as she set herself to the sickening task: "Will he never die, then, the disgusting old man!" He told me this in a voice strangled with fury and tears.[103]

In attempting to explain this reflex, the internationally renowned physician and essayist Charles Richet cited humankind's instinct for self-preservation. Pus and other fetid liquids provoked an invincible disgust. Overcoming this revulsion, he convincingly claimed, required an almost superhuman act of will.[104]

The three deadliest diatheses were such an affront to the senses that they left even the battle-hardened feeling chastened. Describing those with endemic scrofula, one contemporary timorously acknowledged that "one would take them for a cadaver taken out of its tomb. Not long ago . . . I saw appear one of these wretched souls who had every aspect of an Egyptian mummy; one had to make him speak to realize that he was still living; his voice was weak, almost sepulchral."[105] Late-stage tuberculosis similarly conjured up images of unremitting torture and inhuman decay, described by one student as follows:

> the wasting arrives at an extreme degree, the skin desquamates, the hair falls out, all the subcutaneous fat disappears, the zygomatic arches protrude from sunken cheeks, the orbits which have lost their fat appear too vast for the eyes . . . the entire muscular system atrophies and wipes out all of the patient's strength; the spinous processes stick out sharply from the spine; the muscles of the buttocks can be atrophied to the point that one can distinctly make out the configuration of the pelvis.[106]

These evocative yet sanitized images offered this relative neophyte an idiom for mastering his horror. In this retelling, the tendency of all cases to resemble each other was reinforced by the student's description of a generic decomposing body.

The fact that half-dead patients preserved certain human attributes (a voice, memories) made bearing witness all the more distressing. In one poignant example, the mother of an affluent young consumptive observed how "the wasting was extreme, her body resembled nothing more than a skeleton, and, a few days prior to her death, while we changed her linens with a stifled sense of terror, she laughingly told us: 'one could easily perform an anatomy lesson on me.'"[107] Gallows humor aside, her half-submerged anguish captured the cruel reality of the wasting diseases. In the end, even the most privileged bodies ended up anonymous and dehumanized, suitable for display in a hospital amphitheater. This was particularly true of cancer, which epitomized decay and despair.[108] Those who invoked the disease's lasting effects had good reason. One commentator invoked primal imagery, likening malignant growths of the face, urethra, and other intimate regions "to the destruction that rats carry out in the anatomy amphitheaters."[109]

The tone and content of countless medical testimonials should give pause. Physicians were convinced, not unreasonably, that they were less squeamish than the general public, comparably unaccustomed to foul smells and severe suffering.[110] Firsthand experience with misery and social injustice may have also made them more sympathetic to the plight of the downtrodden.[111] Romantic poetry notwithstanding, it is possible that medical discourse—for all its horror and disgust—understated the diatheses' impact on contemporaries. In the absence of some powerful unifying impulse, the de facto response to terminal illness was fight or flight. Faced with diseases that were disgusting, incurable, and possibly contagious, people's judgments were swift and severe, formulated in the most compelling available idiom.

## Terminal Illness and the Nature of Life

The coexistence of radically different representations of consumption is a tribute to the disease's powerful effect on contemporaries. Throughout the nineteenth century and into the twentieth, the medical and romantic vision of the disease overlapped.[112] Across time, however, the former took center stage. That this occurred despite the elite's investment in the latter partly reflects the growing prestige of scientific knowledge. Yet another important issue was also at stake. Doctors' framing of consumption was particularly persuasive because it so closely mirrored conventional morality. Prevailing systems of thought established a direct link between aberrancy and suffering. Literally and symbolically, death by wasting represented the ultimate symbol of personal transgression.[113] In a society reflexively prone to moralization, it was vital that the moral and hygienic lessons of the deadliest diatheses be commensurate with the misery they caused.

Obsessed with order and stability, the social elite liked to believe that the punishment always fitted the crime. Despite the fact that it exculpates people, there was something deeply unsatisfying about ascribing terminal illness to bad luck; one must accept an enormous asymmetry between cause and effect. Randomness also has a terror of its own, as it implies that nothing determines the way our lives unfold. For an insecure elite and an equally insecure medical profession, the notion of biological anarchy was anathema.[114] Consciously or unconsciously, the French of the nineteenth century made a Faustian bargain. In return for the reassurance that there was order in the universe, they accepted the risk that they too might succumb to a stigmatizing illness.

Contemporaries showed an abiding commitment to decoding these disorders. Because they were visible and burdensome, wasting diseases were like a form of public property in which everyone had a stake and therefore had a say. And given that these disorders posed a threat to those around them, rare was the sufferer who could credibly argue, "leave me alone, this is my business." Most obviously, they threatened the well-being of the near and dear. Over time, however, authorities became increasingly concerned that they and other degenerates would undermine the health of the nation. The furor around the issue of national decline exposes one of the many ironies of this story. The tradition of singling out and denying care to incurable diathesis sufferers served to reify their otherness even as it increased their misery.

The critical role that aesthetics played in the construction of tuberculosis, cancer, and scrofula is not unique. A similar dynamic existed around epidemic diseases in early modern Europe; the response to disorders like the plague was particularly virulent because they represented "the visible externalised horror of the transformed body."[115] Yet during the nineteenth century, literary portrayals of the gruesome effects of illness flourished despite declining numbers of such outbreaks.[116] This apparent paradox makes perfect sense if one remembers that wasting diseases were another group of repulsive and contagious conditions whose visibility, if anything, increased during this period.

In the setting of terminal illness, phenomenology and ontology have been and remain inseparably linked. As the philosopher Georges Bataille noted decades ago, decaying bodies are a deep-seated, even archetypal, taboo.[117] As imagery, it has largely been off-limits, as evidenced by Hollywood's highly selective and sanitized depictions both of cancer and cancer deaths.[118] The same is also true of painting, explaining why works like Hans Holbein's *Dead Christ* are so profoundly disturbing.[119] In his brilliant study of Western attitudes toward death, Philippe Ariès claimed that European societies lost all taste for the macabre in the early modern period and that grisly imagery was repressed between the seventeenth and late nineteenth centuries. As far as Ariès is concerned, it was only in the latter period that a new representation of death began to appear, one "improper like the secretions of man . . . the ugly and hidden death, hidden because it is ugly and dirty."[120] Yet Ariès appears to have discounted the extent to which the macabre was a staple of everyday life in a world where consumption was rife. Like another fearsome object traceable to this period, anatomical representations of decayed bodies, wasting diseases triggered considerable unease regarding the nature of life and what it meant to be human.[121]

Of course alienation and accusation do not tell us the whole story. Both rhetorically and substantively, religion was a consolation to many. Further, social behaviors were never uniform. Some individuals outdid themselves, whether out of duty, affection, or because of some particular form of socialization (notably religious training). Nor did physicians blindly demonize the sick; they regularly expressed sympathy towards the dying, even when they found their presence trying.[122] More than anything, the setting of terminal illness was marked by a tug-of-war between sympathy and self-preservation. Yet as with epidemics, one can reasonably speak of scapegoating. Slow death raises deeply troubling questions. In the past, those we now tend to perceive as victims were readily blamed for the personal failings and social pathologies that their predicament brought to the surface. Like insanity, an aura of disrepute hung over them, testimony to people's aversion to agony and decay.

# 5

---

# Medical Attitudes toward
# the Care of Incurables

Shortly before Christmas 1866, Auguste Runeau de Saint-Georges had his physician and his confessor join him for a sumptuous meal. He ate nothing. His condition, worrisome in September, had steadily worsened since. Beyond wanting to make a show of good graces, he had presumably invited his physical and spiritual doctors to thank them for their efforts at assuaging the "atrocious pains of a long illness." The final course completed, a toast to the priest served as the prelude for a touching farewell to his grandchildren. There's little doubt that, whatever the official prognosis might have been, de Saint-Georges had few illusions about the future. Foresight, in this case, was 20/20. He died fifteen days later, on December 29. That grief and sadness apparently didn't give way to reproach suggests that all concerned had successfully risen to the occasion.[1]

We do not know how commonplace a scene like this was, but it clearly corresponded to a vaunted ideal. Throughout the nineteenth century, a series of behavioral norms dictated how the major actors in an incurable illness—patient, family, priest, and physician—were expected to behave. Often, however, one or more of the interested parties failed to do his part. This is not very surprising given the many barriers that impeded the translation of ideals into practice.

Our exploration of the intimate and emotional world of chronic progressive illness and palliative medicine begins by examining physicians' attitudes toward the care of incurables. While their motives were complex, some doctors clearly believed that their diagnostic and therapeutic skills were wasted upon hopeless cases, and their uninterest evoked charges of selfish indifference. The issue was generally more complicated, however, and a historical retelling must eschew simplistic pigeonholing that discounts the complexities of doctors' motives. Doctors' perceptions and practices grew out of an intricate and often conflicting set of instincts, priorities, and experiences. More than anything, they reflected unease with suffering and death, two vivid and distressing symbols of medical "failure." Equating them in this way was not, strictly speaking, chimerical; people were quick to criticize when things did not go as they hoped. Medicine's impotence in the face of chronic progressive disease often bred hostility and distrust, feelings that strained an already fragile and emotionally intricate doctor-patient-family relationship.

In response to a tangled web of influences and imperatives, the players in this drama often engaged in controversial behavior. On the one hand, observers denounced physicians and families for actions they deemed pointless and excessive. At the opposite extreme, many critics accused physicians of sinning by omission, a pattern of neglect referred to and experienced as abandonment.

Certain striking continuities in rhetoric and behavior may leave the impression that this experience is somehow timeless, that nothing really changed over the course of the nineteenth century. This half-truth exposes one of the great challenges in tackling the history of palliative medicine. Historical forces—changing material and social conditions, developments in science and technology, broad cultural and ideological shifts—did have important, if sometimes subtle, effects. Doctors became more attentive to the needs of incurables in the second half of the nineteenth century. Medical discourses around palliative medicine also evolved, suggesting a greater complicity between physician and patient. Still, the available repertory of responses to suffering, physical decline, and slow death were not unlimited. Furthermore, some reactions—particularly personal and professional disinvestment—clearly came more easily than others.

Understanding people's lived experiences requires that one walk a fine line. In myriad ways, incurable illness was a culturally freighted and historically contingent life experience. Yet it also has important continuities. Engaging with these two tendencies, I believe, enhances the heuristic value of this narrative: though it is about a specific time and place, it allows us to better understand the timeless aspects of severe debility and death.

## Between Self-Interest and Philanthropy

Reputedly incurable illness invariably elicited strong feelings among physicians; sympathy, hubris, trepidation, and frustration ebbed and flowed, in lockstep with the disease and the mood of the patient and the household. Had physicians been free to choose, they may have avoided incurables altogether. That they regularly embraced the challenge of caring for them reflected a combination of ambition, greed, and idealism. Paradoxically, chronic progressive illnesses were at once the bane of the profession and among its most inspiring calls to arms.

Acute illnesses' tendency to resolve spontaneously led one insightful physician to assert in 1841 that physicians' skills were most readily and accurately judged in the setting of chronic illness. His views weren't original; Dr. Pierre Debreyne approvingly cited the fifth-century physician Coelius Aurelianus who had claimed that they "are not ordinarily cured whether by chance, nor by the kindness of nature; they formally call for the intervention of a skillful physician, and prepare for him, if he succeeds, a greater and more certain share of glory."[2] Tellingly, various observers expressed concern about the overzealous pursuit of such laurels. A jaded medical student, for instance, noted that those who tried to work miracles almost always did their patients a disservice.[3] In a remarkable mid-century work on medical deontology, Maximilien Simon similarly stressed that "those difficult cases when everything is reunited to have him foresee a deadly outcome" often brought out the worst in people. If "generous impulses" and "humanitarian feelings" partly explained doctors' willingness to pull out all the stops, he rued the fact that "vanity, the desire to strike the public imagination as a result of a not-to-be-hoped-for cure, this unbridled desire for publicity . . . are dangerous counselors, and without practicing Puritanism in matters of therapeutics, one could worry that the physician, who takes [such motives] as a guide, forgets the essential goal of the art."[4]

Simon was a small-town practitioner who spent much of his career in Aumale (Seine Inférieure). Over the course of five decades, he published numerous articles, and his list of collaborators included the Parisian notable Gabriel Andral. He also wrote three books, though neither of his later works was as influential as *Déontologie médicale*. At the time of publication, the coverage in the French medical press was immediate and extensive, including several of the country's leading periodicals.[5] Most were extremely positive; one of the only consistent criticisms was that Simon paid too much attention to doctors' duties and not enough to their rights![6] In an eleven-page review in the prestigious *Revue médicale française et étrangère*, Dr. Louis Delasiauve described the book as "a leading publication of our era."[7] Though critical of Simon's ideas on reforming the profession, Delasiauve felt that everyone should carefully read *Déontologie*, which he hoped would become "the gospel of every practitioner."[8] In 1852, the book was translated into Spanish. Five years later, the Imperial Academy of Medicine awarded Simon the Prix Civrieux.

If curing an incurable could cement one's reputation, another mid-century work on ethics and professionalism noted that even failure could occasionally be rewarding. Early in his career, Charles-Polydore Forget cared for a prominent individual whose illness, he quickly concluded, was both fatal and incurable. Rather than regret the patient's demise, a senior colleague confided, he should relish the publicity that came with attending the social elite![9]

In an era of rising incomes and expectations, the chronically ill had much to recommend them. Numerous and desperate, they were avid consumers of medical products and services. Many contemporaries observed that both charlatanism and the newspaper business lived off promising them relief. One vocal critic of patent-medicine palliatives, for example, insisted that he couldn't begin to count the syrups that supposedly made consumptives' cough disappear.[10]

Though united in decrying the commercial exploitation of incurables, many aspiring young doctors promoted unorthodox panaceas or dubious curative systems.[11] Even those critical of such ruses admitted that a subset of incurables was commercially interesting. In an 1885 address, Dr. Adrien Coriveaud acknowledged that "among the various sources from which we draw our honoraria, one of the surest and most abundant can be found precisely in the treatment of very drawn-out illnesses . . . a physician called to the side of an incurable patient, especially if this patient is wealthy, is perfectly entitled to experience a feeling analogous to a merchant beginning what he considers a good business deal."[12]

Coriveaud was quick to stress that money was important mostly because such patients need spare no expense in pursuing a cure. Others, perhaps uncharitably, insisted that doctors cared about little else. In a widely read advice book that valorized self-help, Dr. Audin-Rouvière parodied the pretentious behavior of the medical elite. One setting he singled out for satire was that of an affluent incurable who asked his treating physician to request a consultation with another illustrious colleague. Though they might be visceral enemies, divided by personal animosity and competing medical systems, Audin-Rouvière insisted, "Do you wish to know the point which unites them? It is around the question: *is it a nice place? Will we be paid well?*"[13] His work clearly found a loyal readership; it went through sixteen editions between 1823 and 1863. In targeting doctors' venality, Audin-Rouvière definitely knew of what he spoke. The historian Matthew Ramsey has described him as "one of the most prominent pill merchants of early nineteenth-century France."[14]

Patients, however, also complained that everything took a backseat to professional fees. In a letter to the famous actress Rachel (born Elizabeth Rachel Felix), whose tragic struggle with tuberculosis was followed closely by the French press at mid-century, an embittered businessman wrote, "Believe me, mademoiselle, doctors today no longer practice the art of curing, but that of enriching themselves at the expense of those who suffer."[15] While clearly an exaggeration—doctors would have loved to cure everyone—such outbursts were the most visible manifestations of a fear that haunted many sick rooms: the belief that doctors put their interests first.

The deontological dilemmas must have been formidable. Peddling panaceas was potentially more lucrative and generally a lot easier than devoting oneself heart and soul to chronically ill patients. Those who resisted the temptation understandably wanted to be rewarded for their time and effort, ideally handsomely. Yet while promoting their financial livelihoods, self-respecting professionals didn't want to appear to be rapacious profiteers. In an effort to appeal to more exalted principles, physicians increasingly portrayed palliative medicine as a near-sacred duty. Explicitly distancing themselves from Hippocrates, who recommended sending incurables away, physicians after mid-century increasingly singled out incurability as the ultimate test of whether one was a good doctor.

In 1855, an obscure practitioner captured this ideal when he wrote that "the poor soul who suffers without hope has a more sacred claim to our compassion, than he in whom the perspective of being cured renders his suffering less bitter."[16] Arguably the most vocal spokesman for an ethos of sympathy, Max Simon repeatedly stressed that the care they provided benefited both doctor and patient.[17] As the century advanced, various acclaimed practitioners showed an interest in the dying process. The internationally acclaimed North American physician William Osler, for example, took a holistic view of palliative medicine, care that for him epitomized practitioners' ethical engagement.[18] Framed consistently as a moral duty, palliative medicine's rising prominence paralleled the growing concern with issues of social welfare. Mirroring claims that society had an obligation to help the helpless, physicians increasingly proclaimed that the care of incurables was a singularly sensitive ethical barometer.

The form and content of these apologetics suggest a growing psychological complicity as empathy slowly and unevenly eclipsed pity and noblesse oblige. Nowhere is this more apparent than in the words of a respected cancer surgeon who in 1911 wrote that "to come to the aid of these poor souls is certainly one of the most gentle and noble tasks of our art. It is worthy of great hearts, which are often worth more than great minds. . . . Only those who have hitched themselves to this hard task know what one must give of oneself to keep these disabled ships afloat, but they also alone appreciate the quiet joy and profound satisfaction that a simple grateful look of one of these poor patients bestows."[19] Without questioning their sincerity, physicians have long shown an affinity for stylized, celebratory self-presentations.[20] More importantly, lofty sentiments weren't enough to generate widespread enthusiasm. Even eloquent apologists recognized that it was easier to be a self-interested dispenser of tonics than an empathic philanthropist who remained at the patient's side until the very end.

Georges Daremberg's 1905 analysis of relations between doctors and consumptives vividly illustrated how formidable the challenge was. In a particularly candid moment, he stressed how "we have preached authority and vigor to the physician of curable tuberculosis patients; we preach weakness and indulgence to the physicians of dying ones. The physician who wants to be of use to consumptives must be in turn a master or an apostle, a man of science or of the heart, and especially must not reduce his role to that of a dosing machine."[21] These were inspiring words that demonstrated why "consolatory medicine" was always a tough sell. Well aware of the weighty burdens, physicians also knew that the satisfaction it offered was oblique and elusive. Each practitioner had his conscience as a guide, and even the most dedicated presumably didn't always live up to their ideals. Doctors' natural affinity was for the authority, vigor, and science of "the master."

## Professional Identity and the Spirit of Scientism

In an observation both sincere and unoriginal, a book on chronic disease decried the embarrassing gaps in contemporary understanding of them, ascribing it to "the indifference with which [they] have been studied."[22] As the diagnostic techniques of the Paris School became increasingly routine, the chronically ill lost much of their semiotic appeal. Not only were their outward signs of disease painfully obvious, but one's diagnostic virtuosity had little impact on the unfolding of events.[23] In outlining how to detect subtle signs of early, curable tuberculosis, Joseph Grancher told Paris medical students in 1890 that, in cases of well-established disease, "we auscultate patients out of duty, but without scientific curiosity, without a hope of finding anything on this examination of any inspiration for treatment. When they have arrived at the moment when they resemble each other, consumptives cease to interest us."[24] Other testimony suggests that incurables' suffering was also, medically speaking, uninteresting. Addressing the issue of breast cancer pain in 1894, a leading surgeon noted, "Later on, pains due to the compression of nerves appear; but they are then of as little interest to the physician as they are cruel for the unhappy patient."[25] In the only contemporary text devoted to incurable cervical cancer, surgeon Joseph Récamier Jr. candidly admitted that both hospital physicians and their underlings generally considered such cases totally banal.[26]

To most minds, curing illness was medicine's highest calling and acute disorders the test of one's mettle. Directly contradicting earlier statements about chronic disease, a prominent early-century practitioner demonstrated that acute, relatively benign, conditions were central to doctors' professional identity. For it was in this setting, Dr. De Montègre insisted, that the practitioner had to be far-sighted "like the pilot at the helm, guiding his boat with confidence through the reefs which he identified; the storm is menacing, but the currents are favorable; his eye always fixed on his path; he raises or lowers the sail, varying their size according to the impetuosity of the wind and the resistance of his vessel, and soon, happily restored in the port, he all but forgets the dangers he ran."[27] Strikingly, a work devoted to incurable illness defined medicine as "the art of treating, directing, and curing disease."[28] Taken alone, this slip seems inconsequential. Yet it accurately betrayed the profession's affinities and priorities. Physicians were always happiest discussing medicine's strengths, its scientific credentials and therapeutic achievements.

Admittedly, they had much of which to be proud. In the decades after the anatomic-pathological revolution, developments in statistics, medical chemistry, microscopy, and physiology suggested that they were protagonists in a scientific project of unprecedented nature and scope. Late-century society, in turn, exhibited a growing faith in medical science. By the 1880s, even modest practitioners were benefiting from the knowledge-power dyad.[29] They basked in the glory of discoveries—notably Pasteur's dramatic triumph over anthrax and rabies and Koch's discovery of the tubercle bacillus.[30] For these important events seemed to prove that medicine was beginning to demystify and conquer disease.

In a world fixated upon progress and success, incurables as a group fared poorly. Some observers suggested that science's rising prominence actually worked against their interests. While perhaps overstated, contemporary researchers clearly disliked negative findings. Incurable illnesses left physicians feeling humiliated, both as individuals and as a profession.[31] Their distaste for revealing "the secret of their impotence," Dr. Jaumes observed, explained physicians' reluctance to publish observations that chronicled their defeat.[32]

Such scruples partly explain why a member of the Academy of Medicine warned that officially acknowledging cancer's incurability would stifle research on the disease.[33] One physician who devoted his career to finding a cure for cancer and tuberculosis touchingly recognized the importance of success, however modest. Jean Barrier wrote that he experienced such cruel setbacks in 1847 and 1848 that he considered abandoning the field altogether. As he noted, however, "a few satisfying results came to raise my hopes, casting me back into the field of experimentation almost in spite of myself."[34]

In a different vein, Max Simon's careful scrutiny of the language of contemporary science led him to suggest that a growing fascination with research had undermined physicians' sense of compassion. In settings where they had little to offer, he was alarmed by the paucity of sympathy "for the suffering of humanity; it would seem that for a science without a soul, they had become a simple object of natural history. . . . There are even some of these works in which one would not only search in vain for some ray of human sympathy that naturally springs from the heart of the physician, but where you will find in its place a sort of half-concealed joy, in the presence of the fatal event, which permits to verify an uncertain diagnosis." Despite occasional disclaimers, Simon clearly believed that science divorced of moral (that is, Christian) tutelage dehumanized both doctors and patients.[35]

Though his concerns were likely exaggerated, questions of professional identity and personal preference did place incurables in an unenviable position. It is hard to imagine that doctors were more interested in the autopsy than the patient. Everyone, however, was painfully aware of the meager satisfaction such cases afforded. Calling it a thankless struggle, Coriveaud spoke volumes when he admitted that "here, none of the immediate and flattering successes which the cure of acute illnesses at times procure for us. It is an indefinite succession of infinitely small victories, which barely compensate for the repeated defeats."[36] Effusive apologetics aside, negative perceptions remained the norm. Tuffier, for instance, refused to speak out against surgeons' indifference toward inoperable cancer patients. The "condemned," he admitted, didn't even allow the illusion of victory.[37]

It is little wonder that palliating incurables remained a low-status activity throughout the nineteenth century. Edouard Auber began his 1865 analysis of physicians' duties to patients with the observation that "the physician must know that his role is not restricted to curing, but that it consists also of prolonging the life of those with incurable illnesses and of rendering them bearable. This is assuredly not the most glamorous part of his art, but it is a delicate task which has all the merit of a good work and a pious act of charity."[38] On both sides of the Channel, "comfort care" was considered banal and routine, though passing comments suggest that it left physicians feeling vulnerable and in need of peer support.[39]

At century's end, an expanding repertory of palliative treatments encouraged physicians to be more engaged and involved. Despite that, consolatory medicine remained largely a moral and custodial duty.[40] In a highly revealing turn of phrase, a passionate advocate for the treatment of curable tuberculosis recommended that bare-bones dispensaries and hospices could see to the "useful and unglamorous" task of assuaging the rest.[41] Amid various transformations in theory and practice, such duties remained the antithesis of heroic medicine, unappealing and unavoidable. To an outside observer, doctors' reflexes were so deeply ingrained that they appear instinctual. Yet before condemning them outright, it is important to appreciate how difficult it was to do the right thing.

## Of Professional Precarity and Radical Uncertainty

The preface to a modest health primer (1864) captured a misgiving that, for all the wonders of the age, gnawed away at everyone: "if it is true that the medical sciences have entered into an era of progress . . . why are there still so many reputedly incurable illnesses? Why such a frequent lack of success when it comes time to combat them? Why, in a word, are there so many errors in medicine?"[42] In a society where arrogance and cynicism were common currencies, this question spoke volumes. Physicians certainly knew that their track record with chronic disease was a real liability. In addressing an 1862 conference on this issue, Hermann Pidoux observed that "it is a thing most worthy of note, Sirs, that Medicine, whose science so long ago left the Middle Ages, still remains mired there as a profession. On this score, it has made almost no progress; and Molière's sarcasms rain on her with all their acidity."[43]

Taking up the great dramatist's mantle in the 1830s, the brilliant French artist Honoré Daumier satirized the quixotic struggle of competing medical luminaries to brilliantly expose one of the profession's worst-kept secrets: learned airs notwithstanding, their patients succumbed disturbingly often. With a remarkable economy of expression, a lithograph produced in the late 1860s reveals much about the contemporary healing business. It suggests that "the cure" was a collective fixation. Physicians, one can reasonably surmise, took their cue from the rest of society, valuing that which everyone around them prized most. Yet it also partly explains doctors' ambivalence toward incurables. For, like Daumier, patients and families tended to be harsh judges. In an attitude presumably informed by faith in Nature's beneficence, most were apparently convinced that "every regrettable symptom is the product of the remedies, and when the illness worsens, it is always the doctor's fault. The public knows no other criteria than the result."[44] This was certainly true of the small army of unlicensed healers; what counted was success, not titles or diplomas.[45] Yet even as they complained about unfair expectations, doctors promoted a therapeutic vision that subverted their interests: Nature seconded by the "right" medicine was potentially omnipotent. The downside, of course, was that if Nature wasn't to blame, who was left?

Certain physicians' reputations as miracle workers served to fuel misgivings. One mid-century observer noted that Joseph Récamier was among those to whom "patients superstitiously addressed themselves when they believed that they had nothing left to expect from the medicine of doctors."[46] Récamier must have experienced many setbacks. Yet the perception

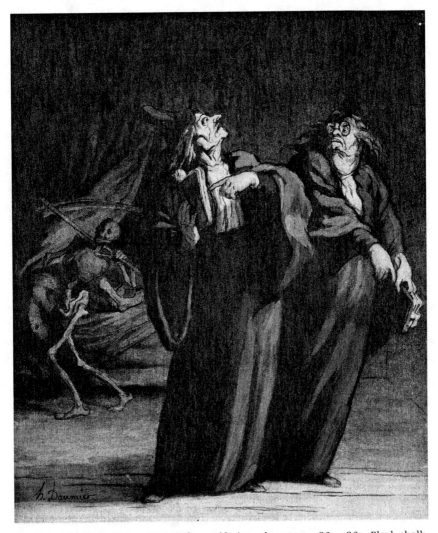

FIGURE 5.1. Honoré Daumier, *Les deux médecins et la mort*, c. 1865–1869. Black chalk, watercolor, and gouache on paper. 27.7 x 23.1 cm. From the Collection Oskar Reinhart "Am Römerholz," Wintherthur. Reproduced with permission.

that physicians were not all created equal would have made life particularly difficult for the mere mortals.

Accusations that regularly surfaced from within the profession further encouraged cynicism and mistrust. In an age of high conflict and low credibility, professional animosities regularly made their way into discussions of chronic progressive illness. The professionally marginal frequently singled out (un)happy outcomes to promote their interests and attack their colleagues. One obscure Italian national, for instance, warned the ailing actress Rachel that French doctors' notorious ignorance was putting her life in danger.[47] Desparquets, for his part, spoke glowingly of his therapeutic system while suggesting that the medical elite indifferently allowed incurables to die. In a moment of rhetorical flourish, he admitted, "We cannot hide the temerity it takes to claim to cure afflictions that the faculties and academies have declared incurable; but this reproach cannot stop us . . . it is according to the data of our personal experience that we affirm that we obtain results that the members of this learned body regard as impossible, they being too distracted from their medical duties by the preoccupations of vanity and ambition."[48] His 1855 book on reputedly incurable illness was part of an established and expanding literary genre, best described as medical protest literature. Nonelite physicians, struggling in obscurity with the demands of an ordinary medical practice, increasingly used these disorders as a pretext for a withering assault on the status quo.

Nearly all decried the audacity and incompetence of their professional superiors. Clearly resentful and presumably envious, they mercilessly criticized their mishandling of such cases. Audin-Rouvière, for instance, was adamant that

> it is not through incriminations, but by actions, that you must refute the practices of those you don't even deign call adversaries; do better than they and you will no longer need to be believed, to lavish insulting epithets, loud words, and insignificant phrases in such profusion. It is at the foot of a dying patient's bed, who you alone have cared for, that you rail against so-called charlatans, who in spite of having less adept hands (according to you), previously had the pleasure of relieving their first pains or of bringing him back to life![49]

While not limited to this period in history, the backstabbing was particularly vicious in the first half of the century, largely because of professional overcrowding in the most lucrative markets.[50] Rising incomes and social status in the decades after 1860 encouraged medical collegiality, marked by an increasingly cohesive esprit de corps.[51] In the earlier period, the corrosive effects of financial competition and professional jealousy were also densely overlaid with questions of politics and ideology. With every change in regime—Empire, Restoration, July Monarchy—professors' heads rolled (at least figuratively), spawning lifelong animosities.[52]

Assaults on status relations and rival "systems" often served as a pretext for a personal settling of scores. Nowhere was a writer's intent more transparent than in an 1826 article on the treatment of cancer. One case related the story of a young patient who, encouraged by her family, refused Dr.

Faneau Delacour's offer of surgery, citing a colleague with opposing views of cancer's nature and prognosis. After noting how he had forcefully outlined the implications of her decision, his account betrayed more than a trace of vindictiveness. Like any good morality tale, his narrative ended with a chastening lesson: "Mlle. D . . . died a victim of her confidence. Some time before this moment, she wanted to see me: I would only give some sterile consolations, feeble resource against a mortal affliction."[53]

Even those who didn't have as sharp an axe to grind admitted that clinical science left much to be desired. Consistent with conventional wisdom, one mid-century practitioner reminded his colleagues that it was sometimes exceedingly difficult to distinguish true and false incurability.[54] Other than warning against laxity and carelessness, Jaumes's advice was "if there is a shadow of a doubt, beware of renouncing a radical treatment."[55] Decades later, Coriveaud observed that diagnostic errors meant that some patients were still being misclassified as incurable. Given the tragic implications, he felt that it was imperative to be "careful, even modest, in our declarations. Let us not forget . . . that this or that fatal prognosis, though based on the most categorical and conclusive reasons; on diagnostic signs which were long verified and mediated upon, have often been contradicted by an unexpected cure. Oh! diagnostic and especially prognostic errors . . . what harm they can cause us."[56] Not surprisingly, second opinions from senior colleagues were always a popular safeguard. Although they carried the risk of contradiction, such consultations served to increase one's credibility and dilute one's responsibility.[57]

It was widely known that the public had zero tolerance for prognostic errors, and an aura of disrepute surrounded stories of recovered incurables.[58] In a letter to the practitioner whom he credited with saving his life, one erstwhile consumptive wrote of "having been the victim of the errors and the ignorance of a great number of doctors for four years."[59] Even less jaded accounts were tinged with irony. In her second letter to the dying actress, Elisa Pin informed Rachel of her unexpected cure from "incurable" tuberculosis, writing, "I said in my first letter that M. Andral, of Paris, had condemned me, I name for you here M. Barrier and Bouchacour; at Hyères, M. Laure; at Montpellier, M. Bouisson; at Allevard, M. Chatin. It is distressing for science, but it is fortunate for me."[60] Another correspondent, a former notary, spoke of a mineral water spa that specialized in hopeless cases. Describing the marvels he had witnessed there, he stated that "during my stay at Celles, I saw many patients struck down with *grave pulmonary afflictions*, reputed to be *incurable* by the princes of medical science, and all recovered their health. Many had even been sent to the doctor as a *challenge* by confreres in the capital."[61]

Marvels such as these were an integral, if problematic, part of the collective folklore. The majority of chronically ill patients died or didn't get better. Yet exceptional cases of recovery made it difficult to openly admit defeat. Making matters worse, many licensed and unlicensed healers denied that any patient or illness was irrefutably incurable. Nineteenth-century societies showed considerable tolerance for such "charlatanism"; the warning e caveat emptor was often the only limit placed on their publicity campaigns. Diagnostic errors, urban myths, and a lack of prognostic consensus together ensured that the "Truth" of incurability remained contested. Little wonder that so many people refused to give up, even in the face of the obvious.

## Therapeutic Excess

Hope, uncertainty, and suspicion had important implications for mortally stricken patients. Doctors often felt pressured to do something, rather than merely watch them slip away. In suggesting ways of handling this situation, Max Simon admitted,

> It is often difficult for the physician to remain an inactive spectator before events whose progress must inevitably lead to death: the love of science, of humanity, the incessant obsession of a family in tears who do not admit that art has its limits, all come together to do violence to his prudent circumspection, and to push him in a line of conduct in which uncertainty is still a form of hope. The physician must have enough firmness and independence of spirit to resist such suggestions. . . . is it also not his duty to spare the dying person the tortures of useless medications?[62]

He was neither the first nor the last to express such concerns. In 1817, H. F. Ragonneau criticized those colleagues, alas all too numerous, who stopped at nothing to keep dying incurables alive. He was clearly one of the conscientious observers who "were painfully witness to efforts at unnecessarily prolonging the torments of poor patients by reanimating their nearly extinguished remains, stirring the combat between life and death, useless combat, as the dying patient could not escape death." Incurability alone, he insisted, should dictate whether one stood quietly beside a dying patient or mobilized all available resources to prolong his life.[63]

Responsible physicians, he maintained, let incurable illnesses run their course with the help of a few palliatives. Dismissing reported cures of end-stage aneurysms, phthisis, and cancer, he also sanctioned practitioners who believed that anyone who was still alive could potentially be saved. In Ragonneau's mind, this was "an erroneous opinion much talked about at a certain period that has been reduced to its just value."[64] He apparently spoke too soon, as ambiguous statements about end-stage phthisis still figured prominently in the fifth edition of Broussais's *Histoire des phlégmasies chroniques*, published in 1838. After extolling the virtues of palliative remedies, the author cautioned against doing anything that might impede recovery, as, in his words "we must rarely despair of a man who is still breathing."[65]

Whether it was appropriate to subject dying patients to painful treatments remained controversial beyond mid-century. Always circumspect, Jaumes insisted that accurately diagnosing incurability was exceedingly important, as one could thereby avoid various annoying, unpleasant, or dangerous curative treatments.[66] Such concerns were not idle; for even on people's deathbeds, "some physicians, and especially the common people, have recourse to violent means that serve to maintain people's failing sensibility, to prolong the action of the great organs of life; ammonia, combustion, mustard plasters."[67]

An article from 1849 suggests that doctors still hadn't sorted out their ideas, let alone reached a consensus. While expressing concern for their physical comfort, Dr. A. Lagasquie nonetheless recommended using any and all means to revive dying patients, admitting "why, some might say, prolong the torture of a dying person? . . . it is not simply a question here of doing what our heart invites, it is experience that teaches us that some dying people have been brought back to life, and, however rare these happy exceptions (especially in chronic illness), it is always advisable to conduct oneself as though this unexpected success were possible."[68]

A half century later, some physicians still had trouble admitting defeat.[69] Many had apparently learned their lesson, however. If they agreed to intervene in exceptional circumstances—such as in dying patients who hadn't settled important financial matters—doctors increasingly spurned violent measures.[70] Addressing the Academy at the end of a long career in 1875, Pierre-Adolphe Piorry argued that comfort should come before all else. He felt that such views were worth defending publicly since

> I have seen (in earlier times it is true) people *employ in the most empiric, absurd and even cruel way*, painful interventions that weren't sanctioned by good sense or by science; for those who had recourse to them, knowing nothing of the anatomical causes of the accidents that caused death and guided by a freakish imagination, inflicted such tortures on the dying person that civilization and humanity would not allow to be carried out on criminals, such as the application of a burning hide to the feet, cauteries to the vertebral column, horribly painful operations etc. . . . Let us allow him to die without increasing his pain, surrounded by the affectionate care of his family, his friends

and ourselves, without hastening his final moment; science demands
it and philanthropy enshrines it as a law.[71]

Nineteenth-century orators like Piorry often invoked the therapeutic absur-
dities of the past as part of an "ode to progress." Such interventions were
also the logical outgrowth of doctors' affinity for highly visible, unpleasant,
heroic interventions. As well, medicine's rising prestige may have made it
easier for doctors to admit that there was nothing left to be done. Yet his
evocation of "torture" suggests certain primal instincts.

At the very least, loved ones' hopes were probably inseparable from a
powerful fear—that of their own death. Yet that which appears useless, even
punitive, may well carry even more sinister overtones. In light of the accusatory discourses surrounding chronic progressive diseases and the suffering
they elicited in others, one thinks of one explanation for the early modern
witch hunts.[72] It is possible that, on occasion, mortally ill patients were (un)
wittingly punished for the discomfort they caused in those around them.

## The Terrible Challenge of Caring

Though better than being labeled incompetent, invoking the natural limits of science was by no means straightforward. Even elite physicians, who
presumably knew it wasn't their fault when a patient died from cancer or
tuberculosis, were often on the defensive. Speaking of a notoriously refractory and ominous manifestation of late-stage tuberculosis (diarrhea), Pierre
Louis asked, "Must one thus remain a simple spectator in the face of a
symptom that can bring about the death of the patient?"[73] His question captured doctors' worst fear, that of being a bystander, helpless in the face of a
desperately ill and suffering individual. Their discomfort elicited reactions
that on the surface are difficult to reconcile. Many doctors, probably most,
were troubled by what they witnessed; some responded, paradoxically, by
dehumanizing the victim.

Incurable illnesses' devastating complications, casually described as
humiliating or revolting, made it hard to identify with the stricken. Certain
incurables were almost beyond sympathy. Coriveaud laconically observed
how "a senile hemiplegic, a cancer patient, a podagrous or dyspeptic victim
of gout, a scrofulous, dartrous or tabetic patient" had "nothing very attractive, or poetic, to them." Though it wasn't easy, doctors needed to remind
themselves that "delicate souls view them with horror, selfish ones run from
them even as they pretend to pity them, cynics await the tardy moment
when, death having finally done its job, they will be able to take the place
and the worldly goods of the poor devil who stood in their way. The physician
does not and cannot belong to any of these classes of stupid and villainous

people."[74] Nowhere was the experiential and aesthetic chasm starker than when illness capped off a life of hardship. Economic realities made personal dignity a luxury denied to many, while contemporary class relations ensured that the "better sorts" rarely cultivated such illusions.[75] When they afflicted the deformed, the depraved, and the poor, incurable illness was another reminder of the distance separating society's winners and losers.

Unfortunately, this was more the norm than the exception in a socioeconomic order where most people were poor. The underfed and impoverished were also particularly vulnerable to scrofula and tuberculosis. Deprived of basic physical comforts, to say nothing of expensive palliatives, lower-class incurables suffered terribly. Their misery usually provoked an awkward mixture of sympathy, revulsion, and helplessness, leaving even well-meaning individuals asking, "Where am I supposed to start?" With wealthy incurables, various forms of care helped spare everyone's sensibilities. The poor, on the other hand, had it so bad that their situation was almost beyond pity.[76]

Occasionally, physicians questioned whether such lives were worth living. A late-century thesis on uterine cancer outlined a leading gynecology textbook's criteria for evaluating surgery's usefulness. Immediately after noting that the time to relapse was the only way to judge the value of an intervention, it underscored that "once the relapse has occurred, the patient is considered condemned, and it is of little importance whether or not she drags herself along in her painful existence for some time more."[77] Others reached similar conclusions about consumptives. Quick to sing the praises of palliative medicine, Daremberg nevertheless placed a different value on the lives of the curable and the incurable. In the introduction to his highly regarded book, he wrote, "If the prolonged use of medications was satisfied with quickening the end of incurable consumptives, we would not have very violent reproaches to make of them; for the life of an irremediably lost tubercular is neither gay nor useful enough to not allow all liberty with regards to them." He also criticized young incurables for being a burden on the public purse and a threat to public health.[78]

A thoughtful late-century article gives valuable insights into the psychological underpinnings of this mind-set. After suggesting that disfigurement and alienation dominated the clinical tableau, Émile Tardieu noted that the chronically ill all but inevitably "lost that which most attracts others: joyfulness, triumphant optimism, strength." He went on to observe that "he's among the vanquished; his arms broken, he no longer has anything to propose, to undertake; he no longer has anything to offer, except his remains, which he furiously defends . . . but this indigent holds his hand out to everyone; shameless beggar, with greedy manners he absorbs the time, the assistance, the compassion of those who are willing to look after him; never is he given enough."[79] One can readily appreciate that neediness, not ugliness, was what troubled everyone most. Rather than being the culmination of a formulaic process of dehumanization, the belief that incurables were better off dead more often reflected resentment at the guilty feelings they provoked.

Despite encountering legions of dying people, nineteenth-century physicians were anything but desensitized, and their anguish often found its way into print. One sensitive student noted that well-intentioned physicians were always deeply troubled when they approached the bed of a patient preyed upon by a chronic illness. The problem was that "worn by worries and profoundly altered by suffering, [such individuals] implored a relief that it is not within his power to grant."[80] Having singled out incurable illness as a cause of suicide, the staunchly Catholic psychiatrist Alexandre Brierre de Boismont suggested that doctors rarely forgot the physical tortures they'd witnessed. This was the prelude to a surprising admission from a man of his convictions: "it is very easy, in effect, to say to the man who suffers: have courage, be patient, your ills will pass. These banal consolations have but a mediocre influence on he whose days and nights pass without a moment's rest. . . . The immense majority of men feel an invincible aversion for pain. . . . Run away from the pain, that's humanity's instinct."[81]

More than almost any other disorder, advanced cancer vividly demonstrated the discrepancy between medicine's limits and humanity's near-limitless capacity for suffering. Insisting that he knew of nothing more cruel or ghastly than breast cancer relapses, Alfred Velpeau acknowledged that seeing such patients "every day or every week, not knowing what to tell them, which words to use to console them, which drugs to prescribe so that they might be patient, which look, which countenance to adopt to keep them from sensing the despair with which we are penetrated, is a veritable nightmare!"[82] Another experienced physician who had specialized in the treatment of incurables tellingly insisted that if he'd had the chance to start over, he'd rather be spared "this chalice of bitterness."[83]

Though moral convictions were a source of fortitude, the company of incurables was clearly unwelcome. Given the frequency with which the term *revulsion* was applied to suffering humanity, it isn't surprising that healthy people, out of defensive selfishness, withdrew from the sick.[84] Tardieu was convinced that everyone reflexively recoiled from the chronically ill, insisting that "whether we beseech him to sacrifice his entire existence, many years, or if it is a simple call for aid which steals away a day, an evening, a minute, a simple gesture, the first natural, instinctive movement is refusal, a minimization of effort."[85] It was clearly the emotional costs that led physicians everywhere to conclude that incurables weren't worth the trouble. In a particularly candid moment, the late-century American physician Austin Flint observed, "It is trying to a physician to continue to visit patients when he feels that the resources of medicine are powerless and to witness the closing scenes of life," a feeling echoed by his French colleagues.[86]

## The "Abandonment" of Incurables—Rhetoric and Substance

Among the highpoints of Desparquets's book on incurable illness was his censure of those "who, not appreciating their mission, are disheartened or remain idle spectators, neglect their patients or abandon them! In such cases, the interest we carry for them in our hearts must increase."[87] Though most of his testimony was suspect, this accusation was tellingly ubiquitous. Wounded pride and personal discomfort together encouraged a pattern of neglect widely known as "abandonment."

Dr. Tirat de Malemort, an erstwhile Parisian professor who peddled an herbal cure for incurable diseases at mid-century, published a self-celebratory monograph in which he repeatedly alluded to this type of professional misconduct. Madame Levasseur, for example, had been "abandoned as an incurable chest case" by three famous physicians.[88] "Condemned" by all who examined her, Madame Claverit had also been cruelly abandoned by several physicians, including a professor of medicine.[89] Importantly, this turn of phrase also figured prominently in letters asking, or thanking, de Malemort for his counsel. One distraught father wrote to him "requesting your advice for my son, who is in such a grave position, that all the doctors have abandoned him as a chest case."[90] A colleague from Paris's faculty of medicine, on the other hand, marveled at the remarkable cures he had obtained in "poor patients abandoned as incurable."[91]

Although the medical elite were no strangers to self-promotion, accusations of abandonment generally came from the profession's lowest reaches. In offering his services to Rachel, a self-described "modest practitioner" wrote that he had successfully cured "a young girl of eighteen years, abandoned and reduced to a severe state of malnutrition."[92] A hypnotist wrote to the famous actress's doctor to tell him of "a new curative means, which for forty-six years has never failed, even among patients abandoned by their doctors."[93] Writing in the 1870s, an herbalist insisted that his remedy—copied from Nature herself—targeted the legions of sufferers "abandoned by regular medicine."[94]

Such accusations were clearly a popular rhetorical device carrying connotations of personal and professional mediocrity. As advertising, they'd have played strongly to the fear, resentment, and disappointment of those who no longer mastered their own destiny. That moral indignation was exploited to selfish ends is, in itself, not noteworthy. Its ubiquity suggests that people found it compelling, though. In fact, considerable evidence supports Desparquets's claim that doctors' misbehavior in hopeless cases ranged from idleness through neglect to outright abandonment.

Doctors often directly or tacitly acknowledged that they acted as though there was nothing left to be done. Once they'd decided that someone was incurable, physicians often "desire[d] to no longer have to look after them, and the rare visits which they make have no other goal than that of saving appearances by appearing to fulfill one's duty."[95] Various offhanded remarks suggest that the profession frequently responded to hopeless cases with passive indifference. In the case of stomach cancer, one physician mentioned in passing, "It is always wrong to abandon these patients, for lack of being able to cure them; one must always seek to relieve them and one is often able to do so."[96] In an equally telling moment, another doctor reminded his colleagues that "although cancer of the liver is incurable, one must seek to alleviate the suffering of the patient."[97] Several decades later, in the early twentieth century, strikingly little had changed.[98]

Such attitudes and behaviors were not cancer-specific. Doctors regularly reminded themselves that, even though they couldn't cure consumption, they nonetheless needed to be diligent about treating those with the disease.[99] It was also common knowledge among poverty-stricken consumptives, one late-century authority noted, that "chest cases, at the hospital, are almost always abandoned, happy when they are kept in the service until their fine death."[100] French doctors, not surprisingly, were not the only ones who were guilty of the practice. Article 5 of the American Medical Association's 1848 Code of Ethics asserted that "a physician ought not to abandon a patient because the case is deemed incurable" before outlining, in high-minded language, the conduct that was expected of its members. The form and content of this injection strongly suggests that American physicians were subject to similar temptations and had recourse to the same moral suasion as their French counterparts.

Carefully scrutinizing their physicians' gestures and behaviors, the chronically ill referred to them in emotionally laden terms. When they were given certain diagnoses, patients spoke of having been "condemned." "Abandoned," on the other hand, captured patients' frustration at seeing their complaints ignored and their suffering unassuaged. This must have been quite frequent, given doctors' commitment to telling white lies and maintaining a cheerful disposition. In their daily dealings with incurables, Joseph Récamier Jr. insisted that "if it is useful to reassure the patient and to appear confident before her, the patient, who senses that the situation is serious, must see that the physician also judges it to be so and acts accordingly. Otherwise she will suddenly lose confidence in him, and think that, like the popular expression says, her doctor has abandoned her, and then there would be nothing left to do but change medical attendant to give her a bit of courage."[101] Often enough, the hollowness of their gestures left little room for doubt. When chronic illnesses continued to worsen despite their best efforts, physicians tended to shorten the consultations and become impatient with the awkward demands of a patient who did not yet realize that his case was hopeless. Stripped of the role of miracle worker, physicians' prescriptions went from being carefully reasoned instructions to mere "formal scribbles."[102] In other words, if doctors rarely refused to see incurables who were willing to pay their fees, their nonchalance was often depressingly transparent.[103] On occasion, the abrogation of duty was so flagrant that those in positions of authority spoke out publicly. This happened most often in three sets of circumstances: when patients were poor, difficult, or on the verge of death.

In 1806, Marc Antoine Petit noted with sadness that patients who had been surrounded by students because of the pedagogical interest of their case generally found themselves abandoned as they lay dying. Rather than giving in to such inclinations, he called on everyone to be resolute: partly because everyone's clinical judgment was fallible, mostly because this was what one human being owed another. In an assertion reframed by a steady stream of successors, he emphatically insisted, "Above all, do not go away, as long as he that requested your help preserves enough awareness to sense your having abandoned him: the laws of humanity, the respect that we owe to the dying . . . make this a duty."[104]

If dying hospital patients arguably ran the highest risk, poor Parisians were often abandoned weeks, even months, before they died. In 1856, seven years after the establishment of a new system to oversee the city's medical and hospital services, the director of the Assistance Publique sent a circular to the mayors of Paris's *arrondissements*. Echoing grave concerns that recently enacted reforms had sought to remedy, he wrote of having been informed of "several physicians, who otherwise acquit themselves of their duties with devotion, [who] neglect to go see patients afflicted with chronic diseases, when their care will be impotent at preventing a fatal outcome." He was particularly distressed by their willingness to sign prescriptions and write observations in the treatment record despite not having visited the patient. Beyond questions of strategic planning and "quality assurance," he was most disturbed by the fact that, for the patient, this premature abandonment "becomes an indicator of their imminent demise, and, with their confidence, strips them of the little strength they possessed to fight against the progression of their disease. The Administration has to expect more zeal from physicians who accept the mission of looking after the poor; in cases where a cure appears impossible, the physician can still give counsel and consolation, and his poor client must be visited by him until his dying day."[105] Even though his successor claimed that such behavior was a thing of the past, far more evidence suggests that old habits died hard.[106]

Physicians were obviously more attentive to affluent incurables. Yet even here, their actions weren't above reproach. A commonplace and controversial behavior was to recommend a trip to a spa or thermal station. Doctors' eager use of hydrotherapy as a last-gasp measure led one well-known hospital physician to protest against a "barbarous practice," that of submitting "individuals in a state of marasmus, barely having a breath of life, to all that is most-distressing about hydrotherapy, when the obvious course of action is to simply let them die in peace."[107]

Such exotic treatments were tempting for at least two reasons. Healthier patients may well have benefited physically and emotionally from a change of scenery and the renewed sense of hope that came with "taking the waters." Yet, following the adage "out of sight, out of mind," the attending physician was arguably among the principal beneficiaries. They may have even projected their own sense of relief when evaluating these treatments' usefulness. At the very least, the spa trips were often proposed without specific therapeutic indications. In a particularly angry moment, Max Simon insisted that "it is impossible to not recognize the frivolity, even the cold-hearted cruelty that one sometimes detects in such conduct, if not a more damnable calculation. . . . It is undoubtedly distressing to visit a patient each day simply to record the impotence of the medical arts, yet this is less distressing than to have to hesitate in answering the formidable question . . . : have you, through an imprudent consul, co-operated in shortening a life?"[108] Forty years later, Coriveaud voiced one of the profession's darker secrets. In a conspiratorial tone, he alluded to those "specters returned from some voyage, as far-flung as it was pointless, that they were recommended with the sole goal of ridding ourselves of them for a few weeks? Who among us, Sirs, could not in this regard perform a little, or a great *mea culpa*. . . . But let us not insist."[109]

One prominent contemporary made no apologies for exactly such behavior. Alluding to certain consumptives "whose difficult character [was] a source of anguish for those around them," the respected Parisian professor Benjamin Ball told his underlings that "nothing seems to please them, everything seems to ruffle them: most often we get rid of them by advising them to make a prolonged sojourn in the Midi."[110] This was clearly not something he was ashamed of, as his teachings were reprinted in the French periodical *L'Encéphale*. Ball himself was editor in chief.

## Conclusion: The Blame Game

Had they been forced to defend the profession against accusations of systematically mistreating incurables, physicians would undoubtedly have responded with objections of their own. First there was the ingratitude of patients and their families, a term that at least partly meant reneging on the bill.[111] In the next breath, they might have mentioned patients' disloyalty. In an observation that was particularly apt in chronic progressive illness, Dr. Petit noted that "changing doctors is for many people an act of the greatest indifference." The problem was that "attaching themselves to no one, no one becomes attached to them; and when the hour of danger comes, they will search for a devout friend in vain."[112] Loyalty, in other words, was a two-way street.

More than one also complained about the superhuman patience such cases demanded. Evoking the chaos of the sickroom, a medical student bemoaned the fact that prescriptions were often modified, ignored, or delayed by loved ones, when they weren't "terrify[ing] the patient with stupid stories" or "repeating the judgments that they heard pronounced about his condition." This diatribe followed a heartfelt discussion of the average country doctor's sad lot. Were his "arduous and repulsive studies" not bad enough, he faced a life marked by "the inclemency of the seasons, the continuous fatigue, the irregularity of the meals, the sleep deprivation; to live in the midst of suffering and pain, in the middle of miasmas and contagion; in the countryside, to have to cover long distances on horseback, exposed to cold and to storms; confront all dangers to speed to the aid of someone who suffers: these are the sad circumstances of his profession."[113] For most of the century, law was a far more attractive career than medicine.[114] It was also much safer. Between 1825 and 1846, the mortality rate for medical students was over 50 percent higher than for those studying law.[115] Other demographic indicators suggested that doctors died much younger than members of other liberal professions.[116] Worn out physically and emotionally at the best of times, incurable illness must have been the straw that broke many a camel's back. This was particularly the case as incurables had an annoying tendency to blame doctors for their predicament. Those whose life was slipping away apparently had "an almost constant tendency to burden the physician with what is the product of the impotence of the medical arts themselves." Many apparently went to their grave without showing any signs of appreciation.[117]

Doctors rarely responded with equanimity. One authority could think of no better way to describe the public than as "a judge most often radically incompetent, demanding and thankless, proud and absurd, frivolous and cruel." A few pages later, Dr. Forget angrily denounced the readiness with which people blamed the doctor for bad outcomes. The problem most often, he insisted, was that the prescriptions had been poorly executed or ignored.[118] In these difficult circumstances, feelings of mutual suspicion and hostility often strained relations to the breaking point. In 1905, Georges Daremberg noted how "if things go badly, it is the fault of the doctor, of the climate, of nature and of mankind. They accuse everything, the elements and living beings; while they should accuse only themselves, they who made themselves sick by their obstinacy or their insouciance, and who are not cured because they do not want to listen to any advice."[119] Often enough, about the only thing doctors and patients agreed on was that it had to be somebody's fault.

In retrospect, this unhealthy dynamic was partly the product of factors beyond everyone's control. The period's daunting health needs and social problems made it reasonable, if cold-hearted, to assign a low priority to the incurably ill. Besides, it is not as though doctors didn't do anything. In turning to the substance of contemporary palliative efforts, it is clear that they were always pressured to do "the right thing." One might add that patients were as well, as neither suffering nor impending death absolved them of their duties toward those around them.

# 6

---

# Medical Strategies, Social Conventions, and Palliative Medicine

Prognosis has long affected patterns of social behavior and is justly deemed a critical determinant of something now known as patients' "illness trajectory."[1] It should come as no surprise that nineteenth-century society had weighty expectations in the setting of chronic progressive illness. Physicians' behavioral blueprint essentially consisted of three healing gestures: trial and error, morphine, and deception. Yet this enumeration belies the richness and complexity of the palliative encounter. Incurable illness was an intricate form of performance in which the idea of tragic predestination was omnipresent. People's line of conduct was also subject to rigid conventions and norms. Yet for various reasons, this social encounter was marked by considerable, and generally unwelcome, improvisation.

Although opiates were in many ways the cornerstone of care, other palliative practices played an equally important role in shaping this experience. Both the form and content of these customs highlight contemporaries' single-minded commitment to sustaining hope. A combination of tradition, "hard" science, and social consensus ensured that most saw this as a therapeutic objective worth pursuing at all costs. It is obviously tempting to view doctors' white lies as an egregious form of medical paternalism. In fact, it reflected an intriguing, multidirectional dialectic among patients, healers, and families, each acting in accordance with perceived self-interests and within the limits of various constraints. More than anything, deception was an integral part of the culturally driven and socially acceptable language of caring.

At an abstract level, fostering hope was unproblematic. Translating theory into practice proved much trickier. Like most delicate social interactions of comparable importance, palliative practices engendered almost as many dilemmas as they solved. For this reason, physicians regularly complained about the shortcomings of their therapeutic culture. Among the things that troubled them most was that, in attempting to stage-manage incurable illness, the line between "good" and "bad" medicine was disquietingly fine, subjective, and easily crossed.

In attempting to provide a full reckoning of nineteenth-century palliative medicine and end-of-life customs, I'll pay particular attention to the cultural specificities of the dying phase of incurable illness. Though it was often easier said than done, everyone who moved within this social space was expected to act in accordance with some perceived greater good. Importantly, patients and families remained deeply committed to the dominant action model, mostly because it assuaged certain forms of distress without putting too much strain on social ties. Physicians, of course, also had their own reasons, noble and ignoble, for being single-mindedly committed to having things go "well," that is to say, according to plan.

## The Therapeutic Ethos of Deceit

When they suspected the worst, doctors choreographed the diagnostic process lest a careless word or gesture let the cat out of the bag.[2] A reassuring diagnosis was thus always preferred. In an 1846 lecture, the eminent physician Auguste Chomel initiated students into the art of double-speak. He was well-placed to lecture on the issue of medical decorum. Descended from an illustrious medical family, his career had been brilliant. An accomplished anatomist, he replaced the recently deceased René Laënnec at the Academy of Medicine in 1828. A fervent Orleanist, he was rewarded with a professorship in 1830 before being named consultant to King Louis-Philippe in 1832.

The thrust of Chomel's lecture was that if diagnostic acumen was critical to earning patients' trust, it was not to come at the expense of their morale. Nowhere was this balancing act more critical than in chronic illnesses, "which pass for incurable in the minds of most people." As he noted, "If you establish the diagnosis as you're convinced you should, you will destroy the patient's hopes and do irreparable harm." It was preferable to tell consumptives they had chronic bronchitis; chronic gastritis would similarly substitute for gastric cancer.[3] Any doctor inclined to second-guessing could invoke tradition to justify his behavior. The first tradition was "common sense"—common to both sickly New Englanders who liked the term chronic bronchitis and the French working class who often referred to chronic lung ailments as *rhumes négligés*.[4] There was also the wisdom of the ages; centuries before, Michel de Montaigne had insisted that "a means of assuaging illness often consists of sweetening the name"[5]

Doctors had to be just as careful with the deployment of remedies; one didn't want to treat a consumptive with the same treatments he'd seen used unsuccessfully on others.[6] In the 1880s, one authority called for the abandonment of a therapeutic mainstay for consumption, donkey's milk. Better to use cow's milk, he insisted, as it didn't carry the connotation that the patient was a "chest case."[7]

Linguistic and therapeutic contortions, while essential, were only the start. The challenge of managing patients' expectations was even more formidable. A deceptively simple question exposed a terrible conundrum: "should we tell the patient the truth or hide it from them? In the latter case, you will be accused of having been wrong, in the former, you are discouraging the patient."[8] In the end, most went no further than vague pronouncements. It was understood that one could be more candid with the patient's entourage, though complaints surfaced about "servants or ignorant friends" whose loose lips had spoiled everything.[9] Unfortunately, even darker fears sometimes haunted the issue of truth telling. Particularly when money was short or social ties tenuous, caregivers risked concluding that terminally ill loved ones weren't worth the effort or expense. A late-century apologist for what he called "relative truth" warned that "often one must also sustain hope in the hearts of his assistants until the end, so that a patient receives the necessary care."[10] In an oft-cited work on medical ethics from 1883, the American physician Austin Flint similarly observed that "the effect of the abandonment of all hope, on the minds of nurses, relatives, and friends is bad. Their cooperative efforts are thereby relaxed."[11]

In an effort to tame his protégés' ardor for full disclosure, Chomel recounted two memorable experiences. In the first instance, youthful forthrightness prompted accusations of insensitivity and incompetence. The second, involving a terminal cancer patient, was more chilling. After another consultant matter-of-factly told the husband the truth, he apparently "took a pistol and repeated to his wife what the doctor had said, and offered to kill her saying he would then kill himself. Upon his wife's refusal, the man, out of his mind, blew his brains out in front of her and their daughter."[12] For all their singularity, horror stories often have long and rich lives of their own. They also clearly serve an important social control function.[13]

If distraught families were bad enough, incurables who suspected the worst were an even bigger headache. Some apparently pointedly asked, "Do I have a chance of being cured or not?" while others used the question "Do I need to get my affairs in order?" to probe their doctors' feelings.[14] Even the young and inexperienced understood that lying outright could irreparably harm their reputation.[15] Seasoned practitioners, for their part, favored hopeful ambiguity.[16] In those who could face "pseudo-bad" news, Chomel suggested the following response: "a wise man never leaves home without having seen to all his affairs; one never knows in the morning if one will still be alive that night. . . . If you have arrangements that need to be completed, you should think about doing it as soon as your illness has passed."[17] Though the aim was similar, a mid-century American physician proposed a somewhat different answer: "it is difficult to decide that question. Perhaps it is not proper for me at this stage of your case to attempt to do it. You are very sick, and the issue of your sickness in known only to God. I hope that the remedies will do so and so (pointing out somewhat the effects ordinarily to be expected) but I cannot tell."[18] Presumably out of respect, physicians tended to be more forthright with those juggling complex or weighty dynastic concerns.

Instances of willful transparency were rare, however. More often, physicians complained about patients' incredulity. Those with medical backgrounds were obviously in a class of their own. As one student observed, it was hard to assuage someone who knew that hope "is only the deceitful sweetener that coats a vessel filled with bitterness, or rather, the fine veil used to cover the terrible precipice which will swallow him up."[19] Yet this tendency to know/suspect/fear the worst was apparently commonplace. In the 1840s, one observer noted that consumptives who understood the gravity of their illness were often "consumed, sad and desolate, long before the disease has run its course." This was not some trifling concern, for as Dr. Lauvergne noted, "The number of these martyrs is immense, especially in our era, as learning has imparted to all classes an exact knowledge of the dangers that a 'ruined chest' runs."[20]

Those with close relations who had succumbed were understandably terror-stricken, like one young woman who had nursed an aunt who had also died from breast cancer.[21] Sadly, lies were generally least effective when needed most. No matter what the doctor said, someone who had lost their entire family to consumption was inconsolable when they too fell ill.[22] Critical of the status quo, the occasional practitioner asserted that "mystery too has its inconveniences: many patients are more tormented by doubt than they would be by the knowledge of reality, no matter what it is!"[23] Others recognized that laying it on too thick often backfired.[24]

Notwithstanding such scruples, extreme circumspection long remained the norm in both France and the Anglo-Saxon world.[25] Deception was central to physicians' handling of chronic disease until the turn of twentieth century at which point, in "curable" tuberculosis at least, there was a sea-change in attitudes. Telling patients their diagnosis, it was widely assumed, would encourage compliance with the long, arduous treatments that remained the norm in the era before antibiotics. A small but determined group of English practitioners tried to extend this courtesy (unsuccessfully it would appear) to all patients, even the mortally stricken.[26] Scornfully dismissed by one French commentator, the country remained hostile to the democratization of despair.[27] In defending their position, traditionalists invariably cited the precepts of moral physiology.[28] Hope and faith, they insisted, encouraged recovery, while fear and worry made a bad situation worse. One cannot begin to understand contemporary customs without examining the physiological laws that made "the truth" so dangerous.

### Thou Shalt Not Eat from the Tree of Knowledge: Mind-Body Medicine and the Physiology of Hope

Articulating a belief traceable to antiquity, François Broussais emphasized that external physical forces—cold, dampness, and so forth—and moral forces had similar effects, noting how "the pleasures and pains from moral causes are felt in the same organs as the pleasures and pains of a physical origin: all are genuinely physical for the physiologist as he sees a modification of the living tissues resulting from them all."[29] Though most of his ideas fell into disfavor, the belief that emotions were visibly inscribed on the body remained uncontested until the early twentieth century. It was only then that leading French psychiatrists, notably Pierre Janet, began to suggest that psychosomatic symptoms were not the product of a specific lesion but a stylized and symbolically charged response to intrapsychic distress.[30] In keeping with earlier views, a representative 1889 thesis still stressed the conventional view that the "depressive passions" "diminish the energy of the organic functions, lower the vascular tone by slowing down the heart, cause the digestion to slow and even affect the deep-seated nutrition of the tissues . . . Their effects vary in intensity according to whether the moral impression is sudden and forceful or slow and repetitive; they leave traces that are that much more durable according to the duration of their baleful influence."[31] Although acute, intense fear occasionally acted as a salutary form of shock therapy, sadness, fear, and worry were understood to be extremely injurious.[32] Without careful and concerted effort, mind and matter became locked in a downward spiral. No matter how desperate the situation, it was essential to effect an air of calm nonchalance.[33]

Positive thinking, on the other hand, supposedly worked wonders.[34] In a critically acclaimed book on the physiological effects of the passions (1844), Felix Descuret wrote that "the hope of being cured is the first step towards regaining one's health . . . we daily see grave and resistant afflictions which, to a great extent, owe their happy outcome to the hope which one ably succeeded in awakening."[35] In the mid-1870s, Amédée Bertrand similarly insisted that with tuberculosis "all hesitation is baleful, all uncertainty and groping about can lead to death" and concluded that "a patient convinced that his cure is probable is certain to be saved."[36] Bertrand, who practiced at the interface between mainstream medicine and quackery, could reasonably be accused of hubris. Yet this was not such an extreme view. For even as medicine embraced innovative paradigms such as bacteriology, the long-standing belief in the power of mind over body was being given a new and forceful lease on life. Two prominent social happenings—Charcot's highly public lessons on hysteria and the surprising events at the Catholic healing shrine Lourdes—vividly reconfirmed that hope, faith, and willpower could work miracles.

Charcot, whose views on psychosomatic medicine dominated late nineteenth-century thought, remained committed to a lesion-based conceptualization of mind-body relations.[37] In proposing a reconceived system for diagnosing and explaining hysteria, he defended the view that the mind could engender an array of somatic symptoms and physical stigmata. And as well as holding the key to understanding many illnesses, the mind also possessed remarkable therapeutic properties.

Late in life, Charcot turned his attention to Lourdes, where growing numbers of incurables came away miraculously cured. Like most high-profile opponents, his interest in the shrine was both political and therapeutic. Anyone who has read "Faith Cure" understands that his account of the pilgrimage experience had two objectives: firstly, to undermine the Church's legitimacy by demonstrating that Lourdes's cures were natural, not miraculous; secondly, to provide an account of the "neuroscience" of faith healing with an eye toward harnessing its therapeutic potential.[38] For only the most doctrinaire anticlericals denied that a trip to the grotto had powerful effects. Surviving narratives show that many pilgrims were transformed by it. Intense prayer, ritual immersion, and the care proffered by attendants and believers helped sufferers transcend the fetters of illness and experience what they perceived as divine grace.[39]

Given the poisonous atmosphere that prevailed in fin-de-siècle France, it is surprising that so many physicians kept their political agendas and therapeutic obligations separate; freethinkers who vehemently attacked superstition sent incurables to Lourdes when all else failed.[40] Though generally tinged with condescension, tolerant eclecticism had long been a feature of the palliative landscape.[41] Medical humanism at its best demanded no less. In one example of many, a mid-century essay on medical ethics by Charles Forget insisted that "it has been wrongly alleged that medical studies are by themselves a school of atheism." To his way of thinking, "the religion of the physician is gentle and tolerant; it adopts no sect, and excludes no faith; it closes its eyes on impiety even, its role being to radiate on all men, without the pretence of censoring or guiding consciences. If the physician has the misfortune of being an atheist, he should be careful to not reveal his convictions, less out of fear of reducing his public esteem, than so as to not sow bitterness and despair in the spirit of patients who, upon his word, might come to see only nothingness in death."[42] This was at most a half-truth. The Paris faculty was a hotbed of anti-Catholic materialism; some hospital physicians were known to actively impede the bedside ministrations of pious friends and priests.[43] Forget's work also appeared at an exceptional moment, as a rainbow coalition of reformers was enthusiastically welcoming the Revolution of 1848. Yet even as relations between secular physicians and Catholics deteriorated, concerns about incurables' physical and moral well-being united many members of these otherwise hostile factions.

Physicians' responses to a high-profile petition in 1906 vividly illustrated that, for most, moral duties trumped all else. Jean De Bonnefon, a virulently anticlerical journalist, tried to mobilize the profession into pressuring the government to close Lourdes on public health grounds. Presumably even he was surprised by the chilly reception he received. Across prevailing ideological fault lines, his opponents invoked three higher-order principles: firstly, "republican" concerns with individual liberty and freedom of conscience; secondly, evidence that suggested that Lourdes posed no greater threat than the innumerable spas and climactic centers to which consumptives also flocked; finally, many respondents invoked the therapeutic imperatives of the doctor-patient relationship. Politics and ideology simply had no place in the sickroom. Dr. Albert, for instance, believed in scientific progress, not miracles; he was nonetheless adamant that "as long as scientific medicine is impotent at curing certain illnesses, the medicine of charlatans, in Lourdes and elsewhere, will remain a RELATIVE BLESSING."[44] Others, like Professor Renon, were more openly conciliatory. Rejecting the idea of impeding the movement of pilgrims, Renon insisted that "any freethinking physician worthy of this title, free of confessional or political agenda, would respond in the negative without hesitation. No, we givers of hope, we the eternal cradle rockers of human suffering, even if we believe the contrary, have no right to say to our fellow, 'We can do nothing for you. Your life is over, really over. Don't look anywhere beyond.' To break the moral fiber that gives hope is more than cruel, it is almost a crime."[45] Critics, French and foreign, happily pointed out that miraculous cures were as old as civilization itself. What they didn't appreciate was the extent to which "superstition" had become a legitimate and destabilizing topic of scientific debate; to varying degrees, Lourdes undermined scientists' confidence in some of positivism's basic assumptions.[46] Today, it is difficult to fully appreciate the pervasiveness, heterogeneity, and popularity of these various medico-religious "sects."[47] Considered alongside the contemporary epidemic of hysteria and railway spine, the late nineteenth and early twentieth centuries were in some ways the golden era of psychosomatic medicine.[48]

Various healing cults proliferated in both Europe and North America, including mesmerism, mind-cure, Christian Science, and Christian mysticism. Disparate explanations circulated about whether they were effective and why. The scientific mainstream saw proof of the power of the human mind. This tenet of scientific rationalism also helps explain why an all-but-unassailable consensus existed around the issue of deceit. Reflecting the dominant view, one earnest young student accorded it the status of a moral imperative, writing, "There is no practitioner who does not make every effort to appear calm and full of hope before his patient until the end . . . he who is unaware of the marvelous advantages that this admirable force furnishes the art of *healing*, of *assuaging*, of *consoling* mankind would be unworthy of practicing medicine."[49]

Morality, reason, and precedent thus dictated the behavioral do's and don'ts in the setting of incurable illness. Yet doctors' faith in hope's therapeutic power also reflected their own needs. Beyond allowing them to tell themselves they'd done the right thing, this belief system was a counterweight to futility and impotence. The power of the mind held up the promise, however precarious, that one could still help the hopeless. Efforts to control the moral experience of the stricken were thus salutary for both patient and physician, for whom it was a rudder with which they steered a sinking ship.

Physicians' efforts to raise incurables' spirits were thus inextricably linked to struggles with the question "How useful am I?" While trying to convince themselves that their efforts left patients better off, many were uncomfortably aware that the art of palliation generally meant mediocre damage control.[50] When they stood back to discuss the plight of incurables, physicians were often hostage to their own form of hopeful ambiguity. Despite knowingly giving the impression to patients that things were not as they seemed, they were partly taken up in this conspiracy of belief.

## "Maybe, Just Maybe?" Understanding Palliative Medicine

Rare was the physician who was content simply to lie to incurables before abandoning them or shipping them off somewhere. Some actually insisted that palliative medicine was a source of professional pride. Likening it to a military campaign against an unbeatable opponent, Adrien Coriveaud told his colleagues that "the true physician, far from getting discouraged in the face of incurability . . . learns to be content with incomplete victories."[51] In the vocabulary of chronic progressive disease, successful palliation and incomplete victory were synonymous. Yet despite its apparent conceptual clarity, the terms *palliation* and *palliative* referred to several different therapeutic achievements.

Consistent with today's definition, palliatives were understood to be anything that reduced suffering. Depending upon a patient's social class and diagnosis, doctors used a host of interventions. Over the course of the century, physicians and industrial manufacturers repackaged existing remedies and developed novel detergents, sedatives, tonics, and analgesics. Others developed innovative "therapeutic aids," like a waterbed invented at mid-century by Dr. Demarquay to prevent and cure bed sores. The objective was clear-cut—the reduction of physical distress—and success was measured in terms of patient satisfaction. When the Academy of Medicine discussed Demarquay's invention in 1862, it was noted that "the best argument which pleads in favor of the invention, as with all others, is the enthusiasm with which patients speak of it and the difficulty one has trying to take it away, once their bed sores are healed."[52] As a last resort, surgeons also increasingly performed "palliative surgery." Emboldened by surgical anesthesia, hundreds of colostomies, tracheostomies, and gastrostomies were performed in the late 1870s in an effort to assuage suffering.[53] With the development and spread of asepsis, cancer surgery entered a new era. By the early twentieth century, palliative procedures had become routine. In 1911, Théodore Tuffier wrote, "I can no longer count the number of gastro-enterostomies and entero-enterostomies which I have performed in [incurable cancer]. The relief afforded patients, their prolonged survival, is no longer doubted by anyone."[54] Despite high operative mortality and potentially "disgusting" consequences, desperate times called for desperate measures.[55]

Yet whether they intervened medically or surgically, physicians were chastened by the modesty of their ambitions. Palliating incurables was essentially the professional scraps left over when curative efforts had failed.[56] Beyond their distressing predictability, incurable illness also exposed the inadequacies of the palliative repertoire. At the beginning of a tellingly short section on palliating consumption from 1882, one elite physician admitted, "As much as one must have hope, courage, audacity, and initiative . . . in treatable forms, we can only despair in untreatable ones."[57]

In the latter part of the nineteenth century, however, there was increasingly an undercurrent of optimism amid the gloom. Nowhere was an orator's intent more transparent than in an address on uterine cancer by the respected gynecologist Amédée Courty (1871). After highlighting the therapeutic value of diet, tonics, hydrotherapy, and local treatments, he concluded that "one cannot imagine the success at relieving patients and prolonging their existence by a treatment that appears first and foremost to be simply palliative."[58] Courty's message was clear: palliation meant more than indifferently managed distress. He and other apologists insisted that palliative treatments could prolong, occasionally even save, patients' lives.

Under the heading of palliation/palliatives, most writers willfully conflated providing relief, arresting disease, extending life, and creating the illusion of a cure. Like Dr. Jaumes, everyone's first priority when palliating incurables was to "obtain as great longevity as possible in mortal afflictions." Only later did Jaumes add that it was also important to "soften the harshness of the symptoms."[59] Another author eschewed concerns with relieving suffering, defining palliatives simply as "apply[ing] in medicine to all means that we employ to delay the distressing outcome in illnesses recognized as incurable."[60]

Doctors consistently likened themselves to doomed soldiers who continued to fight the good fight. In a typical example, Maurice Raynaud noted that when hydrotherapy failed, "the last duty of the practitioner . . . is to hold back as long as possible the invasion of cachexia. Once this last period has arrived, there remains the painful mission of sustaining the patient's strength as best he can, and to continue to fight without illusion, but without cease, against a fatal denouement."[61] For some, the cure remained the focus until the end; a leading hydrotherapist adamantly insisted that "it is the physicians' duty to not despair as to their salvation, and to not remain an inactive spectator before their suffering; it is their duty to try, until the last moment, all means which are not manifestly condemned by science and by reason."[62]

Rather than simply lacking scruples, many who resorted to polypharmacy, panaceas, or electromagnetism probably shared their patients' desperate hope that "something just might work." This seemed reasonable given three features of the nineteenth-century medical credo: firstly, the conviction that no disease was inherently incurable; secondly, people's faith in the healing power of nature; thirdly, the therapeutic power of hope. Finally, in an era when some still spoke of the uniqueness of each person's illness, prognostic notions remained fluid, not absolute.

In retrospect, *palliation* could best be defined as "that which one could still accomplish when others concluded that nothing could be done." Unexpectedly curing the patient was the most meritorious; convincing them that there was still hope, the least. When judging the fruits of their labors, practitioners were free to decide whether a pure palliative had been sort of curative. It is tempting to dismiss such distinctions as trifling. Yet it is altogether human to want to frame one's efforts in the best possible light. Most comfortable working toward a cure, doctors refused, in its absence, to eschew the importance of being useful. Strikingly, both patients and doctors resorted to almost anything to put off the nightmare scenario: openly admitting defeat.

### "Everything but the Kitchen Sink," or the Pragmatism of Despair

Contemporary narratives written by and about the chronically ill are pervaded by equal measures of pragmatism and desperation. Like moths to a light, they attracted "the famous and the obscure, the fanciful and the dogmatic, the extremists, charlatans, and lunatics," who invariably arrived "radiating infectious optimism, official dispensers of hope that they express in hyperbolic phrases destined to raise the stakes over the tired refrains proffered by their predecessors."[63] For those willing to try anything, the railways were a godsend. They allowed growing numbers access to various prized destinations, be it the American West or the south of France.

In Europe, hydrotherapy proved increasingly popular among those who had all but given up hope. In 1856, Napoleon III's personal physician complained that too many people still viewed it as a last resort.[64] A year later, another leading hydrotherapist, Philibert Patissier, similarly noted that "thermal establishments are the rendezvous of all the patients who, after exhausting all pharmaceutical preparations without benefit, come to the mineral springs requesting relief that ordinary medicine refuses them."[65] The case of Count Henri de Béarn was in many ways typical. After watching his health decline for months, he went to take the waters at Trouville three days before he died. He had barely arrived when the intensity of his symptoms led him to return immediately to Paris without having had a single bath, only to succumb the following day![66]

Hydrotherapy's growing legitimacy and the country's growing affluence set the stage for large-scale expansion. Leading spas like Vichy and Aix-les-Bains became popular vacation spots; the key to success was a pristine location, adequate capital investment, and railway access. The most exclusive resorts were lavishly appointed, with state-of-the-art bathing equipment and a multitude of leisure activities. Spa holidays also allowed the socially ambitious and upwardly mobile the chance to learn the art of living from their social superiors. Yet for a social class still uncomfortable with unbridled consumption, the austere, medically regimented bathing rituals served as a reassuring counterpoint to pleasure. It afforded the guilt-free enjoyment of an experience that, sybaritic delights notwithstanding, was "good for them."[67]

Rapidly changing mores explains why an authority on chronic disease noted with relief in 1874 that thermal stations were no longer "haunted only by lazy rich people or by desperate patients."[68] Available statistics certainly speak volumes, as the number of bathers went from 90,000 in the 1840s to 800,000 in 1900.[69] Spas nonetheless remained beacons for those with nothing left to lose. In 1879, one physician noted that the excited buzz surrounding his establishment ensured that "all the incurables, all of medicine's desperate cases decided to head this way. We saw numerous examples from our rural clientele around the years 1874, 1875, 1876. Many came despite our advice, and returned embittered and disappointed."[70]

Those who couldn't afford such luxuries still pressured their physicians to do "something." The usual response was to substitute one curative remedy for another. Contemporaries also weren't above prescribing inert treatments, if only to avoid being accused of not having done everything possible. Despite dismissing most traditional remedies for tuberculosis, the noted skeptic Pierre Louis nonetheless allowed that it was often necessary "to give in to the wishes of patients and especially their families, for in the treatment of a distressing disease, it is important to avoid regrets, which while without foundation, would be too cruel just the same."[71] Mindful that people would simply turn elsewhere, doctors even indulged patients' fanciful ideas. One seasoned clinician, for instance, acknowledged that "I have adopted the principle of permitting the usage of useless or absurd remedies, so often obsessively demanded by patients, to the extent that these treatments are without inconvenience. Allow hemorrhoidal patients to carry chestnuts in their pockets and gouty ones to sleep with brooms made of birch bark; even allow hydroptics to take a bath in cow's blood, no matter how revolting the means, if only to convince patients of their extravagance."[72] Patients were also pressured by their entourage. A family intimate noted that two days before Prince August de Broglie succumbed to tuberculosis in June 1867 he "consented again to have recourse to homeopathy, though he was without much hope, but rather out of duty and to be able to say he'd tried everything."[73]

Inert medications were understood to be harmless, though symbolically laden diversions that simultaneously proved the case wasn't hopeless and the doctor still cared.[74] As one careful observer noted in 1849, "There are [incurables] who absolutely want to be treated pharmaceutically. All other therapies seem to be a decoy and testify to their doctor's lack of zeal. This disposition is an indication for treatment that must be respected. Write prescriptions, if it makes the patient happy."[75] If placebos had the advantage of being risk-free, similar justifications were mobilized to defend cancer surgery. Prognostic uncertainty made it hard to identify candidates for radical intervention. The resulting chaos was described in an 1874 article that noted that "a few years ago in the hospitals, one could follow patients who, refused at La Charité were accepted at Lariboisière, or had addressed themselves to l'Hôtel-Dieu. It is that the surgical temperament varies like their methods, and the interpretation of contraindications to surgery is influenced by various factors."[76]

Panaceas, placebos, and palliative surgery remained integral elements of the nineteenth-century therapeutic arsenal. They were nonetheless highly problematic and a source of considerable unease. Exposing the uncomfortable territory into which such practices dragged the profession, one commentator observed, "One must not confound this sage behavior with charlatanism, which employs this magical quality of remedies to exploit patients. The [honorable] practitioner deceives the patient, this is true; but it is to tear him away from the terrors of the imagination, and thereby save his life."[77] Among the challenges confronting the medical mainstream, few had as corrosive an effect on professional identity as embracing the methods of the nostrum peddler.

## Incurable Illness, Mainstream Medicine, and "Charlatanism"

Given its importance in the lives of incurables, it is essential to have some understanding of the murky world of charlatanism and its place in the contemporary medical marketplace. French doctors—like those in every other country—consistently portrayed it as an evil. Such Manichaeism, of course, grossly oversimplifies a complex phenomenon. As historian Matthew Ramsey has noted, even the labels used to distinguish between "medical orthodoxy" and "medical fringe" are freighted, subjective, and contingent.[78] He makes an excellent case for applying the term "medical outsider" to the disparate mass of unofficial healers. As I see it, the term should also be applied to anyone (licensed or unlicensed) who practiced "nonstandard" medicine. One can even consider nonelite physicians outsiders, albeit in a narrower sense.

Several features distinguish French experiences from those of the United States and other European countries. There were specific and draconian laws against the "illegal practice of medicine" (that is, without a diploma) and the selling of "secret remedies" (that is, without disclosing the ingredients). Pharmacies and pharmacists were also theoretically bound by strict rules. The most important was the prohibition against compounding or selling anything that didn't have an official seal of approval, namely inclusion on the list of conventional remedies known as the *Codex*.

In practice, there existed a panoply of nonstandard practices and practitioners, most noticeably in the poorest neighborhoods and the vast countryside. The first and most widespread was medical self-help, expertise transmitted both orally and through an expanding array of health manuals. Certain individuals (wise or cunning folk) were believed to possess particular skill at preparing remedies and healing amulets. Some also cast spells. Most cantons also possessed an array of paramedical healers with specialized skills such as bone setting, dentistry, or midwifery. They were tolerated, even embraced, by official medicine, except when they went beyond their area of expertise (something they apparently were prone to).[79] Partly because controls were lax, pharmacists also regularly gave advice and treatments without a physician's involvement; some also flouted the law banning secret remedies.[80] They were not alone, as many merchants and grocers also sold medicines on the side. Complicating matters further, a broad cross-section of the population—including artisans, merchants, priests, landowners, and farmers—offered various medical services, including surgery! Most were generalists who treated a range of internal and external maladies. Others focused on specific illnesses (notably skin diseases and cancer) or a specific type of diagnostic/healing practice, be it magnetism, urinoscopy, or sorcery.[81]

In terms of legitimacy and institutional power, none rivaled the nursing sisters who provided much-needed nursing care throughout the century. They were also officially sanctioned to prepare and distribute a range of basic remedies from the *Codex*.[82] In theory, they were only allowed to treat indigent patients using supplies from the hospital pharmacy or local dispensary. In practice, they used this privilege (and the pricing power that came with buying in bulk) to reach out well beyond. Their fees varied according to the remedy's complexity, quality, and the patients' ability to pay. Business was brisk and profitable. The proceeds were turned over to the order or used to subsidize other activities, particularly teaching.

Until late-century, nuns provided much of the country's medical care, particularly in staunchly Catholic rural areas. In this, they were aided and abetted by both the Church and local authorities. During the Catholic renaissance (ca. 1815–1870), and particularly after the passage of the Falloux Laws on education in 1850, thousands of nuns infiltrated the countryside with an eye to educate, heal, and proselytize.[83]

Several factors explained this state of affairs. The first and most obvious was that no doctor was available in much of the country; even the group of second-class physicians known as health officers avoided the poorest areas.[84] Everyone's fees were also prohibitively high. Health officers' comparably modest ones rose dramatically whenever a house call was required; charges were levied according to the (often considerable) distances involved. Nursing sisters, on the other hand, typically worked for free, thanks to wealthy donors and profits accrued from selling medicines. Other "outsiders," most of whom had another occupation, carefully priced their services according to what the market would bear. Perhaps most importantly, the treatments offered by doctors weren't that different, nor necessarily more effective, than those of their competitors. The latter were equally at ease (and sometimes even more aggressive) with the lancet, purgatives, and other heroic interventions. It wasn't until late in the century, in fact, that the medical profession successfully laid claim to a unique, and increasingly efficacious, amalgam of knowledge and practice.[85]

One could also speak of a cultural divide between educated, self-consciously scientific physicians and the more rustic elements of the population. Many Frenchmen were devout Catholics, superstitious, or both. For them it was natural to entrust both body and soul to a nursing sister. The Church's promotion of various healing cults and miracles, it goes almost without saying, actively encouraged this reflex.[86] Unorthodox healers, for

their part, were keenly aware of the power of thaumaturgy. Many incorporated rituals, phrases, and objects that were familiar elements of popular
piety. Such practices were partly a backlash against mainstream medicine's
embrace of philosophical materialism. At the same time, their enduring
appeal demonstrates the ongoing vitality of mysticism and antiauthoritari-
anism in an era of aggressive rationality.

Ongoing efforts at controlling the medical marketplace had, at best,
limited results. The state established a process for evaluating new therapies,
entrusting the duty to the Royal Academy of Medicine (founded in 1820). The
medical profession also launched increasingly pointed attacks on the nursing orders. This rarely translated into sanctions, however, partly because
the sisters enjoyed the support of the population and local notables (many
of whom were staunch Catholics, all of whom appreciated the cheap man-
power). The legal system also turned a blind or indulgent eye.[87] Individual
physicians also had to tread carefully. Via a feminine network of contacts
and connections, sisters influenced people's health-seeking behaviors,
including their choice of doctor. This spirit of tolerance was also partly
driven by certain features of the French legal system; the harshness of the
laws on secret remedies, the practical challenges of enforcement, and concerns about property rights ensured that they were rarely enforced.[88] In fact,
despite the profession's best efforts, even the two most vulnerable groups of
outsiders rarely felt the full force of the law. The first—itinerant healers who
read urine, laid on hands, or dispensed potions and panaceas, usually with
carnavalesque flair—enjoyed the relative advantage of being highly mobile.
The other—a relatively small group of brazen, iconoclastic, and commercially
successful practitioners—frequently enjoyed a cult following. There were
admittedly a few high-profile court cases involving individuals who brazenly
flouted the law banning the sale of secret remedies and the illegal practice
of medicine (sometimes with deadly consequences).[89] Even when they were
successfully prosecuted, however, the net result was often increased popular
hostility toward doctors.[90] Some prominent defendants were even lionized
as popular heroes.[91]

When physicians discussed charlatanism's popular appeal, many blamed
a combination of credulity and irrationality. In his "psychological study" of
the phenomenon published in 1867, Dr. Benjamin Verdo described how
"men of most outstanding judgment" fell into this trap; at a certain point, he
insisted, "reason is vanquished, and there is then nothing to do but to call
for the charlatan and swallow the panacea."[92] Others framed the issue a bit
differently, insisting that desperation was the main motive force and incurables the principal victims.[93] In light of this image, it is not surprising that
an aura of disrepute hung over the field of palliative medicine. Two leading
etymologists, for example, explicitly equated it with deceit, defining *palliate*

as "curing an illness in appearance only."[94] Another elite physician similarly observed that "palliatives are, in the hands of charlatans, powerful means for deceiving [people's] blind credulity; with such medication, they succeed in promptly soothing some symptoms, and in thus procuring for themselves an ephemeral triumph, from which they always shrewdly extract a significant profit."[95] As one would expect, medical insiders were always most comfortable playing the expert, aggressively denouncing charlatans' exploitation of incurables. But this pyramidal model—desperate incurable and charlatan at the base, worldly physician looking on from above—was simplistically polarizing. Although there were certain rules of good conduct, the line between charlatanism and respectable medicine was disquietingly thin.

If they ferociously attacked unlettered *guérisseurs*, many critics also gave their colleagues a failing grade. Aware of the difficulty in distinguishing benign and malignant growths, Gaspard Bayle and Jean Cayol nonetheless insisted that the uncertainty surrounding cancer treatment reflected "conceit, a desire for fame, which speculates on that which is most dear to humanity, a shameful weakness that keeps one from admitting that remedies were unfruitful."[96] Even someone quick to defend his colleagues recognized that many engaged in "honest charlatanism." Some wrote prescriptions in Latin to make mundane treatments more impressive, a practice some experts considered acceptable when done in the patient's best interests.[97] Physicians also exaggerated an illness's seriousness to make the patient's recovery appear more extraordinary. Even the medical elite weren't above using deceit, machinations, statistics, and other ingenious lies to promote specific surgical procedures or proprietary treatment systems.[98] It is presumably no accident that legislative solutions to quackery took certain forms and not others. Physicians had every interest in sanctioning the illegal practice of medicine and secret remedies but leaving aside other questionable forms of behavior.

Occasionally, members of the medical elite admitted that charlatans played a useful role on the fringes. Reflecting de facto policy, Marc-Antoine Petit suggested that the hope charlatans offered incurables was a boon to humanity, before insisting that their ministrations "become opprobrium and a scourge when applied to the ordinary ills of life, when it then merits all the animadversion of the law, and the surveillance of the magistrates."[99] When it came to their health, nineteenth-century Frenchmen were both open-minded and pragmatic. Fortunately or unfortunately, they had a dizzying array of questionable therapeutic options at their disposal.[100] Yet in a setting where nothing worked well, even skullduggery arguably did less harm than good.

That desperation made for strange bedfellows is vividly illustrated by the adventures of Jan Hendrick Vriès or *le Docteur noir*, a self-trained physician who rose to prominence in the late 1850s. According to the best available biography, Vriès came from Surinam and landed on the shores of the Seine after an unsuccessful stint in London.[101] While presenting himself as the prophet of a new Christian sect, he peddled an exotic treatment for humanity's worst diseases, something he called "the quinquina of cancer."[102] After testing his panacea on France's leading dermatology ward for a year to no avail, he briefly enjoyed a lucrative private practice.[103] His career peaked in 1858 when word got out that he'd cured several incurables, including a member of Parisian high society. Adolphe Sax, the inventor of the eponymous musical instrument, had been diagnosed with and unsuccessfully treated for a fatal lip cancer by several Parisian *princes de la science*.[104] Offered radical surgery that involved the removal of part of his face, he summoned Vriès. When the tumor fell off, as predicted, *tout Paris* began to take notice. Desperately ill patients turned to him in droves.

Concerned by his growing notoriety, two prominent hospital physicians allowed him to treat seventeen terminally ill cancer patients for six months. In February 1859, a strange story became even stranger when police raided Vriès's home demanding his diploma and confiscating his remedies. The efforts of several "honorable people" and an unspecified "august intervention" allowed him to continue his experiment. No stranger to controversy himself, Sax gave a sumptuous banquet-concert in Vriès's honor at the posh Hôtel du Louvre; the guest list included a fascinating cross-section of high society, including the composer Hector Berlioz.[105]

After a controversial two-month stint at La Charité, Dr. Alfred Velpeau ended the trial, announcing that Vriès's exotic extract was an inert placebo. Several months later, *le Docteur noir* was charged with illegally practicing medicine and fraud.[106] In January 1860, Vriès appeared before the judge. His hearing lasted two days and included depositions from dozens of witnesses. Aware that his colleagues' reputations were at stake, the pathologist Charles Robin nonetheless testified that Sax had never suffered from cancer. His tumor was a benign fibrous growth.[107] On January 11, 1860, Vriès was found guilty, fined, and sentenced to fifteen months in prison.[108]

He wasn't the only one who came away bruised and battered. A physician sympathetic to Vriès testified that he'd been branded an enemy by the entire medical community.[109] In defending his actions, he excoriated hospital authorities for stopping the experiment prematurely and for the racist harassment Vriès experienced. Velpeau, for his part, deeply regretted the whole affair. Even as he was putting an end to things, he found himself defending his actions before the Academy of Medicine. Clearly ill at ease, he admitted that had he known more about Vries's past, "I would never have taken the trouble to examine the pretensions and affirmations of a man of his stamp; but, deprived of this information, and willing to admit somewhat to the good faith of the protagonists, I had a lapse in judgment."[110] At his funeral a decade later, a friend and colleague noted that this episode remained, in Velpeau's mind, a humiliating blemish on an otherwise extraordinary career.[111]

Better than any testimonial, this episode demonstrates that desperate credulity didn't only color patients' judgment, it made a fool of experts. Its subversive effects on socioprofessional distinctions was truly extraordinary; an internationally respected surgeon opened up the most jealously guarded academic enclave to a flamboyant huckster who addressed his patients in halting, broken French.[112] In the midst of all the controversy, Charles Fauvel valiantly defended his mentor, asserting,

> We live in an era exempt of scientific prejudices, and medicine, when
> it is impotent, generously raises towards it, without overly worrying
> about who they are, any man who tells it "I cure those whom you allow
> to die." But, if in the interests of humanity, science exposes itself to
> frequentations which are unworthy of it, it is its duty, as soon as it has
> acquired proof of the deceit and lies with which some would abuse
> it, it is its duty, I say, to proclaim to patients who anxiously await
> the results of experiments upon which their life depends: Stop! You
> are being deceived; this man is neither a messiah, nor a benefactor
> of humanity, he is an impostor who pitilessly exploits the thing that
> honest man hold most sacred, the suffering of his fellows.[113]

In setting the record straight, he struggled to make a shocking embarrassment seem like an example of professional probity.

Whether to have recourse to unproven or exotic wonder drugs was one of many ethical dilemmas practitioners faced. In an unusually forthright celebration of medical salesmanship, Dr. Guneau de Mussy suggested that physicians had much to learn from their disreputable competitors. In a lecture on phthisis, he invited students to embrace their methods, as they were experts at "acquir[ing] patient's confidence and speak[ing] to the imagination! Also, by virtue of the effect they produce on the patient's spirit, it is rare that the latter, for some days at least, do not experience a type of improvement that he attributes to arcane treatments, the gestures of magnetism and other turpitudes. . . . Do not abandon, sirs, these powerful means to charlatans, know how to use them while investing it with an honest form, in the interest of the medical art and of humanity."[114] Even an austere positivist such as Paul Broca acknowledged that it was sometimes difficult to draw the line between cancer doctors and quacks and admitted that proffering lies and placebos was one of the most painful medical duties. His apologetic included an important disclaimer, however: "each will find in his own conscience the excuse for such conduct, which differs from charlatanism as much as charity differs from cupidity. That which the empiric does out of ignorance or deceit, the honest and learned practitioner must sometimes perform out of a sense of humanity."[115] In a setting without hard and fast rules, the difference between respectable and illicit was less a question of substance than intent.

Outside of certain behaviors, the distinction between licit and illicit interventions in chronic illness was largely an issue of branding and of standing. At one extreme were physicians whose credentials and social position underwrote their credibility. Entrepreneurial quacks that brazenly promised the moon and demanded payment up front like Vriès occupied the other. In struggling to survive, the great mass of physicians had to choose between a comparably strict moral code and various forms of "honest charlatanism."

The paucity of patient narratives does not permit a full accounting of incurables' interactions with so-called quacks, but the commercial success of the patent medicine trade suggests that those who felt abandoned or condemned placed hope and dollars in their words.[116] The nostrum peddlers exploited their freedom from the rules that restrained their competitors. Above all, they offered hope when all hope was lost. Medical outsiders' popularity did not of course prevent patients from turning back to hospital physicians; indeed the growing frequency with which they did so indexed the growing allure of medical science. Yet end-stage or terminal disease was particularly problematic in that it left doctors and patients with little choice but to face facts and find the strength to accept the inevitable.

## What Now? Attitudes and Behaviors in the Terminal Stage of Illness

Few physicians would have disagreed with Hermann Lebert: the best way to manage an illness like tuberculosis was to keep quiet and let the disease do the talking. Addressing this professional quagmire in the 1870s, he stressed how "when you have made your prognoses extremely circumspect, the progress of the illness takes on the duty of gradually diminishing the illusions of the entourage and the patient himself. You have prepared the family without taking away hope; now it has disappeared little by little on its own."[117] Many dying incurables feared the worst, having "read the terrible sentence that science has pronounced on the faces of near relations."[118] Others needed no outside cues; in late-stage tuberculosis, worsening anorexia and vomiting left little to the imagination.[119]

Though denying the obvious is rarely easy, many physicians insisted that a stronger dose of lies was the best solution for worsening distress.[120] One fervent advocate insisted that "outside of absolutely exceptional cases, one must maintain the hopes to which the dying person clings, like the grasses to which a drowning man's fingers cling. It is a fine thing to lie with assurance, and to allow them to foresee a possible cure: and no one is more authorized than the physician, who must at the same time remain completely unimpressionable, as the dying patient tries to read the true verdict on his features."[121] Often, however, choreographing the dance of hope became well-nigh impossible.[122] When they couldn't stretch the truth any longer, doctors generally preferred to leave breaking the bad news to someone else. Describing it as one of the most unpleasant set of circumstances for physicians, Forget concluded that "sometimes, perhaps, he would do well to restrict himself to warning the family, engaging them to entrust to the religious minister this painful mission that is essentially within the attributions of the doctor of the soul."[123]

Others were more categorical. Reflecting both therapeutic and religious convictions, Max Simon insisted that "to declare . . . that one's remedies are useless, is to cast despair into the spirit of a poor unfortunate, and such a mission would become, only in rare cases, that of the doctor."[124] At a time when the secularization of death was becoming a fait accompli, the instinct to off-load this duty remained strong. In a late-century article on terminal care, a fervent Catholic physician suggested that doctors limit themselves to platitudes like "the matter is serious, but I have seen people come back from worse, we will do all we can . . . ," while leaving discussions about the patient's affairs to someone else—a family member, the parish priest, a nursing sister, or some pious family friend.[125] If they less often had the luxury of summoning the priest, English and American physicians nonetheless concurred that this definitely wasn't their job.[126]

In Catholic countries, the duty long fell to the confessor. Their arrival was so portentous that one medical student suggested that a priest be summoned at the start of every illness, serious or no. Otherwise the terror they instilled could have disastrous, even fatal consequences.[127] Given this, it is not surprising that most families who were told to call the cleric assumed the undertaker was next.[128] In a richly documented study, historian Thomas Kselman has shown that tensions sometimes arose between confessors and families, often around the issue of inheritances.[129] That some clergymen resented being systematically used as the bearer of bad tidings has gone largely overlooked.[130]

Like other aspects of life, the act of dying was increasingly secularized over the nineteenth century. Religious indifference and science's growing prestige together ensured that priestly duties increasingly fell upon physicians. In 1883, a leading physician of his generation offered up the following apologetic: "It rests with the physician more than to any other to possess and to inculcate in others in the strength of character and the spiritual tranquility that can stand up to all the ill treatments of fate. There is room for him either beside or for lack of a priest. Amid the diversity of beliefs one encounters common principles, discernible even in the absence of any particular faith. Common sentiments, in which physicians are freer than pastors, can be made to speak to some moral value [dear] to the patient."[131] By late century, even Catholic doctors conveyed a religiously neutral message whenever they were uncertain about a patient's convictions.[132] Unthinkable even a generation before, a late-century reissue of a clerical handbook allowed that doctors were generally the best judge of what course of action to take in the presence of the dying person.[133]

Physicians responded idiosyncratically to these newfound responsibilities. Anticlerical physicians sought to banish superstition from the sick room; in 1865, the attending physician at La Charité Hospital fought to prevent the administration of water from La Salette, a Catholic healing shrine, to a terminally ill patient.[134] Most, one suspects, struggled with mixed emotions. Proud to be the center of attention, they would have felt the weight of the added responsibility. They were presumably happiest when patients demanded little from them and quietly slipped away. Yet often enough, doctors faced angry or distraught people in whom only death could bring an end to their misery. It was then that Max Simon asked them to relinquish the title "man of science" and humbly become "men of charity." Many refused. None, however, could have ignored that this was the essence of good palliative medicine.

## Conclusion

One can readily equate deceit with paternalism. If the doctor-patient relationship was as lopsided as some have claimed, incurable illness would have worsened power relations: as patients became more dependent, physicians alone remained "in the know," demigods left to wield complete authority.[135] There is, of course, some truth to this. Nineteenth-century doctors were paternalistic and social inequalities were definitely part of the story. Yet this was not simply a matter of "doctor knows best." Patients and families played a critical role in establishing and sustaining this social system.

Encouraged to suffer in silence, people were rarely that docile. Incurables pursued the proven and the exotic, changing doctors and hospitals in pursuit of a cure. On one level, suffering put people in the driver's seat; patients with intense or protracted pain often forced their doctors to rapidly move from one remedy to the next, sometimes without waiting long enough to see if they were effective.[136]

Physicians occasionally spoke openly of the emotional pressures placed upon them. After refusing to operate on a breast lump he concluded was benign, one surgeon noted that the woman, her mother, and her husband wouldn't stop harassing him, holding him personally responsible for any-thing bad that might happen.[137] Despite its dismal track record, incurable cancer patients often pushed surgery because they simply couldn't accept doing "nothing."[138] Incurables' peregrinations to far-flung shrines and spas demonstrated the lengths they'd go to get what they wanted. Frustrated and impatient, they were singled out as demanding, selfish, and angry.[139] In many ways, this clinical encounter calls to mind a mountaineer dangling over a cliff, secured by the failing grasp of a fellow climber. Incurables had a strong personal and emotional claim on those around them, a power they under-standably sought to exploit.

Market forces also played a role in discouraging truth telling. Medical services were a commodity and unsatisfied customers took their business elsewhere. It was self-defeating, in other words, to be excessively frank when those around you offered soothing words and empty promises.[140] Interest-ingly, when doctors began to systematically reveal the truth to tuberculosis patients that they deemed curable, many patients and families refused to believe it.[141] Ultimately, the politics of revelation, like individual treatment decisions, reflected a dynamic, multidirectional interaction between doc-tors, patients, intimates, and "charlatans."

Yet doctors' single-mindedness strongly suggests that their own inter-ests were being served. Beyond narrow economic incentives, hiding the truth offered emotional breathing room and a gratification of sorts. Sparing patients was one of several healing gestures that symbolized their concern. A leading mid-century book on cancer noted, "There is no better coun-sel to give in the treatment of chronic diseases than to properly regulate [patients'] hygiene."[142] Hermann Lebert didn't believe that this was terribly useful. Mostly it allowed the doctor to show he cared.[143] Guilty feelings, on the other hand, partly explain the profession's rhetorical commitment to treating incurables indulgently. Unlike curable ones who had a duty to obey, here the flow of obligations was inverted. Beyond tolerating therapeutic insubordination, lying was perceived as the least one could do.[144] In the end, superfluous treatments and emotional manipulation were the burnt offer-ings that physicians offered to those they were powerless to save.

Invariably depicted as an expression of concern, this code of silence was intimately linked to fears of being a "mere spectator." Medicine, after all, is the art of being useful. Cast in the role of directing a tragedy they knew by heart, physicians focused on the effort and dexterity required to successfully veil reality. This was more than a game of cat and mouse as feeling useful encouraged them to remain engaged. It was when they believed that there was really nothing left to be done that the temptation to abandon patients was particularly strong. For almost all concerned, truth telling was a Pando-ra's box that risked turning a bad situation into an intolerable one. Beyond forcing everyone to confront futility, it opened the door to an emotional spontaneity that most contemporaries preferred to avoid. This carefully scripted process ensured that feelings were successfully straitjacketed, just as the stylized and genteel dances of the period allowed disturbing sexual instincts to be channeled into less threatening social forms. In the end, a shared commitment to therapeutic illusions served the interests of care-givers and patients alike.

# 7

## *Ecce Homo*

### Opiates, Suffering, and the Art of Palliation

Opiates have inspired several distinct literary traditions. Physicians and poets have celebrated their medicinal virtues for millennia, while (non) fictional accounts of their pleasures and pains have proliferated since the nineteenth century. Long intrigued by famous habitués, historians have progressively broadened the scope of their reflections. A range of studies, spanning countries and eras, explore concepts such as intoxication and addiction, criminality and repression. The sheer number of works devoted to "drug problems" and "problem drugs" speak to their interest as historical objects. Few other social artifacts, in fact, give such purchase on important aspects of human culture and social relations—art, genius, deviance, virtue, geopolitics, colonialism, racism, class prejudice. The most compelling accounts follow changing patterns of drug consumption and their impact on perceptions, attitudes, and responses to "the problem."[1] The focus here, however, is deceptively simple, namely opiates' role in alleviating human misery. The topic merits careful consideration, though, because it offers a unique perspective onto two complex and interwoven social behaviors: suffering and palliation.

In the late nineteenth century, hypodermic morphine was simultaneously an indispensable wonder drug and a dangerous sociobiological menace. The prevailing French and Anglo-American historiography suggests that recreational abuse, real and imagined, played a central role in the drug's vilification and in society's heavy-handed response. This analysis highlights the critical and largely underappreciated role of incurables in the construction of addiction. Given their substantial and (theoretically) legitimate use of the drug, this was no simple matter. Yet as will be seen, they were central actors in an increasingly harsh web of suspicion and censure.

With the advent of hypodermic morphine, doctors found themselves on the horns of a dilemma; they were caught between their duty to alleviate suffering and the obligation to reserve this dangerous substance for those who "truly needed it." Understanding physicians' behavior requires a thorough understanding of both the contemporary culture of adversity and the competing priorities that they (and society at large) struggled to reconcile. The French case is particularly interesting in that contingent social and political concerns ensured that narcotic consumption/addiction quickly came to be viewed as an urgent public health issue. Leading sociomedical authorities consistently expressed concern about the grave dangers of addiction among incurables. Hard-nosed ambivalence toward morphine and suffering, already discernible in the late 1870s, became increasingly pronounced in subsequent decades.

In tackling this issue, I'll explicitly address a bias that permeates the historiography of pain and palliative medicine: that religion (that is, Catholicism) was an impediment to progress because it celebrated the spiritual value of suffering. In fact, there's compelling evidence suggesting that religious scruples played little part in the genesis of the morphine scare. Devout Catholics also played a vital and largely constructive role in assuaging the sick. Rather than single-mindedly laying blame, I'll explore the impact of emotional and deontological concerns, technological innovation, and sociopolitical trends on physicians' hardening attitudes. In retrospect, it is clear that suffering, palliation, and addiction were not narrowly conceived "worlds unto themselves" but interconnected elements of an elaborate moral system. Codified in the lexicon of "good patients" and "good deaths," society articulated an ideal of terminal illness in which the relief of suffering was part of a broader struggle to minimize the personal, existential, and societal fallout. The next chapter takes up these related notions, as they provide the soundest framework for understanding palliative practices and the experience of dying in the nineteenth century and arguably today.

## Between Failure and Fear: Perceptions and Usage of Opiates in Incurable Illness

The best French history of opiate use has appropriately framed it as a series of intertwining narratives.[2] Simultaneously examining the writings of literati, doctors, and social commentators, *Les poisons de l'esprit* details the creation of a novel category of deviant behavior (drug abuse) and of deviants (drug abusers). The work includes two important observations about the nineteenth century. First, contemporaries recognized several patterns of opiate use: recreational, "medical," and psychiatric. Second, explosive growth in the (mis)use of hypodermic morphine, a practice introduced into France in 1859 by Dr. Louis-Jules Behier, fueled fears that it was both causing and symptomatic of France's progressive "degeneration." Far more debatable is historian Jean-Jacques Yvorel's suggestion that opium use in chronic progressive disease was peripheral to the "morphine problem." In characterizing contemporary practices, he cites Dr. Guimball (1891), who insisted that "morphine prolongs existence, calms the pain and especially puts to rest the moral suffering. By virtue of this we could advise its use even in intensive doses, as those physicians accustomed to prescribing it do today." Depicting him as a medical Everyman, Yvorel claimed that "such an attitude would have been inconsequential if the only conditions concerned were cancers, consumptions, and other tabes," suggesting that recreational abuse single-handedly drove concerns around morphine mania.[3] English and American authorities were also primarily concerned with the nonmedicinal use of opiates by undesirables. Despite this, historian David Courtwright has justly observed that chronic disease long remained a leading proximate cause of addiction.[4]

One admittedly finds innumerable nineteenth-century endorsements of opiates' palliative virtues. In 1833, a medical student noted that "opium is often like the last word of an art whose mission is to console and to assuage, when it is impotent to cure. No agent . . . can pretend to render as useful a service."[5] The hospital physician Démétrius Zambaco spoke in similar terms a half-century later at an international medical conference (1882), reprinted verbatim in the French medical journal *l'Encéphale*. Speaking in the alarmist language typical of this period, Zambaco nonetheless allowed that for those

> in rooms on whose frontispiece we read in large letters the fatal condemnation of incurable . . . for those condemned without appeal, without the least glimpse of hope, not only to death, but also to cruel suffering without cease or mercy to their dying breath; for those poor cancer patients especially, it is certainly permitted to use morphine injections in a continuous and daily fashion. It is even a humane duty to bring them some relief with morphine, which puts them to sleep or stupefies them, and helps them forget the sad fate that the tortures of pain constantly remind them.[6]

If such testimony stands on its merits, one needs to distinguish between lofty statements of principle and the messy realities of daily life. For buried amid the panegyrics was much awkward soul-searching. The gloom surrounding the "palliative enterprise" only began to lift after 1860, as a series of technological innovations transformed incurables' illness experience forever. Yet amid universal acclaim, hesitation and ambivalence quickly surfaced. Rather than being peripheral to the growing vilification of narcotics, incurables vividly illustrated their destructive properties. Ultimately, when one speaks of the physical, moral, and social hazard of drug abuse, incurables were subject to (essentially) the same censure, suspicion, and surveillance.

## Somewhat Better Than Nothing?
## The Palliative Use of Opiates ca. 1800–1850

Opiates were a mainstay of the nineteenth-century pharmacopeia and were dispensed in a broad array of preparations. These included pills, lozenges, powders, plasters and liniments, as well as enemas. Probably the best known was laudanum, a liquid composed of opium dissolved in tincture of alcohol. Opium was also one of the active ingredients, along with alcohol and later cocaine, in various patent remedies, tonics, syrups, and cordials—a number of which were marketed as soothing preparations for infants and children.

Intrigued by its remarkable properties, turn-of-the-century researchers began to study opium's chemical composition. Working independently, Charles Derosne, Armand Seguin, and F. W. Sertürner identified its principal active element. Sertürner proved particularly adept and christened the powerful crystalline substance he isolated *morphium*. Soon after, the French pharmacist-chemist Robiquet isolated another of opium's medicinal alkaloids, codeine. The importance of these discoveries was appreciated immediately, and Sertürner was awarded a prestigious prize by the Institut de France in 1831. Spurred by the development of a novel process for obtaining morphine, English, Scottish, and German companies began commercial-scale production in the 1820s and 1830s.[7]

For much of the nineteenth century, however, the reliability of the opium supply was a major concern.[8] Commented on in France as early as 1819, an 1839 alert illustrated the magnitude of the problem.[9] It observed, "A mass of opium, furnished to the central pharmacy, having been recognized of a fraudulent nature, seizures were carried out in the depots of the supplier and at several Parisian druggists."[10] Given the "tiny proportion of morphine that it contained," this adulteration "transformed an eminently active medication that is endowed with an incontestable efficacy, into a material without effects, whose administration could have the most deplorable effects."[11] A decade later, it was emphatically asserted that cancer care, already difficult enough, was complicated by the fact that "many pharmacists' narcotic extracts are only coal and starch."[12] Fraud and adulteration appear to have occurred at every stage of opiates' torturous journey from peasant farmers in the Middle East and Asia to retail druggists and shopkeepers.[13]

In an 1855 report questioning the feasibility of establishing a domestic poppy industry, Hector Aubergier observed that "the proportion of this alkaloid is far from being identical in opiums, reputed to be of good quality, which commerce supplies for medical usage. The variations that they present are within such wide limits so as to not fail to seriously preoccupy practitioners."[14] Calling to mind the catastrophic consequences of sudden changes in the purity of street drugs today, Aubergier observed that "often the proportion prescribed by the physician is exceeded, and frequent poisonings have been the result. . . . Furthermore, the physician orders a mixture of oils and of laudanum, and as the mixture is imperfect, the proportion of active medication varies with each rubbing."[15] Guaranteeing opiates' integrity remained a pressing problem until tools for analyzing their composition and concentrations were gradually improved and applied. It was only in 1877 that observers noted that their adulteration had become so difficult that defrauders had more or less given up on it.[16]

One immediately understands, then, why contemporaries took opiates to be as much a poison as a panacea. Popular with suicide victims because of its perceived gentleness, accidental overdoses were also quite common. The risks were particularly high with children, and middle-class reformers regularly denounced the ignorance and cupidity of working-class mothers, wet nurses, and child minders.[17] Among adults, dispensing errors occasionally had tragic effects. The lion's share of poisonings, however, were caused by users who simply took too much, mixed opium with alcohol, or inadvertently overdosed after a period of relative or absolute abstinence.[18]

The relatively indiscriminate use of the drug led one elite physician to complain in 1819 that ignorant practitioners "harm the reputation of this precious medicine, uselessly offering prodigious amounts and often in direct opposition to what is required," noting "many patients become fearful at the very mention of the word opium, fearing that they will fall asleep forever."[19] It is less clear whether such scruples were uniquely French. Opium was widely, even casually, consumed throughout the century in England by rich and poor alike.[20] Far less is known about consumption by France's lower classes, though some evidence suggests that it was considerably more modest. The issues may simply have been accessibility and cost.[21]

Alongside perennial concerns with acute intoxication, other anxieties increasingly surfaced toward mid-century. Lower-class opiate consumption began to attract attention among English public health reformers. And decades before doctors started pontificating about addiction, the drug's association with intoxication, incurability, and death ensured that, in France at least, "most lay people dread opium, which they know to be a poison and whose terrifying effects they have heard spoken of. . . . We can dissimulate opium under the name of *extrait thébaïque*, laudanum under that of *teinture thébaïque*, and the salts of morphine under those of *acétate* or *chlorhydrate thébaïque*, designations known to pharmacists whom we can warn of our intent."[22] Their untoward effects on cancer patients led to calls for careful dosing, lest families conclude that they had shortened the patient's life.[23]

Such concerns were not completely idle. In 1817, a student who'd been witness to "dubious" behavior on the part of his teachers asserted that "the physician who has recourse to [high-dose opiates] must do it with much prudence, and constantly remind himself that he is there principally to console and prolong life."[24] Keenly aware of the temptation, a mid-century treatise on medical deontology vehemently asserted that no degree of suffering gave physicians carte blanche to knowingly administer lethal doses.[25] Three decades later, incurables apparently regularly pressured physicians to put them to sleep forever.[26]

If oral opiates' undesirable effects were always taken seriously, they were generally considered minor given the illnesses they were used to treat.[27] A far more pressing concern was the refractoriness of patients' symptoms. Referring to consumptives' cough, one well-known expert observed, "If it is strong and disturbing, it will be countered with calming preparations . . . opiates, stramonium (either in pill form or in cigarettes), fumigation with an infusion of this plant or an analogous one; if these means do not succeed, we will have recourse to large emollient poultices, to mustard plasters . . . even to blisters."[28] Before the arrival of hypodermic morphine, unassuaged suffering was doctors' overriding concern. To their credit, they improvised as best they could. One popular technique consisted of applying opiate poultices directly to painful areas. They also combined them with sedatives like belladonna and created abrasions or used lancets to administer them under the skin.[29] Desperate patients also turned to a variety of alternative healers whose arcane methods (which frequently included opiates) held up the promise of relief when all else had failed.[30] Given the challenges, physicians were understandably pleased when they managed to soothe suffering incurables, however briefly.[31]

Physicians were helpless whenever suffering was intense or protracted, however.[32] Those for whom palliatives were an unaffordable "luxury" obviously had it worst of all.[33] Given that poverty-stricken cancer patients were better off in hospital, Herman Lebert's stark description of the "lucky few" speaks volumes. He noted that as they became increasingly frail and bed-bound, "these patients require an effort of their reason and their will to see to their needs, and the little strength they have serves to experience and express their suffering."[34] Mind-numbing torment figured prominently in the (terminal) illness narratives from across the class divide, however. Intimates spoke of affluent incurables whose suffering was "unutterable" or "unheard of."[35] Mme. Joséphine Brulé, for instance, apparently suffered "all that it was humanly possible to suffer" while "the pains of all the patients of Paris combined (apparently) could not equal those of Mme. Pierson."[36]

There were thus two parallel discourses about palliation and incurable illness. Abstract discussions celebrated opiates' virtues, while doctors' case notes and clinical vignettes spoke of abject misery. While not the intention, one brief passage captured both the aspirations and limits of contemporary medicine: "in how many unfortunate consumptives have we quieted their pains, calmed their despair and prolonged their lives with this precious morphine syrup, which in some cases they decide on their own to take fabulous quantities, to procure a feeling of wellness and some restorative sleep that brings them at least a temporary reprieve from their suffering and suspends their sense of imminent demise."[37] If these drugs were a godsend, doctors' poetics clearly reflected a desire to play up every victory, however incomplete or ephemeral. The careful and insistent celebration of opiates' virtues was also partly pedagogical, part of an effort to counter fears that the remedy served to make a bad situation worse.

The late-century discursive shift supports the idea that professional vulnerability encouraged earlier generations of physicians to sing opiates' praises and downplay their drawbacks and limitations. As industrial-scale production of purified morphine forever transformed the palliative landscape, fear eclipsed exaggeration. The belief that incurables couldn't be trusted led to calls for careful control, lest they fall victim to an evil nearly as pernicious as their illness. Medical discussions no longer focused on opiates' magical qualities, but on the failings of those seeking relief in the arms of Morpheus.[38]

## The Ecstasy and the Agony of Hypodermic Morphine

In 1891, hypodermic morphine was hailed as the most useful innovation of the nineteenth century.[39] Credit for its development is shared between Drs. Wood (Edinburgh), Rynd (Dublin), and particularly the London-based surgeon James Hunter, who first recognized that the drug's effects were general rather than simply local.[40] Quickly transported across the Channel, this wonder drug was readily embraced in France where it too at first "counted only enthusiasts."[41] Doctors' wonder and elation at instantly relieving suffering was poignantly described by one observer who noted how "the physician, possessing a truly marvelous means to diminish or suppress pain was unable to resist the patients' prayers begging him for relief, and sometimes gave in too readily to the pleasure of accomplishing veritable miracles."[42] A symbol of nursing sisters' devotion to the terminally ill, hypodermic morphine epitomized modern, scientifically sophisticated, care.[43]

If doctors relished its potential, misgivings quickly surfaced about morphine's physical and behavioral effects. Notwithstanding the ring of novelty, depictions of the highs and lows of chronic opiate use had long circulated.

The European reading public was well acquainted with Thomas De Quincey's 1821 classic, *Confessions of an English Opium-Eater*, and would have heard spoken of its ravages in China.[44] Tellingly, Benedict Morel included opium on his list of poisons responsible for the progressive decay of the species.[45] In defending the liberal use of oral opium, one mid-century professor insisted that it produced none of the horrifying effects seen among oriental opium smokers.[46] Late-century practitioners would thus have known that there was, strictly speaking, nothing new about humanity's penchant for opiates. Yet its arrival in hypodermic form had seemingly unleashed a terrifying new disease: "morphine mania."

Though scattered reports had appeared earlier, notably by the well-known English physician Clifford Albutt in the *Practitioner* (1870), Edward Levinstein's book *Die Morphiumsucht* (1875) ushered in a new era.[47] Citing 110 addicts whose detoxification he had overseen, Levinstein carefully described the ravages of addiction and the horrors of withdrawal. His central argument was that morphine mania was a distinct neurosis in which desire for euphoria produced a litany of physical, behavioral, and "moral" problems.[48] An overnight success, the book was translated into both French and English in 1878 and became a standard reference for a generation of European and American physicians.

If it shared certain affinities with another passion, "dipsomania" (alcoholism), the syndrome had its own decisive features.[49] Some habitués were initially intrigued by the idea of "getting high" or used it to combat psychological distress. Most sought relief from physical pain. Certain problems, like constipation and skin abscesses, developed immediately. But it was only after regular use, often unsupervised, that a full-blown morphine habit was acquired. A select few consumed stable amounts with few ill effects; the archetypal morphine maniac became caught in a downward spiral. Increasing consumption caused severe, refractory anxiety and insomnia. Ultimately, life consisted of acquiring and consuming, with predictably devastating effects. Likened by many to premature aging, one expert observed that addicts' "eyes gloss over, their faces tend to become an immobile and expressionless mask, the skin yellows and takes on an ever more sickly tint."[50] Oblivious to all other concerns, those who didn't die of an overdose "slowly wasted away and died, consumptive or cachectic."[51]

Its behavioral effects were depicted in equally stark terms. From naïve self-indulgence, the passion proved so seductive that users stopped at nothing. Most became pathological liars, demanding no less from loved ones.[52] Some turned to crime, stealing, even murdering, to satisfy their cravings. As one 1877 article put it, the morphine habit "rapidly led to the total perversion of the intellectual and affective capacities, leading to a veritable state of mania."[53] The choice of the term "perversion" was obviously not innocent.

The leading French expert, psychiatrist Benjamin Ball, summed up contemporary judgment with the statement that "most often, the patient expires in a state of advanced marasmus, in a state of complete physical and moral cachexia."[54]

Though contemporary rhetoric was almost farcically hyperbolic, commentators' concerns should not simply be dismissed. For many, the horrors of addiction were fact, not fiction. And as one thoughtful review article recently suggested, this was not simply an issue of social construction.[55] Yet in a country that saw itself on a slippery slope, the dramatic rise in morphine consumption and addiction couldn't have come at a worse time. Reeling from its humiliating defeat in the Franco-Prussian War (1870–71), France was "objectively"—demographically, economically, militarily—falling further behind its rivals. Domestic affairs were scarcely more encouraging. Workers' growing militancy terrified the bourgeoisie, who sensed the class hatred that had led to the death of thousands during the Commune (1871).

The country's unique social configuration partly explains why opiate addiction was especially culturally visible in Belle Époque France.[56] Statistical estimates of the number of Parisian addicts, the best known of which were overinflated best guesses, shined a disturbing light onto this shadowy practice. There was of course also the notorious penchant of well-known literati like Charles Beaudelaire, Jean Cocteau, and Guillaume Apollinaire, along with a host of more minor literary figures. Some, like the writer and editor Édouard Dubus, died from highly publicized overdoses. The bohemian poet Adelsward Fersen was involved in a high-profile court case involving polysubstance abuse and the homosexual seduction of young men.[57] These and other so-called decadents chased after ever more intense and refined sensations at the expense of their own health and, many reasoned, society at large.[58] Opiate addiction also figured prominently in less flamboyant fictional and poetic genres, particularly in writings by and about colonials, soldiers, and seafarers.[59]

Importantly, this crisis erupted at a time when public health reform was thought to hold the key to salvation. The importance of the parallel struggle against dipsomania cannot be overstated. It provided both a conceptual framework and vocabulary for depicting addiction and deviance.[60] It also offered a troubling example of the dangers of ignoring the problem. The language and methods of the war on drunkenness were also readily adaptable to other drugs. And though alcohol consistently remained public enemy number one, social reformers had reasons to be deeply concerned about morphine.[61]

Alcohol was and remains a fixture of French life and an integral part of most important social rituals. Furthermore, consumption of reasonable amounts was tolerated, even encouraged, opprobrium being reserved for drunkards. Hypodermic morphine, on the other hand, seemed the antithesis of alcohol, an antisocial substance par excellence. Experts consistently warned that even innocent sampling was perilous, that it was impossible to consume it in moderation.[62] Addicts were solitary figures, moving away from prying eyes to indulge themselves. About the only thing "social" about morphine abuse was its apparent contagiousness.[63] Writers and artists were notorious apologists. Women were also frequently implicated in its spread; proselytizers ranged from high-class *mondaines* to simple garment workers and prostitutes, particularly those living in port cities.[64] Accusatory fingers were also pointed at family members and careless or unscrupulous doctors and pharmacists, some of whom were themselves under its thrall.[65] One alarmist suggested that addicts' propensity to corrupt others justified their all being preemptively interned.[66]

People's embrace of a "poison" foreign to traditional patterns of socialization also raised troubling questions about human nature. It suggested that desire made a mockery of moral strictures and people's fear of needles. Beyond its violent overtones, repeated injections also destroyed the organ associated with beauty and sensuality, the skin. In extreme cases, the habit created freaks that some compared to lower life-forms.[67]

As with other sanitary reforms, physicians led the charge against morphine. They had good reason to be alarmed. It was widely known that they (and their wives) were astronomically overrepresented among addicts, even allowing for the limitations of contemporary statistics.[68] In his free-fall into decay, the bourgeois addict relinquished all claims to superiority. In one of several high-profile lectures on contemporary social scourges, Dr. Paul Regnard warned that "the abuse of morphine does not merely destroy the body, but also perverts the spirit and the conscience. The doctor, the well-bred man, learned, socially connected, lied like a naughty school-boy, and beat his wife like a drunk."[69] The respectable addict's fall into vice and immorality also spawned a macabre visual and rich literary tradition.

By late century, the wasting associated with chronic intoxication carried a double stigma: moral (addiction) and material (physical decay). Through the effective juxtaposition of visual images, authors like Regnard suggested that high-bred European addicts were indistinguishable from the emaciated coolies languishing in opium dens.[70] That the habit caused one to descend down the scale of humanity was one of the complex links between the Orient and opiates. On the one hand, travelers, novelists, and aficionados were drawn to opium smoking's exotic allure, with its elaborate rituals and ornate paraphernalia.[71] There was also European guilt at its shamefaced promotion of opium (ab)use in the Middle Kingdom. England successfully waged not one, but two Opium Wars against Chinese authorities (1839–1842 and 1856–1860) with the view to securing diplomatic equality and the unrestricted entry of Indian opium into the country.[72] France played a leading role in the second of these campaigns and profited from the habit's introduction into its Indochinese colonies.[73] These actions precipitated modest internal dissent in France, though nothing remotely comparable to England's Quaker-dominated Society for the Suppression of the Opium Trade.

Concerns with opium and the Far East were intimately linked to the issue of domestic consumption, and the reigning discourse seamlessly melded racism and hygienism. Despite being present in exceedingly small numbers, the idea that cruel, cunning Chinamen had set up a network of opium dens in East London emerged as a persistent fear in the decades after 1870. In France, on the other hand, blame was laid upon those whose activities made them go-betweens between the world of the Self and the Other: colonial administrators, soldiers, seamen, and prostitutes. In both countries, however, moralists were quick to proclaim that the nation was reaping what it had chosen to sow. Perhaps most significantly, these discussions' lurid imagery helped stoke the moral panic around opiates and degeneracy, both individual and collective. European societies struggled with the fear that, despite their racial superiority, they risked finding themselves reduced to the level of the Chinese.

Beyond its highly troubling leveling effects, morphine's physical consequences prompted various warnings like one issued in 1877: "in the evolution as much as in the symptomatology of uterine cancer, tuberculosis, or cancer of the stomach, the clinician has to consider the contribution of the cachexia inherent to the affliction and to the maramus that prolonged morphine treatment inevitably brings in its wake."[74] Beyond evoking a troubling dilemma, this passage hints at incurables' importance to the imagery of addiction. More than anyone, they illustrated the rapidity with which the drugs' beneficial effects ebbed despite ever-increasing consumption. One of Professor Michel Peter's popular medical school lectures (1880–1882), went to the heart of the issue. While allowing that traditional "knock-out doses" kept some consumptives from coughing, "he awakes narcotised the next morning, and has lost his appetite, is plunged into a nauseous state, and his sweats have increased; you have committed harm. Alternately, you give morphine at similar doses. Then tolerance is established; you double the dose, you triple it, and you do more and more harm."[75] Invoking a long-recognized "quirk"—patients' progressive physical tolerance—Peter illustrated how people's reading of it had completely changed; a "therapeutic disappointment" was now a grave form of iatrogenic harm. For this natural process was now seen as the first step on the road to ruin.[76]

In a brief and accurate passage, Dr. Jules Rochard described the physiological and emotional mechanisms underpinning the problem. For him, chronic pain and misguided sentimentality were equally responsible:

the abuse of morphine almost always has, as its point of departure, a painful illness for which the physician believed he should provide a hypodermic injection. In such cases the relief is so prompt and complete that the patient cannot find words to express his content-ment and recognition; but, at the end of a few hours, suffering comes back to the fore, the patient demands another dose of the drug that so marvelously offered him relief, and the doctor hasn't the courage to refuse. Soon, it becomes indispensable to give injections more often and increase the dose for there is no remedy in which tolerance develops as quickly. One rapidly arrives at having the patient absorb quantities that one regrets administering.[77]

Rather than peripheral to the morphine scare, the experiences of the chroni-cally and incurably ill were central and decisive. In Levinstein's landmark 1875 study, nearly two-thirds of abusers suffered from a painful chronic ill-ness.[78] In the first French publication from 1876, two out of six cases occurred in late-stage cancer patients. In each instance, the patients paid a high physical and moral price.[79] The most vivid example was that of a sixty-four-year-old woman whose "cultivated spirit" gave way "to extremely violent and disturbing scenes" whenever anyone tried to confiscate her morphine or dilute the dose.[80] No one dared resist her, and she eventually gave "herself over to an abuse without bounds" before ending her days in an "artificial physical and moral state" that precluded meaningful contact with those around her.[81] The risks and temptations were so high that experts specifically warned that "it is particularly in chronic diseases that one must appreciate how to restrain oneself, under the penalty of having to increase the dose infinitely and thereby arrive at this slow poisoning, at morphinism."[82]

Despite occasional expressions of sympathy, illness was no excuse for immorality.[83] Recreational users were unquestionably most thoroughly vilified, yet the construction of addiction and the image of the morphine maniac largely eroded such distinctions. In France at least, people didn't substantively distinguish between the desperately ill (that is, who arguably needed drugs) and people whose dependence had other roots. In the final analysis, an addict was an addict.[84]

On this score, Levinstein was categorical: all morphine maniacs, incurably ill or not, were indistinguishable. "Emancipation" also required the same strength of character: "every morphine maniac must, to avoid chronic intoxication, submit themselves to cure via abstinence, even if they suffer from a long-standing, painful, and incurable affliction; other-wise, he deprives himself of the sole remedy that, employed with judgment, is liable to durably alleviate his miserable condition."[85] He also developed a "modified protocol" for weaning the chronically ill, while he and others

wrote of incurably ill "maniacs" who were "cured" or "did better" off morphine.[86] Yet nothing illustrates the indiscriminateness of the concept more
clearly than an 1895 report prepared by Paris's dean of medicine, Paul
Brouardel, for the Justice Ministry that emphasized that "most morphine
maniacs learned about morphine and acquired the habit as a result of a
physician's prescription. Perhaps some physicians give morphine too easily to their patients. We believe, however, that outside of cases of illnesses
that are very painful and fatal over a brief period, one would encounter
few physicians who had consciously allowed their patients to become
morphine maniacs."[87] Everything about the phenomenology of narcotic
(ab)use was intensified and foreshortened in incurable illness: the hope/
desire for relief, the initial wonderment, the abruptness with which the
drugs "stopped working," the patient's insatiable appetite. It was also here
that their capacity to cause harm was most immediately manifest. Physically, opiates could worsen the decay and dehumanization that made these
illnesses so troubling in the first place. For families, the guilt of turning
a loved one into an addict would have increased their torment and loss.
Morphine mania thus added a new complexity and urgency to palliative
medicine, leaving clinicians agonizing over how to "make the best" of one
of life's worst experiences.

## Choosing the Lesser Evil in Manic Times

In calling for a thorough reevaluation of clinical practice, leading practitioners of the 1880s generally invoked the recent past. Benjamin Ball, for
example, insisted that "it is better to prevent than to cure; and, better
informed than our predecessors of the drawbacks which morphine injections carry, we must show ourselves to be more reserved in their usage than
the preceding generation whose errors must instruct us."[88] Such appeals
for swift and concerted action were unprecedented. Traditionally, doctors'
experience and conscience had been their only guide. They received no formal training in the treatment of pain and suffering, and leading textbooks'
palliative wisdom essentially consisted of "do what you can." Predictably, the
result was a lack of uniformity and consistency in opiate use in end-stage
disease.[89] Prompted by mounting concerns with addiction, several authorities put forward a practical philosophy of palliation to help others deal with
an agonizing dilemma: allow suffering or "create" a maniac?

Writings about the most painful incurable illness, cancer, demonstrate
that there were at least three possible approaches. Some exceptional individuals like the novelist J.-K. Huysmans valued mental clarity and moral
freedom. In his struggle with cancer of the tongue, he apparently "ener-
getically refused all morphine injections or other sedatives" on personal

and "ethical" grounds.[90] It appears that few people willingly emulated him, though extreme poverty would have left many with comparably little say in the matter. Herbert Snow, head surgeon at London's Middlesex Cancer Hospital, stood at the opposite end of the spectrum. Brandishing firsthand experience and physiological claims, he defended a laissez-faire approach.[91] Insisting that patients be given an unlimited supply, he contended that morphine dependence was actually beneficial. Supported by several case studies, he emphatically insisted in 1890,

> In the case of incurable cancerous patients, the induction of an opium or morphia habit appears to be the most powerful and useful weapon we possess, not only for the relief of pain, but for the prolongation of life and even for checking the development of the disease. It is understood that the maintenance of this habit is the chief (if not the sole condition) of continued existence at all. There is no question of its possible cessation . . . or he will speedily die, and die in misery; whereas these drugs (and they alone) render life endurable, and even pleasurable, under so heavy a burden.[92]

While offering diametrically opposing views of the good life, both championed individual autonomy. Patients, in other words, should master their own destiny. And though neither "doctrine" was embraced by the French medical establishment, they remain valuable reference points. Beyond illustrating the range of contemporary solutions, they demonstrate that their therapeutic preferences were not somehow inevitable.

In staking out their position in the 1890s, French experts were in some ways ahead of their time. Snow's immediate successors at the Middlesex, for example, proved far more parsimonious.[93] American physicians' attitudes also hardened dramatically in the early twentieth century, as the federal government was poised to pass the highly restrictive Harrison Narcotics Act (1914).[94] Quite early on, French opinion leaders defended a minimalist doctrine far closer in spirit to Huysmans, with three interlocking principles whose overriding objective was avoiding addiction.

The first pillar of their palliative system was "give it as late as possible and only when necessary." Regnard and others were categorical: "the physician should never begin the use of morphine without it being absolutely necessary, to never tolerate regular usage, except perhaps in painful illnesses where the patient is condemned in short order, and where one has a duty to quiet the suffering of their last days."[95] Though most practitioners were presumably not so austere, the message from the top was both consistent and insistent. Even a fervent advocate for inoperable cancer patients, Théodore Tuffier, warned that "one should not use this medication with the dogmatic intention of indefinitely continuing its use and of

increasing the dose until all pain is abolished. . . . It is for this reason that
I have the habit of beginning its use as late as possible. . . . One must limit
the prescription, to times of absolute necessity, under the penalty of seeing the analgesia become insufficient or completely annulled before the
patient's lesions have carried him off."[96] In all chronic disease, particularly
in cancer, one needed to wait until suffering had become "unbearable" and
"intolerable."

A similar mind-set inspired the second, related, axiom: never exceed
a certain daily dose. In 1894, Dr. Daniel Critzman highlighted the competing concerns that tugged at practitioners' heartstrings. He was presumably
unaware of the glaring contradiction in his admonition that "it would be
cruel to leave a cancer patient suffer. Not being able to cure them, the
physicians must offer them some relief. The morphine injections are to be
accorded ad libitum, with the unique restriction of not exceeding a certain
dose."[97] Several works illustrated what theory meant in practice. In the most
ambitious book of its kind, Dr. Joseph Récamier Jr. laid out his formula for
managing incurable uterine cancer. Noting his preference for a single bed-
time dose, he allowed that "when the patient wakes up at night and suffers
around three o'clock in the morning, I give a second injection then, but
while always leaving the day free of morphine."[98] As suffering worsened, he
remained adamant that, as long as patients slept reasonably well,

> we can distract and occupy them during the day and ask them to put
> up with dull and acceptable pain until the evening. The dose of 0.02
> centigrams sometimes maintains its effectiveness for a long time,
> but of course, we are forced little by little to give in; one must give
> a shot around noon to allow them to get through the afternoon, and
> finally one arrives at four shots per day, but never do I exceed this
> number. . . . As soon as we stray from this rule all is lost; the patient
> demands a shot one hour after having received the last one.[99]

Others used a similar recipe, administering two injections per day "except in
the last days of life."[100] Yet Récamier's errant remark suggests that patients
and physicians were often at loggerheads. Patients' insistent requests, one
suspects, simply "proved" that they had neither the requisite knowledge nor
independence to safely use these drugs. The doctor alone could juggle the
competing therapeutic priorities. Achieving a good outcome, in other words,
required professional surveillance and control.

On this, fin-de-siècle physicians were unanimous. Their final guiding
principle consisted of a simple injunction: "we avoid leaving the patient the
care to practice the injections and the means to do so. The physician alone
should carry out this procedure when it is necessary."[101] Another insisted
that "there is no danger, as long as the physician remains master of the

situation."[102] Such oversight was increasingly the cornerstone of a broad reform campaign, and a number of commentators insisted that only physicians should be allowed to even possess a Pravaz syringe.[103] Especially with cancer patients, muscular intervention was required. Récamier, for example, insisted that only an extreme measure—hospital admission—would allow "total control." When aspirin and chloral hydrate no longer sufficed, he insisted that "it is better that the patient be an in-patient, for left to himself, he will rapidly increase the dose of the alkaloid to the point of making it lose all beneficial action."[104]

This was clearly unworkable. Beyond their collective distaste for such duties, the finite supply of hospitals and physicians made it inconceivable that they would be available to assuage all suffering incurables. One either accepted that patients acquired narcotics through official or unofficial channels, or that they needed to suffer "somewhat." Both presumably occurred, though the system definitely encouraged the latter. Beyond protecting society, austerity was the only way to avoid the worst-case scenario: an incurably ill addict who wasn't going to die any time soon.

## "Acceptable" Suffering: Who's to Decide?

Albeit driven by concerns with addiction, the emergence of rigid rules towards morphine use speaks to a pitfall inherent to palliative medicine: the intangibility of suffering. Historically speaking, the "one size fits all" mentality was perfectly compatible with the broader scientific enterprise of the late nineteenth century, an era increasingly committed to standardizing therapeutic practices on the basis of universal physiological laws.[105] With palliation, the alternative seemed particularly stark: accepting the chaos of unbridled subjectivity. Yet in an era of assertive rationality, opinion leaders (un)consciously embraced a form of magical thinking: if you followed the rules, you did no harm, therapeutic or social.

Far from abolishing subjectivity, however, the locus was shifted towards the doctor, who (ideally) alone judged when pain was unbearable, intolerable, or unacceptable. Ironically, this transfer of authority probably increases arbitrariness in the setting of chronic illness: many are less obviously painful than, say, a compound fracture. Making matters worse, each physician would have had an idiosyncratic tolerance for the suffering of others. Each would have given in only when their "emotional barometer" was destabilized, when the spectacle was unbearable to watch or hear. Only shared discomfort, in other words, would have compelled them to act. The choice would have been between increasing the dose (which carried associations of therapeutic sin) or retreating into the knowledge that some suffering was inevitable (something at least sanctioned by tradition).

Ultimately, the French elite's proscriptions reflected an exaggerated asymmetry of knowledge: it was clear that morphine caused harm, but one only decided someone else was suffering enough when one suffered too. This simple observation accounts for people's readiness to give morphine to those actively dying. Concerns with iatrogenic harm not only seemed less material, but a regular injection served to lessen the horror of life's most frightening spectacles.

## Medicine and the Suffering of Others

Contemporary descriptions of incurables' experiences have a grim predictability; suffering, usually severe, was essentially a given.[106] To a degree, the problem was technical; many of the most effective palliative technologies were a century or more away. Yet it is also clear that, as long as it remained within certain nebulous bounds, suffering was "acceptable" or "inevitable." Various factors contributed to this mind-set, which has only been aggressively challenged since the 1950s. Perhaps most obviously, doctors' own proclivity for morphine would have encouraged caution. If strong-willed men of character were this susceptible, imagine the risk for ordinary people.

The need to balance competing therapeutic priorities was another important consideration. If curing, prolonging life, and relieving suffering are not necessarily incompatible, palliation often took a back seat. In the most exhaustive treatise on cancer published before the 1880s, Hermann Lebert reminded his colleagues that it was unconscionable to chase "the cure" at the expense of basic comfort measures.[107] Others worried, however, that people suffered more if they realized they were only being treated with "palliatives." In a medical school lecture that was later reprinted, Auguste Chomel recommended that doctors avoid subjecting incurables to painful treatments. In the same breath, however, he insisted that it was "better to have them suffer a bit than to abandon them to the anguish of despair."[108] As we've seen, collective unease with depression and despondency made it difficult to openly admit defeat. Such scruples were one of several culturally driven assumptions that colored perceptions of and attitudes toward the use of narcotics.

Class prejudice was arguably the clearest source of bias; the socially superior often uncritically assumed that the underclass was inured to pain and privation. In an 1855 speech before the Imperial Academy of Bordeaux, Édouard Morel observed that "the rich man is not sheltered from the buffets of adversity; and in his case the trials, the privations are that much more difficult to withstand according to his standing."[109] Those in close contact with the lumpen proletariat often remarked upon their almost inhuman stoicism.[110] A late century physician-reformer, deeply concerned by France's growing softness, found solace in the fact that those of "a coarse nature suffer less and resign themselves when they must."[111] One wonders whether this impassability was more imagined than real, a reflection of the experiential chasm that separated the haves and have-nots. At the very least, the idea that the poor had never known any differently would have helped assuage bourgeois guilt at not having done more to help.

Class assumptions were a double-edged sword, however, and physicians spoke particularly harshly of certain segments of the upper crust—"nervous" types, excessively refined and sensitive. Those who cried wolf were in many ways the principal battleground in the war on morphine mania. Ball, for instance, emphasized that "we would not refuse morphine to tabetics who are riddled with fulgurating pain, to dyspneics who request relief from their anguish, to neuralgia patients whose pain has taken an unbearable acuity. But we mercilessly refuse these injections to hysterics, to hypochondriacs, to neuropaths who perpetually demand its use without really needing it."[112] Such patients, another authority insisted, were those in whom "we can predict their rapidly progressive and soon insatiable appetite for this medicine."[113] Similar views prevailed in both Britain and the United States. George Beard, who became famous for his popularization of neurasthenia, listed a propensity for narcotic addiction among its noteworthy symptoms.[114]

Not surprisingly, gender figured prominently in these discussions. For despite evidence to the contrary, women were singled out as particularly prone to morphine mania. This was, of course, understood to reflect the weakness of will and immoderate emotionality of the fairer sex. An array of cultural representations reinforced the image of women as idle, irrational, and self-indulgent—ready to turn to the Pravaz syringe in the face of adversity.[115] Two equally unflattering archetypes, each marked by the stain of hysteria, dominated the tableau. One was the Eve-like prostitute who knowingly encouraged drug use among her patrons. The other was embodied by the excessively refined, salon-keeping dilettante in whom a shallow taste for novelty found its ultimate expression in deviant political views, deviant habits, and deviant sexuality.[116] These feminine antiheroes posed a double threat in a fast-moving world: they were the antithesis of the bourgeois ideal of family life even as they subverted an economic order where production, not leisure, was the greatest good. And given the link between the neuropathic type and tainted heredity, they threatened the very future of the nation.

It is thus no accident that the prevention of addiction among incurables, particularly incurably ill women, was accorded such importance and that a forceful and concerted show of authority was deemed the key to success. In one example, Récamier transparently asserted that the surgeon's role was to steady the patient's resolve in order that she "accept the rule as it is imposed and be satisfied with it."[117] Just as with other manifestations of a "diseased will"—depression, alcoholism, or insanity—the doctor alone could keep people from being their own worst enemy.[118] The question of character also underwrote the distinction some authors made between two types of users: "morphinists" who collaborated with efforts to cure them of their habit and "morphine maniacs" who were secretly satisfied with the status quo and thus genuinely insane.[119] Unfortunately, experience suggested that the latter were more the norm than the exception.

Finally, fin de siècle palliative practices were constructed amid growing fears that society was becoming too soft for its own good.[120] An early expression of concern can be found in an anonymous popular song about the drug ether (1847). In satirically hailing this newly rediscovered medical marvel as "the" solution to life's problems, the most evocative refrains from "L'éther ou l'art de mourir sans douleur" laconically invoked Frenchmen's growing distaste for self-sacrifice:

> Formerly we saw, legions of volunteers
> Our valiant soldiers drawn up under their colors
> Cast to the wind their martial flourishes,
> One against five, marching with their packs,
> Swords drawn, contemptuous sneers;
> Martyrs fallen in unequal battles;
> They fell, this gallant army!
> In dying this way we suffer not!!!

> All has changed . . . the furrow of glory
> Dug by them, we have deserted.
> Onto the present, steeped in disappointment,
> The dark sky lets loose its wrath.
> To forget a shameful epoch,
> Let us close the book or read it very low.
> Oh Ether, prodigious virtue!!!
> We die of shame! . . . but we suffer not![121]

Invoking the "Art of Dying" ably reinforced the lyricist's intent. Rich in irony, it wistfully evoked the austere and glorious days of the traditional *ars moriendi*.

Various late-century commentators warned that France, comfortable and hedonistic, was sitting on a precipice. Admittedly, no one wanted to see the return of war, famine, and epidemics; yet stoicism, self-sacrifice, and duty became bywords among cultural critics of all stripes. One particularly assertive spokesman insisted that the school system urgently needed to be reinvigorated with these "virile" values. For him, morphine addiction could only be stemmed if the country "react(ed) to those exaggerations of sensitivity, against the growing faint-heartedness that wear out the foundations of the family and undermine its vitality, against the weakness of character that prevents people from rising to the occasion and standing tall, made manifest in the continuous lapses that one sees in public as in private life, which end up weakening the nation itself."[122] The Franco-Prussian War and a desire for revenge profoundly influenced late-century policy debates even as contemporary trends and happenings were inevitably refracted through a prism of fear—of the future, of the working class, of France's rivals. Without simplistically suggesting that incurables were expected to suffer for the "good of the nation," such anxieties must have affected attitudes toward physical pain.[123] At the very least, worries about the "meaning" of this cultural phenomenon would have fostered a divided allegiance. Whether one invoked moral contagion or "decadence" in an era that lionized self-control, manliness, and militarism, the use of morphine was no longer a private matter between doctor and patient but an issue of collective concern.

## The Religious Politics of Suffering

It is worth carefully considering religion's effect on attitudes toward morphine and suffering, if only because it is widely assumed to have been decisive. Many historians have accused the Church of backwardness, based largely on "Catholic" concerns about surgical and (especially) obstetrical anesthesia. One historian, for example, has suggested that the Church discouraged opiate use. It also cynically portrayed pain as a "vehicle of moral progress and salvation" as part of a broad-based campaign to keep the masses in their place.[124] Somewhat subtler variations remain a stock element of most historical analyses.[125] In a rare Anglo-Saxon discussion, Roy Porter stressed how "Enlightenment sensibilities rejected Christianity's apparent acquiescence in the inevitability of pain, and modern secular outlooks have given high priority to its minimization."[126] But it is in historian Roselyne Rey's sweeping history of pain that the links between religious authority and self-immolating stoicism is most thoughtfully explored.

The basic thrust can be summed up as follows: in portraying suffering as integral to the "divine plan," religion strongly encouraged people to suffer in silence. Belief in an afterlife, which sugarcoated the worst aspects of the human condition, was the main impediment to progress. Rey and others make a final critical assumption: that the Catholic Church had an obvious interest in defending, even promoting, unquestioning acquiescence. Suffering, in other words, was central to its defense of the biological and sociopolitical status quo.[127] Question its desirability, and the credibility of the entire "natural order of things" was fatally undermined. To justify her conviction, Rey points to a theological discussion of Evil (*Le Mal*) that apparently demonstrates "a juxtaposition between political submission to the established social order and resignation to pain."[128]

Beyond its firm stand on the religious politics of suffering, Rey's work includes two important observations. First, a sophisticated tradition of biblical analysis ensured that Catholics were never slavish literalists. Equally importantly, she recognized that the French Church was a heterogeneous institution whose concern with pain operated on several levels. Properly understanding this issue, she correctly suggests, involves examining both the theological foundations and the "behavior of its priests, bishops and nuns at the patient's bedside."[129] All of these supposedly point in the same direction—the Church called for docile acceptance of pain as God-given and desirable. Suffering and care, she notes in an aside, were often exploited to encourage conversions.

The Church's well-documented authoritarian and reactionary credentials give such views a thick patina of credibility. Furthermore, Christianity's celebration of asceticism, embodied most vividly in the practice of fasting and mortification, speaks to the link between physical privation and spiritual perfection. Yet one shouldn't lean too much on this, or any other, analytic claim. Immediately after linking Enlightenment skepticism to mankind's progressive emancipation, Roy Porter backpedals. After noting that "caution was always urged upon the faithful, lest they fetishized pain," he observed how "charity also required the relief of pain. Luke had been a physician, Christ had performed healing miracles, and, finally, what was promised in Heaven was not more agony, but bliss. Hence Christian apologists developed nuanced positions regarding medicine and its potential for pain conquest. Suffering was to be embraced as a gift of Providence, as a blessing indeed. Yet it was also to be alleviated by medical aid and charitable offices."[130] Engaging this ambiguity is essential to avoid exaggerating and distorting Catholicism's role. Religious obscurantism wasn't the only source of the problem, nor can secular rationalism adequately account for the subsequent shift in mentalities.

French Catholics did more than offer up austere apologetics; they also led efforts at assisting the incurably ill and dying. Mid-century Catholic writings also show no evidence of religiously inspired scruples towards opiates. On the contrary, a clear distinction was made between suffering's abstract lessons and the moral imperative to assuage it. Any claim to understand Catholicism must first recognize the critical distinction between ideas and behaviors, theology and pastoral work.

A supposedly incompatible mix of conservatism and solicitude permeates Max Simon's work on medical deontology (1845). While respectful of secular humanism, he nonetheless insisted that Christianity offered the readiest source of moral inspiration. Elsewhere, he stressed that suffering spiritualized patients and argued that "man dies unconsoled when his final gaze does not fall upon the wooden cross that saved the world."[131] Such convictions did not keep him from passionately defending the interests of incurables. Beyond admonishing those who abandoned poverty-stricken ones, he insisted that "who is the physician who has not had occasion to admire the effectiveness of opium at accomplishing this important function [easing the pain of the dying]?"[132]

Rather than being an idiosyncratic view, this was mainstream Catholic opinion. P.J.C. Debreyne, a physician and Trappist monk, wrote several works on matters of mutual interest to religion and medicine. Rey cites his treatise on moral theology and medicine as emblematic of Catholic indifference to pain.[133] One reaches quite a different conclusion if one examines the sum of his works, however. In a popular monograph on chronic disease, he made note of his "immense use of opium" and stated that "we believe that without opium there are no therapeutic possibilities for chronic illnesses. If one were to deprive us of the power of this enchanting medicine, of this gentle and beneficent remedy which we continue to give even when we have stopped all others; tomorrow we would renounce practicing medicine."[134] A mid-century dictionary targeting priests and other Catholic authorities similarly insisted that "without a doubt, the consolations of religion are very powerful, nevertheless they do not suffice as choking spells, cruel pains demand to be relieved, and opium alone has this power. One should have recourse also because it takes away the awareness of the patient's physical ills, transporting him to a perfect world where pain is unknown."[135] Other sources also suggest that solicitude, not austerity, was foremost. Abbé Gourdel argued that good Catholics didn't threaten apostates with hell fires but gently tried "to win the heart by the services that one offers to the body."[136] Alexis Lefebvre, a leading Jesuit and founder of the high-profile Association de la Bonne Mort (1859), stressed that in the sickroom one must attend with care "to order, to silence, to the exact observance of the prescriptions and orders of the physician. Anticipate the desires, know the tastes, and via a thousand means alleviate suffering. Pray, read, as was said earlier, lead the patient gently and with circumspection to desire, to request the assistance of religion in a timely fashion. What would I say? In a word, love! Suffer with they that suffer . . . and everything will turn out well."[137] Another confessor convinced a dying cancer patient to swallow her pride and seek refuge in a public hospice, motivated by the desire to spare her unnecessary suffering.[138]

If one turns to the immediate backdrop of the morphine scare, Catholics and Catholic concerns were also not a driving force. Consistent with the laissez-faire attitude of the 1860s, they viewed opiates with equanimity. None of the hundreds of letters written by rank-and-file Catholics chronicling the experiences of terminally ill intimates voiced the least concern about opiates or addiction. Alexis Lefebvre alluded to the issue once, celebrating Prince Metcherski's remarkable vivacity. Nothing suggests that his consumption of large amounts was morally compromising; without disapproval, Lefebvre noted that "one would never believe that he took morphine and opium to calm his nerves and get a bit of rest. He himself assured me that, according to his physicians, he took enough to poison an entire regiment."[139] Physicians' value judgments about addicts' moral worth and the resulting social perils were also free of all references to "Sin." Most of those instrumental in creating and constructing morphine mania, in fact, boasted impeccable anticlerical credentials. In one telling gesture, Regnard counted *morphinisme* and religious exaltation among the leading epidemic diseases of the human mind. It was only at the turn of the twentieth century, a period of intense religious conflict and Catholic militancy, that concerns about spiritual purity were grafted onto universally shared moral concerns around drug abuse.

Without suggesting that religious convictions were immaterial to the contemporary palliative culture, there wasn't anything peculiarly Catholic about calls for stoicism or evidence of some Church-led, authoritarian end-game. Any discussion of nineteenth-century practices should keep in mind an important observation about mid-century American debates over surgical anesthesia. On the basis of for-and-against arguments and "social profiling" of discussants, historian Martin Pernick concluded, "No single social or professional ideology lay behind these criticisms, they represented the full range of differing, often conflicting nineteenth-century medical, social, and moral beliefs."[140] And though it is impossible to disprove that hard-nosed attitudes in France didn't reflect a deep-seated Catholic residuum, invoking such primal forces carries us well into the realm of conjecture. Rather than monolithic or monochromatic explanations of people's responses to a world in which suffering was rife, one is far better off invoking a rich palette of instincts and imperatives.

As will be seen, Catholics and non-Catholics disagreed primarily over the redemptive power they ascribed to illness. Rather than being cowed into submission, dying Catholics actively engaged in an earnest search for solace. The portrait that emerges of religion's effects on suffering is more complex and less sinister, as the faithful rarely celebrated suffering for its own sake. Like most contemporaries, they struggled to make a virtue of necessity, to find something worthwhile about an experience that threatened to rip apart the "ties that bind." In trying to do the right thing, people of all stripes sought refuge in an elaborate etiquette of sickness. In a society where behavioral expectations ran high, all illness performances, especially the final one, were layered with assumptions about what it meant to be a good patient who had died a good death.

# 8

---

# The Good, the Bad, and the Ugly

## Incurability and the Quest for Goodness

D<sub>r.</sub> Georges Daremberg's 1905 study of tuberculosis included an intriguing ethnography of chronic illness laced with value judgments. His interest in illness behaviors had complex roots. His father, Dr. Charles Daremberg, was a leading medical historian of the nineteenth century, an interest that his literary-minded son also shared. In addition to years of clinical practice, Georges's hard-won insights reflected his own decades-long struggle with tuberculosis, a struggle that ended tragically two years after the book's publication. Ironically, Daremberg's analysis began with the premise that "good" patients followed orders and got better. In the world of chronic illness, successful outcomes were the highest form of praise for doctor and patient alike. A select group of consumptives were cured, he insisted, because they agreed "to deprive themselves of all amusing, distracting, or serious occupations that necessitate a permanent effort, that exhaust the nervous system and render the organism vulnerable to the tubercle bacillus."[1] Equating cure with personal virtue was, of course, neither uniquely French nor specific to tuberculosis.[2] The biggest problem, of course, was that chronically ill people were generally not so lucky. Many, like Daremberg, succumbed to their illness. Yet even when victory remained elusive, the stricken were expected to behave according to tightly scripted norms. Unlike curable consumptives who were encouraged to eschew worldly pursuits, incurables were expected to assiduously sustain ties with those around them. Indeed, the entire palliative system was structured around an idealized image of the good patient who had died a good death. Broadly speaking, two variants of the good death coexisted in nineteenth-century France: the poetic death and the lucid-courageous one.

Physicians were obviously not the only ones who spoke on such matters. Religious authorities and families projected their own expectations and demands; many in France were practicing Catholics who turned to the Church for solace and support. That being said, there existed a common currency of prescribed behaviors that transcended ideological and religious rifts. These core values are interesting in that they demonstrate that dying well was rarely simply a question of dying painlessly. The manner of one's death had broader social and political implications, explaining why everyone was so keen to regulate the behavior of the incurably ill. That many incurably ill patients were themselves determined to comply confirms that they too believed this to be of great social value. In other words, if the ethos of the good death was never hegemonic, it enjoyed broad social, medical, and ecclesiastical support. Unfortunately, dying well imposed various demands and strains, explaining why, when theory gave way to practice, tensions and contradictions plagued many a sick-room.

## Illness as Morality Tale

Though no single group monopolized virtue, certain incurables were regarded more favorably than others. In a late-century article, one physician-essayist insisted that only society's most cultivated members could transcend the fetters of their decaying body. As far as he was concerned, the "unwashed" descended to the level of idiots or brutes as their condition worsened. Only the cultured could rise above bodily corrosion, thanks to various distractions including books, art, and edifying conversations.[3] Contemporaries generally embraced the cliché that one died as one had lived. Given that most Frenchmen came from humble and impoverished backgrounds, only a select few responded to terminal illness with the gentility that bourgeois commentators judged dignified and decorous.

In an interesting twist, however, worldly men were assumed to be "not as good at being good" as either young adults, presumably less bitter and jaded, or women, ever attentive to and respectful of medical advice.[4] The links between femininity and virtue, however, reflected more than docility and obedience. Women were singled out as exemplary incurables because they tended to respond constructively to suffering.[5] Rather than reacting with anger or self-pity, many made a stirring display of self-abnegation and devotion to others. Incurably ill men, in fact, were often encouraged to emulate this ideal of feminine virtue.[6] It was widely assumed that religiosity—lauded by some, scorned by others—helped sustain women's moral fortitude in moments such as these.[7] Yet if Catholic ritual and narrative helped many people deal with devastating illness, there existed two idealized visions of the "good death" that transcended prevailing ideological fault lines.

## Contemporary Models of the "Good Death"

In theory, nothing in the annals of history has been as sublime as dying on the field of honor for one's country, a sacrifice long valorized as courageous, poetic, and patriotic. Over time, soldiers' behavior has increasingly been a source of social meaning, and chivalric ideals have played a role in preserving human dignity. They have of course also helped gloss over and thereby rationalize the barbarism of war. In many ways, the American Civil War set a new moral standard with respect to the army's treatment of ordinary soldiers. Enlisted men, officers, chaplains and civilian auxiliaries struggled to secure a good death for every combatant; unfortunately, mechanized warfare and mass casualties made a mockery of this noble aspiration. In this and subsequent conflicts, large-scale destruction and the contingencies of battle ensured that frightening numbers died ignominiously. Many were even denied a proper burial. The scope of human loss and changing relations between citizen and state ultimately led to new forms of commemoration. In addition to acknowledging soldiers' ultimate sacrifice, war memorials attempted to preserve individual identity from the horror of anonymity.[8]

In Catholic and Protestant nations, civilian life also had its own archetypal "good deaths." In France, lucidity and courage were virtues displayed by self-aware incurables who stoically shouldered the burdens of illness. The second type of good death, the poetic death, was most closely associated with the young, idealistic consumptive. In the only nineteenth-century ethnography of death and dying, in 1842, Hubert Lauvergne approvingly invoked the beguiling serenity of these etherealized heroes and heroines, one of their many touching qualities.[9] Even Lauvergne, hardened by years spent as a physician to one of the country's most notorious prisons, was deeply moved by a dying woman's efforts to keep up appearances and family responsibilities. Such unworldly selflessness and insouciance, he insisted, explained why the void left behind by a select few was so overwhelming.[10]

Both fact and fiction suggest that few experiences were as traumatic for both doctors and families as watching a young person succumb to phthisis. The story of the youthful consumptive possessed all the elements of great literature; despite being the tragic victims of fate, they steadfastly affirmed the power of love and of devotion, to duty and to others. Such personages were all the more captivating because they retained a certain childlike quality. In an unusually tender moment, Daremberg noted, "How much less unhappy are the consumptives who die at the beginning of life? They go off towards the other world without cumbersome baggage, without profound regrets, and their end is so sweet, if a bit of affection gives them the sense that they are pitied."[11] Yet if the innocent consistently won highest praise, all good incurables were expected to find illness instructive and uplifting, the culmination and crowning achievement of their lives.

Beyond its obvious pathos, this illness experience was particularly compelling in that it matched the therapeutic priorities of contemporary palliative medicine. In fact, just as physicians struggled to imitate nature's curative ways, Nature's handling of tuberculosis provided a model for managing incurable illness. The poetic variant of the good death was particularly appealing because it was relatively undemanding; the suffering was "reasonable" and the road to death fairly serene. And despite occasional complaints about insouciant consumptives' indifference toward the last rites, even devout Catholics liked to believe that dying this peacefully was a mark of distinction.[12] As they struggled with their own grief, witnesses to relatively tranquil scenes would have found solace in the calmness of a quiet passing. The other form of "good death," to say nothing of the bad ones, was a far more exacting experience.

## The Form and Function of the Other Good Death

Nineteenth-century society left behind illness narratives that collectively map out the contours of the other archetypal "good death." These narratives demonstrate that it was no easy task to suffer and die well, even for highly motivated incurables. Remaining lucid was essential if one hoped to live up to this ideal. It was one of a troika of qualities—along with courage and will—that distinguished those who graciously accepted the news of their impending demise. Everyone fêted these individuals; the baroness of Pibrac's confessor, for instance, glowingly observed how "living for a long time under the shadow of a cruel illness, she had no illusions about the gravity of her condition and on the sacrifice that would soon be asked of her."[13] Physicians were equally quick to praise the firm and courageous few who rose above "the vain terrors of the imagination, who have not forgotten that life is a gift that one must render, and who can contemplate the idea of their own dissolution without trembling; the man of art has less to carry out with them; he can speak of the danger; it behooves him actually to hide nothing; . . . either by courage or perhaps vanity [the spirit] rises above the tomb and contemplates it without dread."[14] Given the mind's importance in both the Judeo-Christian and Enlightenment traditions, it is not surprising that lucidity was so central to the dying process. In addition to being a prerequisite for a virtuosic death performance, lucidity was also a mark of cultural sophistication. It allowed people of standing to know what was expected of them during life's dark moments.

Yet self-awareness was a double-edged sword in that it exposed the dying person to an array of physical and existential torments. Marie Faucher's family found her passing particularly distressing precisely because she had been "caught in the embrace of a most cruel illness, which leaves people in full possession of their faculties to the very last moment." If it was approvingly noted that Marie tried to raise the spirits of those around her, being this lucid was clearly a mixed blessing.[15] The lengths to which everyone went to deceive incurables about the gravity of their illness illustrates the important divide between what people admired and what they preferred. It also demonstrated that, in real life, scripted endings were often set aside in the name of comfort and convenience. Lucid-courageous death was problematic, mostly because the line between equanimity and exasperation was razor-thin; as one observer noted, "long illnesses tire everybody; one no longer has the courage to lie to the unfortunate soul who is equally irritated by the truth and by lies."[16] In a perilous realm where medicine's inadequacies magnified human frailties, "good" patients were those who sought refuge outside of themselves.

## Religion and the Pursuit of Goodness

For Catholics, a good death had long been equated with the last rites, a series of rituals that provided a clean slate for heading into the great beyond.[17] This remained true in the nineteenth century, as the faithful continued to believe that salvation could be won or lost at the last moment. The importance of these sacraments is evident in the deathbed narratives of members of a confraternity founded in 1859 by a socially connected Jesuit, Alexis Lefebvre. Though organizations devoted to helping people die have a venerable history, this was an odd choice for a man of his energy and abilities. The popularity of such confraternities had begun to wane at the end of the eighteenth century; by Lefebvre's time, many existed in name only. Their decline reflected both changing patterns of sociability and the emergence of new attitudes toward death. The dying process was increasingly individualized as people set aside the rituals that had prevailed when France remained guild-bound and rigidly hierarchical. At the same time, grief and mourning were becoming emotionally charged and intensely private experiences.[18]

Given such long-term trends, it is noteworthy that, on February 4, 1859, the Vatican sanctioned the creation of the "Association of the Good Death" in a Jesuit stronghold in Paris. Taking its name from an eighteenth-century Italian organization, the association had a traditional mandate: *"to teach people to die well* and to obtain for oneself and for the other associates a good and saintly death."[19] Yet in consciously referring to his method as the "science" of dying well, Lefebvre was clearly attuned to contemporary attitudes and trends: the traditional art of dying (*ars moriendi*) had been supplanted by science in an era of aggressive rationality.

Two fascinating literary projects were the centerpiece of his efforts. One was a manual on the "science of dying." Closely resembling a school primer, it included prayers, spiritual exercises, and suitable subjects of reflection to help prepare for life's culminating moment.[20] The other was a collection of letters describing associates' struggles with illness and their deathbed experiences. Lefebvre was deeply committed to this project, likely because it demonstrated the critical importance of religion in people's daily lives. Worldly consideration presumably also played a role. Lefebvre had strong ties to the aristocracy who supplied a disproportionate number of heroes. Predictably, the life stories of poor associates invariably trumpeted the importance of individual virtue. In no case did the suffering associated with poverty and deprivation serve as a vehicle for criticizing the prevailing socioeconomic order.

Rare exceptions aside, entry into the Association of the Good Death was always voluntary. Typically, existing members nominated suitable candidates. Final acceptance required the consent of the nominee, who was then sent a diploma and a votive card bearing an image of the death of St. Joseph. Associates were invited to pray for each other daily, while those in the final stages of illness and the recently deceased were singled out at the Association's regular meetings. As part of membership, intimates were encouraged to provide a prompt account of an associate's journey through illness, agony, and death.

While many followed Lefebvre's advice and joined while they were still healthy, others waited until the last moment. Their medical and spiritual circumstances varied; most latecomers succumbed within a month. A few died suddenly or unexpectedly. More often, the patient or the entourage had seen no need to prepare for death. One example was Mme. Duplessis, a young consumptive who "for some time was stricken with a disease of the chest, that had no hope of being cured, but she cultivated the greatest illusions about her state; it is only since fifteen days that she was part of our Association. On the Sunday eight days before, she confessed and took Communion; she received Extreme-Unction a quarter of an hour before she died, fully conscious of everything around her."[21] In extreme cases, people joined only a day or two before succumbing.[22] Especially for those who had turned their back on the Church, membership provided an opportunity for personal and spiritual renewal.[23] Very often, families used it to broach the sensitive subject of incurability and death, as joining a confraternity didn't have the frightening finality of proposing the last rites.

This collection of narratives clearly demonstrate that dying well meant more than a set of rituals. They also indicate that there was no universal blueprint for success. Strikingly, rare "arch stoics" went out of their way to suffer. Blind for the last fifteen years of her life, Lucille de la Libarde was eventually carried off by a "horrible cancer." Not content with the spiritual benefits of suffering so severe that "not a single fiber in her body remained without pain," she demanded to be placed on a wooden floor to better imitate Christ's passion.[24] Auguste Reneau de Saint George eventually refused all palliative remedies, stating that "if the saints in heaven regretted something, it was to be unable to come back to earth to suffer some more, and so I said to myself: since God allows me to suffer, suffer I shall."[25] Another associate, whose obscure existence apparently "consisted of nothing but suffering" cried out a few weeks before she died, "Thank you God, this is nothing, you suffered far more, and you never sinned. More, more! I want to go to heaven!"[26]

The best-known exemplar of self-abnegation was of course Sainte Thérèse of Lisieux, a Carmelite nun who died at age twenty-four in 1897 after a long struggle with tuberculosis. Her autobiography, which chronicled her slow and agonizing decline, was published soon after her death. In the *Story of a Soul*, suffering and renunciation were celebrated as powerful means to a spiritual end. Enormously popular in France, the book was quickly translated into nine languages. Thérèse's steadfastness, stoicism, and humility inspired Catholics around the world. In short order, she became a popular cult figure and copatron saint of France.[27]

If such stories inspired, they generally found few imitators. Even among members of the association, such behavior was highly unusual. To a person, arch-stoics had experienced severe adversity, including protracted and exquisitely painful illnesses. Presumably overcome by suffering, illness had come to define them, a bit like victims of severe, recurrent, physical abuse who insist that they get what they deserve. Yet at the same time, misery provided the opportunity for a display of personal and spiritual virtuosity. When pain was all that one had left, suffering beyond the call of duty became a psychologically rewarding command performance.

Generally speaking, most Catholics viewed pain the way the religiously indifferent did, as something to be stoically accepted when it couldn't be assuaged. Those who refused were disparagingly described as "pusillanimous" or "fainthearted" by the medical profession. One author vigorously dismissed these antiheroes as "sensitive, irritable, fickle, without moral force, for whom all sufferings seem atrocious."[28] Their failings stood in stark contrast to those paragons of virtue who stifled their distress in an effort to spare others.

These were elite souls who, like the Comte Henri de Béarn, "was so courageous, he so feared causing pain to his young wife and his parents, that he succeeded in hiding his suffering, and only reluctantly consulted his physicians, always without [his family] being aware."[29] In a widely admired form of self-mastery, Georges Blanc "scrupulously and adeptly hid his tears the moment his beloved sister came into his room."[30] Alexis Lefebvre's sister

Sophie also distinguished herself; he noted how "afflicted with the cruelest of illnesses, not only did she never complain, but went so far as to hide her ailment, to spare her sister Josephine, who had been deceived as to her condition. One could almost have believed that she didn't suffer at all."[31]

Quietly soldiering on was thus the preferred modus operandi of terminally ill Catholics. In struggling to find peace and meaning, many embraced an informal arithmetic wherein miseries and rewards balanced each other out. Those with a checkered past found much-needed reassurance in the closing months of life. Joséphine-Elisa Collard "thanked God for having made her suffer so much, and for having prolonged her life, for the expiation of her sins."[32] Mme. de Villeduc's long struggle with heart disease was, in her words, "a great grace of God's bounty that gave me the money to pay my old debts."[33] Others, presumably less troubled by guilt, were convinced that their travails had secured them a place among the elect, like a woman who matter-of-factly told her grieving family that she would pray for them "when I'm in heaven."[34]

If always partly self-serving, suffering was also offered up for others. Often, the goal was conversion. During a decade-long struggle with illness, Marie Marillier "long offered [her pain] for the conversion of someone dear to her."[35] Clémence Marmillot similarly stated, "Ah! if my death could obtain [my godmother's and brother's conversion], I would willingly sacrifice my young life."[36] One young woman's suffering was apparently so bountiful that she offered it up for the benefit of the souls in purgatory, sinners, the Church, and the priesthood.[37] Not surprisingly, such behavior was typically gender-specific. Nineteenth-century women, after all, were encouraged to define themselves by what they did for others. It is also possible that male associates had enough to do worrying about the fate of their own souls. More than any specific detail about their lives, the most remarkable thing about these dying women was that they firmly believed that, even on their deathbeds, they could still be a powerful force for good.

Without supplanting spiritual achievements, people also singled out the personal accomplishments of the incurably ill. A dying countess's confessor, for instance, praised her foresight in arranging a suitable marriage for her daughter before she died.[38] Mme. Normand's husband proudly stressed how, despite severe suffering, she "continued to see to her good works" until her final hours.[39] In Sophie Desmazures's case, the achievements were as modest as her origins. Her young life cut short by an exquisitely painful chronic disease, she was praised for having remained "exquisitely calm and perfectly resigned. She was never heard to complain; kind and charitable toward everyone, she died saying goodbye to her family."[40]

In giving a new impetus to an old tradition, the Association of the Good Death responded in a compelling way to the needs of dying Catholics and their families. Its value and importance were evidenced by its membership, which counted 115,000 several years after it was founded.[41] The movement's success reflected the balance it struck between austerity and hope. Its core message was dreary and timeless: life was best spent preparing for death. Yet consistent with changing sensitivities, death was presented in a personal and optimistic fashion. This was the essence of Lefebvre's genius, captured in the hundreds of narratives he so carefully conserved in the *Annales*. Taken as a whole, they indicate that a good death was an individual experience whose significance was magnified through collective action. They also demonstrate that the sum of one's identity—moral, metaphysical, social, and professional—was deeply and seamlessly annealed. On this and many other important issues, the inspired and the indifferent were in complete agreement.

## Consensus amid Conflict: Illness, Death, and the Edification of Those Left Behind

In medical biographies, professionalism was accorded a quasi-religious importance. Terminal illness comes across as an annoying inconvenience. An account of the life of Louis-Jules Béhier, a "great physician of the nineteenth century," began with the observation that "afflicted with one of those terrible illnesses that pitilessly pursues its course; he fought without cease against it, resting only when his strength completely betrayed his courage." Before listing his many professional accomplishments, his biographer noted that "he felt himself deeply touched by his ailment, but he had the sacred spark, and his greatest pleasure was to give his clinical lesson. I will die one day on a stretcher at the hospital he said one day . . . he wished that his final hour be devoted to his students, and that his final words be those of the teacher. His desire came to pass."[42] Stoicism and devotion to duty also figured prominently in medical eulogies. Baron de Monestrol, for example, was praised for the fact that "until his final moments, this fine man saw to our charitable organization. . . . His patience and resignation were unrivalled despite horrible inner and outward suffering, for his body was one large open sore."[43] Such virtues weren't monopolized by the medical elite; stricken with a chronic illness "that forgives no one," one obscure practitioner valiantly struggled to see patients until the day before he died.[44] Yet medical mandarins placed a high premium on selflessness, compassion, and courage; it was assumed that they would follow their declining health with a cool, stoic, detachment.[45] Almost as much as their scientific achievements and charitable acts, quietly accepting the inevitable embodied personal worth. This trope, one might add, wasn't simply a formulaic routine. Elsewhere, physicians were quick to point out that they were often among the worst (that is, cynical and inconsolable) patients; eulogizers also had few scruples about pointing out when a colleague fell short of this ideal.[46]

Forced to settle upon one word that captured the virtues they esteemed and encouraged, physicians would likely have chosen *stoicism*. In a mid-century article targeting a lay audience, one physician spoke for the profession when he asserted "that which we must recommend to all suffering patients is patience and courage. Discouragement, irritation, transport, anger worsen pain even as it denotes a weak and irritable individual. . . . It is grand to see man impose silence on his pain, express a sense of calm and benevolence, even as he is a victim of cruel torments; and one should not believe that such mastery of oneself is simply an idealized quality that exists only in theory."[47] As an incurable's predicament grew increasingly hopeless, doctors resorted to talking cures in an effort to encourage the desired behavior. When invoking happier times proved insufficient, even students saw it as imperative to "take a more severe tone, be it sad like the thoughts of him that one must cure; you must paint the picture of more cruel ills than his . . . raise up his courage, remind him of his duties as a spouse, a citizen, a father."[48] Despite considerable social and political upheaval, this message remained strikingly constant; a leading late-century practitioner insisted that, when all hope was lost, the only thing left to do was to encourage stoicism, which "submits the slavishness of nature to the dominion of the moral freedom that man carries with him . . . for want of consolation, there is abnegation and self-sacrifice."[49]

Championing these virtues was not disinterested, for stoic patients were a lot easier to tend. In a lecture to students, psychiatrist Benjamin Ball excoriated patients who complained too much, contrasting "the indifference and the security with which a man whose lungs are ravaged sees the end coming" whereas, in a neighboring bed, "a simple hemorrhoidal patient stuns us with his tiresome lamentations. . . . There is such a contrast between the stoicism of some and the pusillanimity of others."[50] Calling to mind doctors' thinly veiled animosity toward hysterics, Hermann Pidoux maintained that consumptives with hypochondriac tendencies were "the most miserable patients I know." It required prodigious skill and devotion, he intimated, to put up with chronically ill patients who never stopped complaining.[51]

Rather than focusing on patient inadequacies, doctors preferred to stress the therapeutic value of a stiff upper lip. In the words of one practitioner, those "who distinguish themselves by the superiority of their reason, by the equanimity and goodness of their character" suffered less and lived longer.[52] Citing the nefarious effects of weakness and cowardice, a medical student similarly asserted that "an iron will is a heroic arm that one can use to advantage against the most tenacious physical ills, the most rebellious maladies."[53] While chauvinism and anticlericalism presumably led him to omit women and Catholics, his list of good patients was otherwise representative; stoic philosophers and soldiers were singled out for their willfulness, courage, and vitality.[54]

As the century wore on, partisans and critics increasingly debated whether devout Catholics made better patients. In the 1840s, a Christian apologist lamented the fact that few incurables died peacefully under Louis Philippe's reign, a time of growing cynicism and religious indifference. Men of distinction were too proud and set in their ways, while the urban proletariat died as they lived, like animals.[55] Only inhabitants of the countryside and surrounding small towns, untouched by modernity, continued to die well.[56] Religious observance held the key, Lauvergne insisted, for "nothing is as typical as the agony full of hope and love of him that conserved a faith in God all his life."[57] Always a point of pride among Catholics, calmness on one's deathbed was a badge of honor for both the individual and the community of believers.[58] Occasionally, it was read as a sign of divine intervention or served as a pretext for criticizing medicine's prognostic inadequacies.[59]

Religious faith was known to be a ready source of sangfroid, and nonsectarian physicians welcomed the foothold it provided in their dealings with the dying.[60] Yet things were never that simple, as even religionists occasionally admitted that fear of eternal damnation could turn the act of dying into a terrifying spectacle.[61] But it was increasingly the Church's most vocal opponents who insisted that freethinkers were far more stoic and resolute than any Catholic. Insisting that religion had only lamentable effects, one anticlerical physician asserted that

> the passage is only truly easy, and is accomplished with dignity only in the case of men who have been able to free themselves, by hard work and education, from the hereditarily acquired general belief in life after death. A philosopher worthy of this name . . . like the sages of antiquity, cast a final and sad look on life . . . and placidly, with regrets sometimes, but always without fear, go off to eternal peace. Terror— for which there is often no remedy—is the lot of them that, fed by religious or metaphysical superstitions, are always full of anguish with respect to that chimerical soul that they believe must outlive him.[62]

Particularly after mid-century, when death increasingly became a source of fierce cultural confrontation, the stakes were high. Catholics claimed victory whenever a high-profile materialist converted on his deathbed, whether out of fear, weakness, or a genuine change of heart.[63] The final disposition of one's earthly remains was another contested issue. Priests' de facto control over churchyards and cemeteries was more and more contested until their official secularization by the state in the early 1880s. Until mid-century, clergymen routinely refused to bury stillborn children, non-Catholics, drunks, suicide victims, and anticlericals on consecrated land, even though this generally meant separating them from the rest of their families.[64]

The founding of the Association of the Good Death was unquestionably tied up with the politics of death and dying. In an era of rising godlessness, membership was a way for believers to help turn the tide. By publishing hundreds of narratives in rapid succession, the assembled *Annales* went from being individual tragedies to a collective celebration of Catholic courage and achievement. In some ways, this work resembled an updated version of *The Lives of Saints*, in which modern-day martyrs defended their faith despite severe suffering and the encroaching antireligious ethos of their world.

The appearance of a Jesuit-run association was also clearly part of a broader strategy to defend the Church's interests. The late 1850s were difficult years that culminated in France's abandonment of the pope during the Italian War of Unification. Suffering and death, unlike many other life events, still largely remained a religious domain. Whatever else they might say or do, many people almost instinctively turned to Catholicism in their hour of greatest need. Eager to strengthen their position in a lonely bastion of authority and tradition, Church authorities decided to change with the times while staying on message.

Aware of religion's ongoing vitality in this realm, militant anticlericals increasingly responded in kind. Blanquist radicals, for example, organized large funeral corteges and presided over explicitly iconoclastic burial ceremonies.[65] In a slightly later period, the atheist leaders of the Parisian Anthropological Society founded the Society of Mutual Autopsy as part of a direct assault on Catholic "superstition." Each agreed to have his brain dissected postmortem to better understand the links between physical form and function. In a direct affront to Catholic concerns with the handling of human remains, the uninteresting parts of the body were to be unceremoniously discarded. Likening these practices to secular last rites, historian Jennifer Hecht has pointed out that "in leaving their bodies to the society, members were repudiating the power of religion to invest purpose in their death. At the same time, they were attempting to invest their death with some meaning."[66]

Rivaling the importance accorded burial practices, people from across the ideological spectrum agreed that a great final illness performance involved discretely accepting the inevitable. From bishop to freethinker, it was understood that incurable illness was a trial in which people demonstrated what they were made of. Various forms of conviction—whether driven by class, professional identity, or ideology—were a ready substitute for traditional strictures about resigning oneself to God's will. Incurables were consistently pressed with the charge that a fitting degree of resignation and courage was the least they could do.

Lionizing stoicism was certainly compatible with a conservative worldview. Yet it was mostly about snatching victory from the jaws of defeat, of preserving a measure of dignity and decorum. For ideologues of all stripes, dying well was ultimately a gift one gave to others. Like the doomed soldier who remained at his post in a lost cause, stoic incurables brought honor upon their profession, their Church, their family, and themselves. Whether one identified with a social or professional ideal, a political cause, or a particular faith, suffering and dying honorably validated both the "man" and the belief system.

If suffering was potentially redemptive, the link between incurability, stoicism, and social norms mostly exemplified the social value that contemporaries accorded to edifying others. Noting its architectural origins, the *Oxford English Dictionary* defines "to edify" as "to build, to construct; to build up (the church, the soul) in faith and holiness; to benefit spiritually, to strengthen, to support; to inform, instruct; to improve in a moral sense."[67] Albeit laden with religious connotations, suffering, like any other performance, could also be personally and socially edifying. Incurables' attitudes and behaviors were truly praiseworthy when they embodied and transmitted core values. The aesthetics of suffering and its pedagogical potential were inextricably linked, a source of personal memories and objective lessons. For Catholics and non-Catholics alike, good patients and good deaths were those deemed worthy of emulation.

Two examples of virtue amid hardship illustrate exactly what it meant to edify others. Eugène Harlé D'Ophove was twenty-nine years old and recently married when he died from tuberculosis. His greatest achievement was that he "forgot his pain in order to look after those around him" and regularly thanked God "for having used the trials of such a long and painful illness to bring him closer and closer" to spiritual perfection.[68] Some years before, a Protestant from a fiercely republican family made a different, if equally fitting, display of virtue. Like most of the medical elite, Laurent-Théodore Biett had his share of weaknesses, rivals, and enemies. During the long, mysterious illness that carried him off in 1840, however, he went beyond the call of duty. As another Protestant member of the Academy of Medicine noted toward the end of his commemorative oration, "The long suffering to which he succumbed, the efforts he made to reach the degree of moral perfection to which man can aspire, were not unavailing. Each day he acquired a greater degree of resignation, of gentleness, and constancy. . . . Truly, this fine life was crowned by a suitably honorable end."[69] Ultimately, it is less important whether such performances were as pristine as they appeared; the sociobehavioral ideals others read into them mattered most. In both religious and secular literature, life was a social, professional, and personal journey, a journey in which the struggle with incurable illness represented the defining moment. Whether one believed in the hereafter or rejected it, how one behaved in the final weeks and months was a critically important part of one's legacy.

## Conclusion: Palliative Medicine as
## Social Control or Social Compact?

Late-century reactions to hypodermic morphine aptly demonstrate how a life-enhancing breakthrough could run aground on deeply held ideals. In the setting of incurable illness, patients and physicians struggled to reconcile two competing tenets: relieve suffering while doing no harm. The problem was that it was often impossible simultaneously to prolong life, minimize suffering, and promote goodness. Sometimes things went well: patients remained blissfully unaware of their fate while requiring little or no morphine. Yet life was rarely so simple. As one authority noted, death among consumptives "does not always present itself with the character of gradual and unselfconscious extinction that poetry has recreated so often." Duty-bound to assuage suffering, doctors were prohibited from using palliatives that might "deaden an intelligence that one must leave master of its destiny to the very end."[70] Although lucidity was as much a curse as a blessing, nothing could justify interfering with a person's mental and moral personhood.

This largely explains why morphine addiction among the dying was so distressing. Like insanity, addiction mocked prevailing norms and conventions. One is hard pressed to imagine a more undignified and unedifying death than that of an incurably ill morphine maniac. Living only for their fix, they lost all semblance of the self-control so cherished in respectable circles. Even starry-eyed consumptives sometimes exhibited behavior bordering on madness. In both variants of the good death, then, patients risked undermining the social fabric they were called upon to strengthen.

One is tempted to characterize such pressures as a form of social control. There is little doubt that the taboos around terminal illness reflected as much a desire to sustain an atmosphere of decorum as a disinterested concern with dying patients' well-being. Physicians' affinity for good patients, as with nearly everything else involving incurables, was closely tied up with their own emotional needs. Tellingly, Daremberg reserved his most lavish praise for patients that were at once affectionate and suitably respectful: "the good tubercular is a man of love. He will praise the doctor. . . . The good tuberculosis patient loves the good doctor for his goodness, but also for his authority."[71]

While acknowledging the constraints to which the chronically ill were subjected, one should not underestimate the destructive potential of bad incurables and bad deaths. If the unrepentant criminal being led to the guillotine publicly embodied death at its worst, the private world of chronic progressive illness also had its villains. Daremberg noted that bad consumptives "love no one; they adore, admire, and care only for themselves. . . . Here are nefarious beings, who absolutely refuse to spit into disinfecting recipients or pocket spittoons. . . . They are nasty, they seek to be disagreeable to all those who care for them with the greatest devotion. . . . Such patients can witness without remorse, without regret, all their entourage perish in turn from hardship or from contagion. They are alive, and that's what counts."[72] Given his glorification of those who successfully recovered from the disease, it is ironic that Daremberg should censure someone for trying to stay alive. His description, however, speaks more to the social dynamics of incurability than to the patient's clinical trajectory. Self-absorbed incurables attacked everyone's Achilles' heel: caregivers' sympathy and doctors' professional vulnerability. Like hardened criminals, the worst patients were antisocial in every sense of the word.

In an insightful observation, the surgeon and essayist Marc-Antoine Petit suggested that incurable illness created a unique social compact in which all parties had mutual obligations. The stakes of compliance were highest for patients; upholding their end of the bargain potentially affected how others treated them. While warning incurables that "all human sentiment is fickle, even in its pity," Petit offered the following admonition:

> Oh you that hear me! if ever malign nature condemns you to incurable pain, learn to stifle your complaints and your cries; think of sparing those around you; do not offer them the constant spectacle of a torture victim; that a smile and some gaiety cross your lips from time to time; prove that you are being given fruitful care; say that you feel well, pretend so if you do not; this consoling avowal will flatter those that serve you, sustain their courage; and the hand of humanity feels gentler and lighter, when the heart can sometimes smile at the happy success of its care.[73]

Edifying others was never simply a matter of pride or personal conviction. It was a social necessity. The incitement to be "good" came with a tacit threat: this is already bad enough for everyone, so don't make it worse.

The boundaries between reasonable expectations and social control were murky, particularly as life reached its close. Yet one shouldn't lose sight of the genuinely noble and compassionate instincts that inspired many caregivers. Then, as now, palliative medicine was also about personal, spiritual, and social dignity. Though many demands were made of incurables, some of them at least enjoyed the luxury of being indulged. Aware that helplessness was among these illnesses' most troubling features, Dr. Jaumes offered up the following sober yet heartfelt prescription:

show yourselves, as much as this can be allowed, to be docile to your patient's tastes, to his caprices even, sustain hope in his heart, raise his spirits, fend off feelings of grief with the help of distractions able to occupy, without tiring, him. . . . After this come words of commiseration, displays of interest that give strength to the doctor's palliative efforts, joining to such shows of friendship, moral and religious consolations, which allow us to counter the despairs of death with a resignation to suffering and hopes for another life. Through the use of these various means, man ceases to exist in the least unfavorable conditions possible, if not content, at least in a state of submission to the supreme force that has made his death part of the natural order of things.[74]

Jaumes didn't sugarcoat things. This was a collective struggle to make the best of a very bad situation, one in which the needs and desires of patients, families, and caregivers regularly brushed up against each other in socially threatening ways.

# 9

---

# The Fate of the Incurably Ill between the Two Revolutions, 1789–1848

Soon after the unanimous passage of landmark pension legislation in 1905, one of the law's framers observed, "It is grounded on the idea that assistance to the elderly, the infirm, and to incurables is not merely a good turn offered up by the collective, but a legal obligation."[1] Coming twelve years after a better-known statute guaranteeing free medical care for the indigent, the legislation of July 1905 confirmed the importance of health concerns within the emerging welfare state. Although a comparable social compact was one of the utopian dreams of 1789, authorities did little in practice to assuage the elderly, infirm, and incurable before the late nineteenth century. The misery that went unaddressed was, of course, appalling.

This state of affairs was not an unforeseen consequence of otherwise well-intentioned efforts but the predictable by-product of a charitable system that limited access to care. Hospice cases remained at the bottom of society's list of priorities, victims of a series of economic, ideological, and professional considerations. Generally speaking, decision makers had little trouble justifying their actions, although more than one struggled with a guilty conscience. Yet despite occasional pangs of remorse, little action was taken during the first half of the century. Partly because they weren't "true patients," incurables were generally left to fend for themselves. It wasn't until the 1870s that the state began taking concrete steps to deal with what was increasingly viewed as an urgent sociomedical problem.

The evolution of charitable discourse and practices reveals much about broader changes in society, partly because French health policy was subject to an unusually high degree of state control. The writings of statesmen, functionaries, and philanthropists thus plainly illustrate why certain problems were more of a priority than others. Their lines of argument also expose the competing concerns that framed responses to the problems of old age, disability, and incurability. Public policies toward incurables, particularly in Paris, were an important element of a larger debate about society's obligations toward its neediest citizens. The incurably ill also raised troubling questions regarding the hospital's role as both a therapeutic space and an instrument of social policy.

Of course, these policy decisions had a considerable impact upon people's lives. Incurables' troubling experiences vividly demonstrate the complex and often dramatic effects that prognostic considerations had on patterns of social behavior, laying bare a dilemma that has long troubled physicians and society at large: the need to balance the twin imperatives of caring and curing. Incurables' experiences also shed a light on important, yet neglected, aspects of the day-to-day hospital routine during this period, particularly with respect to the allocation of scarce institutional resources. Most importantly, however, the intractability of their plight underscores the painfully slow pace at which policies, practices, and experiences coevolved. Together, they are a poignant reminder of both the effects and the limits of sociopolitical change on a complex form of social interaction and a critically important life event.

## The Emergence of "La Machine à Guérir"

Beyond partially destroying Paris's Hôtel-Dieu, the fire of December 1772 stimulated interest in the plight of the sick and destitute.[2] A series of exposés and fact-finding missions reached the same conclusion: the institutions of the ancien régime had done little to assuage the sick. This was partly because of their unwieldy mandate. The massive general hospital system—created by Louis XIV and inhabited by upwards of 15,000 people—illustrated the system's cruel failings.[3] Beyond providing rudimentary care to foundlings, the aged, and the infirm, it was a depot for undesirables; the insane, the chronically ill, and certain criminals were sequestered there. Not surprisingly, conditions inside were austere and medical services almost nonexistent.[4] For all its inadequacies, however, the care proffered was, for many, better than nothing. Generally speaking, these institutions were a valued resource for the indigent, who turned to them as part of a broader survival strategy.[5]

Conditions inside the country's flagship hospital, Paris's Hôtel-Dieu, were definitely most disturbing of all. In addition to housing the acutely ill and injured, it had long been the almshouse of last resort. Widespread poverty ensured that it was always bursting at the seams. In an oft-cited observation, Diderot depicted it as "the biggest, roomiest, richest and most terrifying of all our hospitals. . . . Imagine every kind of patient, sometimes packed three, four, five or six into a bed, the living alongside the dead and dying, the air polluted by this mass of sick bodies, passing the pestilential germs of their affections from one to the other, and the spectacle of suffering on every hand."[6] That sick people avoided the place was a grim cliché, as those admitted with comparably benign ailments often succumbed to infections contracted inside. It was also impossible to provide good care in such a confused and chaotic environment. In an extensive review of Parisian hospitals from 1788, Jacques Tenon observed that one had little hope of recovery in a setting where beds contained four to six patients with a single tag. Medical therapy was, at best, haphazard.[7] If mortality rates were lower and conditions often less grim in hospitals that served smaller cities and towns, most people agreed that drastic measures needed to be taken across the country.[8] The events of 1789 offered a golden opportunity to start from scratch.

The French Revolution ushered in decades of creative upheaval with decisive and lasting repercussions. One of its many audacious ideals was that society was duty-bound to assist those struck down by illness and old age, for whom assistance was a right, not a privilege.[9] In 1790, the chairman of the Poverty Committee of the Constituent Assembly captured the ambitious optimism of the early revolutionary period when he asserted that "public welfare owes the ailing poor assistance that is prompt, free, assured, and complete."[10] Inspired by egalitarian convictions, reformers set about transforming the system of medical and hospital care they had inherited from the ancien régime.

Above all, they hoped to establish a charitable system in which local dispensaries supplied medication while dutiful family members provided nursing care. And while a well-ordered society had no need for hospitals, the committee agreed that the worthy poor without family support could and should be admitted. To ensure easy access, towns with at least four thousand inhabitants would have a small hospice or hospital (with a maximum of 150 beds). Larger towns would have proportionally larger institutions, though for hygienic reasons none would exceed 500 beds.[11] Finally, cities would build small community hospitals and a few institutions specializing in surgical cases, venereal, and contagious diseases. At the nexus of this newly rationalized system would be a form of medical triage that would "sift from the masses of apparently ailing indigents those persons who were really sick and deserved to be admitted for treatment."[12] A few years later, in March 1793, the Committee on Public Assistance presented its own national assistance blueprint. While repeating most of the Poverty Committee's conclusions, its members insisted that the chronically ill also merited hospital admission, as they generally couldn't be adequately cared for at home.[13]

The last Revolutionary-era committee that addressed these issues was the Committee on Health, which had broken away from the Poverty Committee in September 1790. Dominated by physicians from the Legislative

Assembly, the reforms they championed were primarily drawn from a proposal tabled by a leading medical luminary, Dr. Vicq D'Azyr. Less ambitious than its predecessor, committee members argued that access to a trained physician was the key to improving care, a goal attainable via a rational distribution of physicians throughout the country. Members also stressed the need to reform medical education. Beyond combining medicine and surgery in a single curriculum, medical training would henceforth be clinical rather than theoretical; students would spend most of their time getting hands-on experience in large urban hospitals. Finally, the committee highlighted the importance of medical science—anatomical, physiological, and pathological—while championing the need for more research.[14]

Unfortunately, events quickly derailed reformers' ambitions. The decision to confiscate and sell off Church property proved disastrous, as it cut off hospitals' main source of income. The strains and dislocations of the Terror and civil war caused further destabilization even as hospitals faced a massive influx of injured soldiers. Hyperinflation and currency collapse gutted all remaining hopes for the radical overhaul of society. As one authority on this period has aptly concluded, the revolutionary governments "assumed the administrative trappings of a modern state, a habit of national legislation and a steady bureaucratic rhythm which were impossible to conjure up in the political turmoil of the Revolutionary decade."[15] Rather than ushering in a golden era of health and well-being, the years after 1789 were marked by desperate improvisation and growing misery. Napoleon, of course, eventually stabilized the situation. Unlike the Poverty Committee, however, he was primarily concerned with waging war and consolidating power. A mixture of pragmatism and opportunism prompted him to rescind certain divisive measures, like the forced de-Christianization of hospitals and the suspension of nursing orders. More than any other development, the reappearance of nuns, priests, and religious ceremonies symbolized the revolutionaries' failure to sweep away the past.

Though radicals were disappointed, medical care and education were transformed in several important respects. Hospitals were still financed and operated locally but were partially nationalized and placed under the jurisdiction of the Minister of the Interior. Rather than reverting back to private corporations, the largest and most important institutions became public property, accountable to outside authorities. Beyond keeping an eye out for irregularities, the national government would henceforth be free to focus on the big picture: seeing that the entire system ran smoothly.

Convinced that reason and efficiency should guide their efforts, each institution was given a clear mandate. Shorn of their other charitable functions, hospitals would now solely provide medical and surgical services. Large urban institutions would focus upon medical teaching and research. As has been convincingly demonstrated, the medicalization of the hospital was the single greatest French innovation of this period.[16] Yet placing physicians in charge was merely the first step in their transformation. Every gesture and event, from admission procedures to hospital charting to documentation of autopsy findings, reflected a desire to systematize and regularize the process. With an eye to improving efficiency, research capabilities, and patient care, the sick were to be grouped together according to their diagnosis or some other noteworthy attribute. This era thus witnessed the creation of specific venereal and dermatological hospitals, while children, the blind, and the deaf were now housed in their own institutions.

Amid broad consensus, academics have disagreed over the nature and magnitude of contemporary accomplishments. Michel Foucault and other critics of modernity have provocatively claimed that the medicalization of hospitals and asylums was an integral part of a broader program of social control. Foucault was among the first to suggest that the hospital revolution allowed physicians unfettered access to patients' bodies, which they probed in new and disturbing ways. The privileged knowledge they acquired fostered a new set of power relations. Rather than an unproblematic form of progress, the emergence of the "medical gaze" led to a sinister objectification of patient experience. Over time, the medicalization of contemporary life allowed society's masters to gain greater control over more aspects of human experience.[17] Beyond serving their immediate personal and professional interests, science was also used to justify disciplining those it singled out as deviant or abnormal.[18]

The historian Dora Weiner has usefully challenged such views. Rightly insisting that the pursuit of medical knowledge is not necessarily hostile to patients' interests, she has outlined the improvements made to French hospitals between 1789 and 1815. The most tangible was the application of a "one patient per bed" rule.[19] Taken together, early nineteenth-century reforms enhanced hospitals' therapeutic potential, if only because they emerged as less inherently unhealthy places. Her most original claim, however, is that political reform and a concern with social welfare led to the emergence of "citizen-patients." Invoking a commonality of interests between elite reformers and the poor, she maintains that hospital reform was part of a broader egalitarian push to democratize health. Equally important, she suggests that one cannot judge reformers' achievements on the basis of immediate post-Revolutionary experiences. She draws parallels between the Poverty Committee's pronouncements and the U.S. Bill of Rights; even though they weren't all put into practice, these generous ideals were a perennial source of inspiration.

Though this argument is compelling if one takes a long view of history, it probably overestimates reformers' achievements and underestimates their failings.[20] For example, it is not clear that "rationalized" reasonably describes a system that included a hodgepodge of public and private institutions—hospitals, hospices, institutions for the blind and deaf, soup kitchens, dispensaries, welfare bureaus, and English-style poorhouses (*les dépôts de mendicité*). Incurables' experiences also encourage a less sanguine view of the new hospital ethos. Excluding them was certainly not new. The process was enhanced and systematized, however. For these and other undesirables, the early nineteenth-century hospital was a fascinating mix of tradition and innovation. For the first time, hospitals were the center of the medical universe, places where the best and brightest attended to the acutely ill and injured. Yet even in this bastion of medical enlightenment and hope, the poor and indigent were consistently given two stark messages: first, hospitals are for "true patients" only; second, you will shape up or you will be shipped out. Tenon's image of *machines à guérir* elegantly captured both the ideals and the ideology driving form and function.

Admittedly, no nineteenth-century society had the financial or technical wherewithal to meet all the needs of its population. That being said, there's much truth to historian Jacques Leonard's suggestion that the ambitious plans of Revolutionary visionaries were stillborn mirages that subsequent events confined to the dustbin of history.[21] Even reformers' one irrefutable achievement, the hospital's medicalization, was uneven and incomplete. This was particularly true in the provinces where nursing sisters continued to play an active role in the provision of medical services. Perhaps most importantly, the experiences of the chronically and incurably ill demonstrate medicalization's social control function, albeit with a twist. For incurables, the problem was that they weren't sufficiently medicalized. Society confined them to a netherworld of neglect and ostracism. Sometimes, then, it is the "selective medicalization" of human experience that exposes this process's most heart-rending implications.[22]

## At the Crossroads between Ideas and Interests: Understanding the "Charitable Apparatus"

The post-Revolutionary elite couldn't completely ignore the country's social problems. Amid differences of opinion, there existed an agreed-upon set of ground rules. Reflecting a combination of Malthusian, mercantilist, and ostensibly philanthropic ideals, the dominant "charitable ideology" stressed the importance of self-control and self-help.[23] At a time when hard-nosed realism and self-serving idealism were inseparable, the elderly, infirm, and incurably ill occupied a separate conceptual and administrative category: "hospice cases." On one level, this distinction tacitly acknowledged incurable illnesses' devastating effects. Mostly, it amplified incurables' structural disadvantage in the competition for care.

Prevailing social conditions left few indifferent, and a remarkable group of physician-hygienists (including Jean Baptiste Parent-Duchâtlet, Louis François Benoiston de Châteauneuf, and Louis Villermé) painstakingly explored the links between economic misery, chronic ill health, and premature death, factors now known as the social determinants of health. Struck by the rapid transformation of French society, they focused their attention upon the sociomedical effects of urbanization and industrialization. In seeking to move beyond conjecture, they turned to available census and mortality data. Their choice of methodology was no accident. In the early decades of the nineteenth century, investigators from various disciplines began avidly exploring the explanatory potential of "large numbers." Before going on to become conventional wisdom, the results of the hygienists' initial inquiries surprised many. Rather than the expected links to urban topography (elevation, proximity to the Seine, and so forth), disease and death among Parisians were overwhelmingly associated with poverty.[24]

Subsequent studies, notably Villermé's famous two-volume survey of the conditions of textile workers (1840), took these findings a critical step further.[25] In an analytical tour de force, he used vital statistics and detailed observations from the country's leading production centers. Never one to sugarcoat reality, the picture that he painted was somber. Outside of a few noteworthy exceptions, such as the Lyonnais silk weavers, hardship left a large and growing segment of the working class physically and morally stunted. It also reliably carried them off to an early grave. Confronted with this reality, Villermé struggled with a fundamental tension. The factory system, he insisted, was not the root problem per se. While harsh, the working conditions alone didn't explain this sad state of affairs. The main problem was that both worker and master acted in ways inimical to workers' interests. Yet human failings couldn't conceal an even more troubling fact that liberal economic theory generally passed over in silence. Despite working fourteen to sixteen hours a day, workers simply did not earn enough to secure their health and welfare.[26]

Unlike the hygienists, much of the French elite single-mindedly emphasized the role of immoral behavior in the plight of the poor and indigent. A leading Catholic philanthropist, for example, began his 1820 analysis of the causes of poverty by asserting that "indigence is the fault of the indigent—the poor soul suffers, in effect, but it is his own fault. This is the most typical case. . . . Three forces which can act alone, or work together to bring this factitious indigence . . . : this is the lack of foresight, laziness, and debauchery."[27] One of the country's leading liberal economists was equally categorical; in 1842, Théodore Fix asserted that "today the well-being of the working classes in France is the rule and destitution the exception. This destitution has two causes: the usual and most frequent cause is the debauchery and sloth of the workers. Dissolute living is an individual vice that in no way can be imputed to our social organization."[28]

Inspired by Malthus's somber pronouncements, most commentators insisted that the greatest vice was to have more children than one could afford.[29] The resulting high mortality was simply the natural order of things.[30] Yet unlike arch-Malthusians who dismissed charity because it enabled paupers to reproduce, most contemporaries saw it as a force for good.[31] One needed to be vigilant, however, as indigents were quick to abuse the credulity of their betters. It was equally important not to feel too sorry or do too much for the poor, as most simply reaped what they had sowed.

Yet even as they recoiled at the physical misery and moral turpitude that prevailed in working-class households, philanthropists insisted that these same homes could spawn moral and social regeneration. Conveniently ignoring hygienists' arguments about the environmental determinants of health, discussions of poor relief generally sang the praises of home-based care. Successive generations of reformers, in fact, looked forward to the day when the poor would imitate their affluent neighbors. The pervasiveness of this argument hinged on two key points: the belief that one was better off in the care of family and the realization that such a system cost the state a lot less. The mayor of the Tenth Arrondissement succinctly captured one strand of this ideal when he insisted in 1803 that, at home, "everything is done better and to better purpose than in institutions where the sick, the aged and [the] infirm are heaped up, left to unknown and often greedy hands. The aid distributed to families strengthens domestic affections. Hospitals destroy them."[32]

There was supposedly much to gain from keeping these groups at home. Their contribution to the welfare of the household would set a good example for their children and grandchildren. Equally important, caring for them was assumed to create social and transgenerational cohesion. Nowhere was this more pronounced than with the elderly. Forcing children to fulfill their duty protected both family and society. Representing mainstream opinion, Baron De Gerando asked in 1840, "Is not the presence of this old person of the greatest benefit to this family, the duties one owes him, the benediction he brings down on those around him? . . . Ah! let us reestablish and strengthen everywhere those sacred ties, these gentle ties which are the foundation of society, rather than favoring their slackening."[33] This was not a trifling matter, as hospice cases were a central humanitarian challenge throughout the nineteenth century. Many Frenchmen were old, infirm, or incurable; of these, most couldn't fend for themselves.

Few liked the thought of an elderly person living in squalor, although such tragedies were generally attributed to moral failings. Unlike late-century commentators who recognized that low wages, fragile health, and an unpredictable supply of waged labor made it impossible for workers to save for their dotage, their predecessors preferred to invoke imprudence and selfish children. Any solution also risked being worse than the problem. Just as taking in foundlings was associated with illicit sexual activity and parental irresponsibility in the public imagination, state-sponsored elder care was thought to give an equally pernicious message of reckless economic dependence. There was no room for sentimentality in urgent matters of state, one reason why providing a living wage to hospice cases was rejected until the early twentieth century.

Instead, inertia prevailed whereby a fixed sum of money was divided among the socially marginal and medically indigent. Given the burden of poverty, the amounts involved were pitifully inadequate. During the first half of the century, a sizeable proportion of Parisians at any given moment was essentially destitute. Even more lived in squalor. Whenever the price of bread rose above a critical threshold, the majority of workers went hungry. Some starved.[34] Municipal bread lines generally gave small portions to those deemed worthy, just enough rations to keep working families from succumbing. In a country of 35 million souls, between 700,000 and 900,000 people were assisted by the various bureaux de bienfaisance in the years between 1833 and 1850. Administrators had few qualms, however, about rejecting those they judged morally dubious—prostitutes, alcoholics, anticlericals, even the religiously indifferent.[35] In times of crisis, soaring demand strained available resources past the breaking point. Yet even in good years, the aged, the infirm, and incurables competed for crumbs. The intertwining of incurables' administrative identity with that of the elderly affected them in another significant way. It made it nearly impossible to advance a political plan that focused on their specific needs without elder care monopolizing the discussion.

That the amount allocated for charitable relief should be independent of grassroots demand was an inviolable principle of good government until late century. The alternative, a tax-supported system of public charity, was anathema to the ruling elite. A ruthless rearticulation of the status quo greeted an 1836 request from Paris's mayors asking for more money from the national government to redress the city's ills. Despite widespread misery, Louis Philippe's administration was adamant that "relief must help almost everyone and by no means satisfy all needs. If the total amount of available relief was increased, the numbers of those clamoring for it would soon increase. Worse, such action would impede the moral effect of the Charity and bring to France that scourge signaled by Monsieur the Secretary, the Poor Tax."[36] Herein lay a fear that found its way into nearly all discussions of the "social question": the threat of an English-style system of compulsory charitable relief in which rate payers were forced to support paupers from their parish. For the French, the poorhouse embodied the faceless and cruel system that existed across the Channel, a land of bleak disparities and class polarization. Strikingly, groups from across the political spectrum—from Catholic conservatives to socialists—demonized the "English way." Disagreeing among themselves on how to assuage poverty, they agreed that instituting a Poor Law was the wrong thing to do.[37] And although many were primarily concerned with tax avoidance, attacks generally centered on its other baleful effects. By encouraging idleness, anonymous public charity supposedly encouraged the poor to remain poor.

Philanthropists invariably extolled the virtues of private, voluntary charity. Beyond providing an edifying boost in the struggle to save one's soul, getting personally involved reminded the "better sorts" of their obligations toward the less fortunate. Face-to-face giving also permitted patrons to "rehabilitate" the lower classes through useful advice on how to organize and run a household; financial support was thus tethered to moral tutelage.

In the minds of the well-to-do, working-class misery was an opportunity for interclass harmony. Beyond being personally satisfying and spiritually uplifting, private charity was believed to dilute class hatred and attenuate socioeconomic barriers.[38] In 1837, an anonymous French administrator captured elites' view of the difference between the French and English approach, insisting that "while the religious spirit loves the poor person, the administrative spirit merely puts up with him."[39]

One is immediately struck by the distance separating rhetoric and reality. Contemporary French capitalism's main lesson to the poor was that they needed to put in a long day's work if they hoped to survive.[40] The first half of the nineteenth century was a time of monstrous, self-perpetuating inequalities. Primarily because of rapid population growth, Paris became an increasingly violent, despair-ridden, and threatening city.[41] Widespread economic hardship fostered the atomization and grasping that philanthropists so greatly feared. Social tensions were acute, and the moneyed classes generally looked down on their inferiors with a modicum of pity and profound sense of disgust.[42] Yet despite knowing that desperate people were dangerous people, the elite were convinced that it was imperative to limit the availability and attractiveness of charitable assistance.

Moral sanctimony and financial self-interest ensured that hospitals and hospices remained scarce and unappealing. Even those sympathetic to their inferiors clung to the view that hospitals should be places of last resort, not an inducement to laxity. In an early issue of the *Revue d'hygiene*, long the world's leading public health periodical, Villermé insisted that

> hospital establishments should never be numerous or large enough to admit all those who might be tempted to present themselves.

Multiplying them too much is extremely harmful, always more so than not multiplying them enough; for the number of poor increases according to the amount of relief given. . . . Besides, no nation could bear the enormous burden of providing for all those who wish to be fed courtesy of the public purse. The masses [*le peuple*] must never grow accustomed to being received in a hospital or hospice anytime he desires, for his own interest and for that of society as a whole.[43]

This passage points to a fascinating feature of Villermé's life and work. Like the other hygienists, his "social diagnoses" were perceived as radical. The solutions they put forward were anything but. Harshly critical of the utopian socialists, they maintained that only the science of political economy should guide public policy.[44] Issued from the social strata that had benefited most from economic liberalism, they defended its tenets throughout their careers. Foremost among these was the idea that unbridled freedom was the key to prosperity, and the resulting misery was in the natural order of things. Fortunately, enlightened paternalism and gradual reform would progressively blunt its sharpest edges. Outside of banning child labor and certain forms of collective action (notably workers' syndicates), they and other liberals believed that government had no role in regulating relations between worker and master.[45] Charitable relief, both public and private, had to be kept to a strict minimum, lest it interfere with economist Adam Smith's "invisible hand."

Unchecked, welfare institutions supposedly discouraged foresight, encouraged idleness, and corrupted the natural bonds of the family.[46] As one indignant observer noted in 1821, "The greatest inconvenience resulting from the existence of hospitals is disgust for work." In a society organized around capitalist production, laziness posed the single greatest threat to the social order.[47] Rather than a barometer of progress, the existence of a large number of hospitals and hospices was viewed as a symbol of societal decay.[48] The allure of outdoor relief was also thought to be inseparable from the limited appeal of available institutions. Hospices were also criticized for inadequately discriminating between the worthy poor, who by definition loathed charity, and their undeserving neighbors. Self-respecting merchants and craftsmen were often singled out as the main victims of this system. In the 1830s, a prominent citizens' group expressed outrage that aged or infirm paupers could turn to publicly funded institutions while respectable people of modest means, willing to contribute toward their upkeep, had nowhere to go.[49]

Hospice cases were particularly problematic. Beyond being morally pernicious, hospices were indefensible economically. Unlike acute care for the sick and injured, which represented an investment in the country's human capital, they were a pure waste of money. Worse, hospices were thought to support France's least deserving citizens; in 1837, Louis Philippe's interior minister, De Gasparin, charged that hospices were fundamentally "a powerful inducement to laziness and loose living." Rejecting petitions on behalf of the elderly, infirm, and incurable, De Gasparin countered that some of the money currently allocated to hospices should be redirected. Hospices must not, he insisted, "be allowed to grow at the expense of hospitals, as long as the needs of the latter are not completely met."[50] Thirty-five years later, in 1862, the chief administrator of the Parisian Assistance Publique exposed the strong bias that continued to color the vitriolic discussions on the matter:

> without agreeing with those who wish that the Administration work toward making hospice-stays as antipathetic as possible, it is clear that we should not . . . go beyond the bare minimum. As much as it should show indulgence to those it hopes to return to an active and productive existence, so it must be wary, by opening the hospice too liberally, and in developing excessive material well-being, to encourage improvidence and disorderliness in those inclined to see it as a certain refuge in old age.[51]

Even those who concerned themselves with social order and public safety had more pressing concerns. For much of the century, two other scourges, insanity and the foundling crisis, garnered far more attention. The magnitude and social effects of these problems partly account for this; there were approximately 100,000 abandoned babies in 1817.[52] Yet decision makers invariably emphasized other material concerns. In an 1818 report on the kingdom's prisons, hospices, and hospitals, Louis XVIII's interior minister Lainé singled out the acutely ill, foundlings, and the insane as being of greatest interest to the nation. Bringing together two utilitarian arguments, he defended asylum care in the following terms: "humanity and public safety commands that we adopt measures that would immediately allow us to provide asylum to all those who can trouble society, and to ensure that all those deprived of reason receive the care that can restore it or soften the effects of its privation."[53] Two decades later (1838), the July Monarchy went a step further, passing legislation forcing departments to build and operate public asylums.

It was a quarter century before similar legislative solutions began to be proposed for those with devastating somatic illnesses. Despite a growing consensus that something needed to be done, the state did little until 1905. More hopeless and less immediately threatening than the insane, incurables appealed only to an abstract sense of charitable duty. In a tellingly brief section on hospices from 1818, the interior minister presciently grasped the dilemma that faced successive French governments:

if the administration opened establishments in which beggars, supplied with everything necessary to life, can grow old free of care, the equilibrium is soon disturbed. Those reduced to poverty by the natural course of things, continue to plumb its depths; but as the existence of those that came before has been prolonged, the number of poor souls increases, and the establishments created for them become insufficient. . . . Thus, beggars would multiply without cease, and their numbers would invariably exceed the capacity of the vastest establishments.[54]

Experience confirmed that supplying the elderly, infirm, and incurable with life's basic necessities allowed them to drain the public purse longer and deeper. At mid-century, the elderly survived, on average, for four and a half years once they gained admittance to an institution. Even octogenarians survived close to three years.[55] No surprise that, when it came to hospitals, society's overseers sought to leave as little to chance as possible.

### Ordering Chaos: The Central Admissions Bureau and the Modern Hospital System

Unbeknownst to many, a low profile medico-administrative innovation was one of the cornerstones of the hospital revolution. In 1802, soon after the creation of the Parisian Hospital Council of the Seine, a central admissions bureau was set up at the Hôtel-Dieu with an eye to regularizing the admissions process. Urgent cases could still be admitted directly; everyone else was expected to make the trip "downtown." One of the bureau's four physicians would then decide who to admit and where. One upbeat assessment stressed how bureau physicians "practiced a stern medical triage: malingerers now found themselves blacklisted; applicants judged admissible were referred to hospitals and hospices, or—and this is noteworthy—an array of new alternative facilities such as out-patient clinics, infirmaries, dispensaries, and nursing homes, whose success depended on the citizen-patient's collaboration."[56] Yet incurables' experiences highlight the dark side of the "stern triage" that Weiner equates with progress. Besides turning away the able-bodied poor, bureau physicians were given another important task: ensuring that those who wouldn't benefit from hospital care were also kept away.

Barring incurables from Parisian hospitals was not, strictly speaking, a nineteenth-century innovation. When Paris's Hospital for Incurables was founded in 1634, it was seen as an important event mainly because it offered refuge to those excluded from the Hôtel-Dieu.[57] Similarly, many inhabitants of the hospices of the general hospital system were elderly, insane, or incurably ill, that is, people that didn't belong in a real hospital. Finally, members of a leading ancien régime nursing order, the sisters of Saint-Joseph, were prohibited from caring for those with contagious, shameful, or incurable illnesses.[58] In many ways then, article 18 of the admission bureau's policy statement stipulating that "once an ailment has been judged incurable, patients can no longer stay in an institution that . . . is only open to indigents afflicted with illnesses that are susceptible to being cured" simply perpetuated a long-standing tradition: distinguishing between "patients" who required hospital admission and "hospice cases" who mostly needed room and board.[59]

Yet the admissions bureau did more than integrate old habits into a new administrative system. Successive governments made it the lever in the struggle to perfect the science of hospital management. Over the first decades of the nineteenth century, efforts at improving hospital care intertwined with the bureau's evolution in three significant ways. First, decision makers made it the command center for the movement of people and diseases in and out of the hospital; second, a meaningful and lasting effort was made to increase its stature and effectiveness. Finally, it was provided with increasingly explicit guidelines to ensure that both the healthy and the hopeless were identified and excluded.

Among the Restoration's first health policy gestures was to broaden the bureau's mandate and reinforce its ranks. On February 11, 1818, the government tripled the number of bureau physicians from four to twelve. Article 5 added several new duties to their job description. It declared that henceforth "at the beginning of each quarter in each of the hospitals, a visit will be carried out by three of the physicians of the Admissions Bureau, among those not actively on duty." The object of these regular visits, the circular went on to note, was to "verify the status of admitted patients, to send those who are cured or in a recognized state of incurability home, as they must not remain in hospital."[60]

In an equally important gesture twelve years later, the newly constituted July Monarchy government announced that bureau physicians were to be named via a competitive system of *concours* even as it became the mandatory first step in the most coveted medical career—attending physician at a Parisian hospital. With this series of measures, the state demonstrated the importance of this institution, now the headwater of elite medicine. Rarely, physicians' and surgeons' academic careers ended there.[61] Most physicians, however, worked at the bureau for four years before earning a hospital appointment. The tenure of the average surgeon was generally slightly longer.[62] Having the best and brightest triage nonurgent cases was a win-win situation; it allowed the government to claim that no effort had been spared to ensure that only those who "truly belonged" partook of this precious resource.

As a result of these measures, the career trajectory of the medical elite changed dramatically. For them, passage through the bureau would have had several important effects. It became a critical step in their acculturation, schooling them in the system's inner workings. They were entrusted to enforce its logic while serving as the eyes and ears of the administration. Bureau work would also have been challenging professionally, rapidly honing appointees' clinical judgment. Among the first skills they would have quickly mastered was to know when an illness had passed the point of no return.

Though their primary activity was to ferret out and blacklist malingers, bureau doctors necessarily also had to determine the (in)curability of legitimate medical cases. Available evidence suggests that this was a central concern in all Parisian institutions, public and private.[63] Such policies also weren't unique to Paris; incurability was grounds for exclusion from public and voluntary hospitals in much of the Western world.[64] Yet because of the centralized, bureaucratic nature of the French system, its implications are more readily discernible. Local administrators, for instance, were forbidden to use home-care funds earmarked for patients to assuage the suffering of the chronically and incurably ill.[65] Even institutions mandated to provide nonurgent, remedial care were organized around the curable/incurable distinction. The convalescent hospital founded at Vincennes in 1855 was originally built to receive victims of work accidents. Its mandate, along with that of the Vésinets hospital for convalescent females founded a few years later in 1858, was quickly enlarged to include those recovering from illness. These measures were part of a concerted effort to take some of the strain off the hospital system. Strikingly, incurability was among the sole criteria that (theoretically) precluded transfer.

Beyond questions of political economy, doctors had other reasons to prefer looking after those with a reasonable chance of getting better. For one, there was the issue of medical education. In an early report, bureau physicians noted that La Charité Hospital's teaching mandate naturally meant that the cases nobody wanted be sent elsewhere; they stressed how "care is taken to divert eruptive illnesses, smallpox especially, almost all the chronic and interminable maladies, both internal and external, and in general all the ills whose curability is not demonstrated."[66]

By their very nature, hospitals magnify the emotional, professional, and aesthetic challenges of caring; perhaps not surprisingly, physicians repeatedly complained about the deleterious effect on staff morale of having too many incurables. A letter written in year VII (1799–1800) by the attending staff at the Hôtel-Dieu outlined what was at stake. It was written in protest against authorities' plans to replace the existing system of two-month rotations with a system of permanent ward assignment. They argued that some duties, like the lunatic and smallpox wards, quickly wore doctors down. As to the most dreaded assignment, the "chronic ward," which primarily housed dying consumptives from various Parisian hospitals, assigning a physician in perpetuity was nothing short of unconscionable. It was imperative that the planned reorganization not "condemn the physician to the torture of seeing eighty, one hundred desperate cases of consumption every day; . . . if he can sustain six months of such an existence, it would be in our right to think and to say that nature refused him all nature of moral and even physical sensitivity."[67] This issue was a perennial concern throughout the century; whenever doctors discussed the institutional care of the incurably ill and dying, the problem of staff morale came up immediately.[68]

Doctors weren't the only ones troubled by hospice inhabitants; those looking in from the outside left suggestive accounts of the horrors they'd witnessed. In one of several letters to a young heiress who shared his interest in philanthropy (1847), an earnest young reformer insisted that, for the "dregs" of the medical world, public charity "offers special shelters where they can end their days less painfully in the throes of an affliction that only death can relieve. These shelters, which are generally called *hospices for incurables*, have taken the place of the ancient *leprosaria*."[69] Known for his descriptive flair, the novelist and essayist Maxim Du Camp struggled to describe a small but particularly horrible section of the Bicêtre Hospice, home to *les grands malades*. Upon entering the dormitories in which the "paralytics, cancer patients and old dotards were left to wallow," he emphasized how "one is surprised that death should have stopped at the doorstep. The spectacle of useless, unconscious, and immobile existences, disgusting and filled with suffering, which continue despite age and accumulated infirmities, shocks the heart."[70] Such instincts and impulses had important practical repercussions. As one authority noted in 1851, people with displeasing infirmities were at a distinct disadvantage in the competition for a hospice bed compared to the *beau vieillard*; similarly, the existence of a "repulsive affliction" (*maladie rebutante*) or severe infirmity disqualified people from entering a coveted Parisian old-age home, Sainte-Périne.[71] Strikingly, the subsequent development of such a condition was grounds for immediate eviction.[72]

Not surprisingly, the chronically ill and incurable were also subject to expulsion from hospital when other matters became more pressing. In year XII (1803–1804), the partial closure of Saint-Louis hospital created a huge and growing demand for in-patient treatment of skin diseases. The first of six remedies proposed by the admissions bureau was to invite "the Administration to make all incurable individuals leave."[73] Their report concluded by calling for them to be perpetually barred.[74] That no further mention was made of the chronic ward at the Hôtel-Dieu after its early-century reorganization strongly suggests that it was eliminated as part of an effort to "clean up" this institution. Yet the very fact that the bureau physicians expressed the desire to more efficiently exclude incurables confirms what any cynic intuitively suspects: rules were there to be broken.

## Rules, Regulations, and Reality: Incurables and French Hospitals

It would be misleading to suggest that every incurable was systematically and relentlessly excluded from French hospitals. Physicians in Lyon were perhaps unusually lenient because of a shortage of hospice beds. Just the same, one cannot dismiss an 1830 report that observed that "in spite of the rules governing their exclusion, incurables almost always make up 3/5 of the total number of the poor souls received . . . it is not rare that only a tenth of female fever patients have acute illnesses. The Hôtel-Dieu is the providential home for all indigents with incurable maladies, provided they last any length of time."[75] Interestingly, the same physicians who recommended purging Saint-Louis of incurables acknowledged that "the admissions bureau is far from believing that it can justifiably refuse an admission request in cases where a patient's curability is doubtful. Seeing patients only once, and obliged to commit themselves on the spot, it runs a risk of errors in judgment, in a situation where an error constitutes an injustice."[76] Nowhere were the effects of second-guessing more dramatic than with phthisis, which was notoriously difficult to distinguish from comparably curable chronic pneumonias. Consumptives sometimes improved in hospital, occasionally even returned home. "Reputedly incurable" illness thus didn't preclude admission; certain statistics suggest that Parisian hospital physicians were fairly indulgent toward cases tagged with this distinction.

In 1847 and 1848, 48.5 percent (7,553 of 15,587) of those who succumbed to an organic lesion—a category that included all the fearsome chronic diseases—died in a hospital or hospice, not at home. While economic crisis and political upheaval may have encouraged a greater dependence on hospital services during these years, this was not an atypical pattern. Similar data for 1831–1838 demonstrate that 41 percent (9,341 of 22,774) of people whose cause of death was pulmonary phthisis died in an institution, increasing to 49 percent (20,891 of 42,614) between 1839 and 1848.[77] Beyond gravely undermining Philip Ariès clichéd claim that the institutionalization of death and dying is a late twentieth-century phenomenon, these figures suggest that French physicians had a far softer touch than the harsh hospital admission policies would suggest.[78] Indeed, thousands of surviving case reports prove that late-stage consumptives were treated in teaching hospitals until they died.

Interestingly, French doctors regularly insisted that their hospitals' high mortality rates were a tribute to their humanity. If overcrowding was partly to blame, another source of the discrepancy between French public hospitals and English voluntary ones was that consumptives were ruthlessly excluded from the latter.[79] Mirroring claims that private charity was more humane than poor relief, they insisted that French hospitals were actually "better" (that is, more compassionate), appearances to the contrary notwithstanding. Without casting aspersions upon their sense of humanity, there were several other reasons why many French incurables died on public property. Hospices were expected to harbor them and institutions like Bicêtre and La Salpêtrière set aside a small number of beds for cancer patients; some incurables would have also died suddenly or unexpectedly in hospital before they could be sent home. The scientific agenda of the anatomico-pathological school also encouraged researchers to keep them around. Hospitals were the only place where the natural history of complex illnesses could be studied all the way to the dissecting room. When sympathy was lacking, scientific curiosity and ambition offered an incentive to keep the hopelessly ill confined.

Finally, a form of social compact existed during the first half of the nineteenth century whereby hospitals accepted those whose death was imminent. In 1803–1804, bureau physicians noted that they regularly admitted "many patients afflicted with grave afflictions, some are brought almost dying, either after regrettable accidents, requiring operations whose outcome is rarely favorable, or after long delays, often with the specific intent of avoiding burial costs."[80] Despite efforts at curtailing the practice, families continued to abandon the dying on hospital doorsteps well into the 1830s.[81] In 1837, a practitioner at Hôtel-Dieu observed that this institution's exceptionally high mortality rates were still partly driven by this practice. Brandishing evidence from 1806 that showed that 31 percent (786 of 2,368) of patients died within the first three days of admission and 40.8 percent (965 of 2,368) by day ten, Apollinaire Bouchardat insisted that little had changed in the intervening decades.[82] And lest one conclude that the phenomenon was uniquely Parisian, a Strasbourg professor reached basically the same conclusion. While noting that approximately one third of deaths between 1836 and 1839 were from end-stage phthisis, Charles Forget noted that "the clinic is the rendezvous of hopeless cases: our wards are veritable catacombs where the dying come seeking a bit of relief; cadavers a casket, for we have on occasion received cadavers."[83] Only a few female consumptives bucked the trend. In his words, they "dreaded dying in the hospital," presumably out of fear of being dissected.[84]

While providing valuable insights into contemporary cultural practices, these observations also suggest that the location of death does not reliably capture incurables' illness experience. Admitting a dying consumptive or cancer patient as an emergency case is very different from routinely harboring them for months. Some incurables undoubtedly benefited from the good graces of someone in a position of power. Yet deeply ingrained biases worked against them. Those with extensive firsthand knowledge repeatedly complained that the procedures put in place to exclude chronics and incurables worked only too well. In other words, though the exclusion of incurables wasn't airtight, it was effective enough to prompt considerable soul-searching. One can reasonably say that the fate of incurables in the public realm was a story of closed doors and unassuaged misery.

## French Hospitals and French Incurables ca. 1820–1845

In 1820, a careful observer of French charity listed the illnesses that hospitals refused to treat: "darters and other afflictions of the skin, chronic illnesses, and those of children."[85] Some years later, a welfare bureau physician noted that "our typical clientele [is] that class of indigents that the hospital does not wish to accept, either because of the mildness of their morbid afflictions, or because their afflictions have reached the chronic stage or even become incurable."[86] In 1837, a colleague from a particularly poor *arrondissement* observed with distress that "pushed away, after a time, from the hospitals and dispensaries, chronic afflictions overload the welfare services; everyone knows how tenaciously they resist the best combination of treatments, the most favorable hygienic conditions: among our patients, everything is missing, air, light, warmth, food, suitable clothes, moral dispositions; what can we hope to do?"[87]

If the elderly had it bad, everyone recognized that the infirm and incurable were even worse off.[88] Even a committed Malthusian admitted in 1820 that the most urgently needed specialized facilities were *"hospices for incurables.* Such establishments are lacking in many cities, even in large ones like Lyon. The most demoralized beggary thereby finds a pretext for all excesses. . . . We believe it necessary to build hospices for these incurably ill, blind, crippled beggars who fill our streets, where they can be constrained to work as their abilities allow."[89] If only to spare society a disturbing presence, incurables needed to be sent somewhere.

Generally speaking, this mythical somewhere remained their homes. At least on paper, a select group of hospice cases were given special treatment by the welfare bureaus. In a de facto recognition of the hardships they imposed, old age and certain incurable disorders—cancer, epilepsy, paralysis, and blindness—offered the "luxury" of applying for more generous (though still ludicrously scanty) forms of assistance.[90] Those seventy or over, lunatics, epileptics, the blind, and cancer patients also had the right to request admission to a public hospice.[91] Yet the imbalance between demand and supply ensured that these entitlements were more virtual than real. For a start, the tradition of giving a little bit to everybody meant that the sums involved were pittances.[92] Paris's mayors noted in 1837 that even the most desperate cases waited months before receiving anything. The waiting time for hospices often approached four to five years.[93] Though private citizens attempted to shore up the public system, it was widely known that incurables suffered terribly from such neglect.

If there was no easy solution, people generally didn't try that hard to provide one. A physician's account of the system's inadequacies noted that "patients afflicted with cancer of the uterus cannot stay at home; they are refused at the hospital, or, if admitted, are confined to a room without daylight, deprived of warm beverages and narcotic medicines so useful in these mortal afflictions; they only rarely receive a visit from a physician." Rather than criticize his colleagues, Dr. Lemoine threw up his arms, asking, "What are we to do with them? Where are we to put them?"[94]

Some vocal critics, like future mayor Antoine Vée, didn't let the issue drop. Entrusted to prepare the annual report outlining Paris's thirteen welfare bureaus' activities and concerns in 1843, he drew attention to the disturbing gap between society's attentiveness to the acutely ill and their neglect of those in whom

> life will soon be extinguished, whose suffering is agonizing, whose needs unending, whose ills require constant care, yet who can find it nowhere. . . . They are often in the prime of their lives, almost always fathers or mothers of young families, to which their plight brings famine and desolation; and it is after having sold or hawked everything, on a wooden bed without mattress or covers, under an attic or in some dark, unhealthy, ground-floor flat, which the owner has briefly abandoned to them despite a desperate desire to see it more fruitfully occupied, that these poor souls eventually expire, prey to all variety of moral and physical torture.[95]

This and other testimony point to a fascinating feature of contemporary policy debates. Unlike the select few who controlled the country's purse strings or political economists concerned only with abstract notions like the national interest, local administrators witnessed firsthand the consequences of existing efforts. Admittedly, even Vée had no desire to increase spending or create a publicly funded charitable system. He and other liberals mostly wanted to allocate existing resources differently. It was cruel and foolish, they insisted, to give paltry sums to all poor Parisians or allow concerns about efficiency and security to dictate policy. Charity's true raison d'être was to assuage misery that was exceptional, not structural; dying incurables and elderly invalids were its rightful beneficiaries. Such munificence also had few of the distorting effects that economists so greatly feared.[96]

In 1843, Vée and other notables decided to lead by example. Beyond illegally diverting municipal home-care funds, the welfare bureau of the Fifth Arrondissement raised money to assist those excluded from the hospital and neglected by traditional charities. In relating the touching stories of several grateful incurables, he also demonstrated why the status quo prevailed as long as it did. These individuals, he observed, "were those who had elicited the greatest expense," as high as 115 francs in one case, a princely sum by contemporary philanthropic standards.[97] This was clearly not something that could be done on the cheap; one dutiful young woman of modest, though independent means spent 1,470 francs in 1822 to care for an incurably ill loved one.[98] While admittedly singular, a program set up by a single *arrondissement* demonstrated what could be accomplished (even in the 1840s) when a relatively affluent community marshaled the necessary political will. But the costs involved, to say nothing of contemporaries' mind-set against wasting money on hopeless cases, ensured that broad-based initiatives remained a stillborn idea for over half a century.

## "Achievement" Depends Upon How You Define It

Various observations make it difficult to take too sanguine a view of the hospital revolution. In 1837, Paris's mayors insisted that, despite decades of relative peace and prosperity, the fortunes of many charity cases had actually deteriorated. They informed the General Council on Hospitals that "since 1789, even as Paris's population has increased by almost 300,000, the number of [hospice] beds has remained roughly the same, even though this enormous rise in population was mostly due to the expanse of the working classes."[99] Eight years later, in 1845, nothing had changed. Experts commissioned to evaluate Paris's hospitals and hospices similarly concluded that the situation had worsened since 1803; the ratio of hospice beds had declined from one in 108 to one in 180 inhabitants.[100] These administrative bodies admittedly had reasons to look on the dark side; their observations nonetheless demonstrate that no amount of organizational fine-tuning can make up for a lack of concerted action. It also can do little in the face of powerful demographic trends. In the case of Paris, inward migration and working-class fertility created a rising tide of misery and violence.

Rather than a straightforward form of progress, the admission bureau embodied an ethos at once time-bound and ultramodern. It reflected decision makers' desire to reify the idea that modern hospitals existed for one purpose only: caring for the acutely ill and injured. The rest of suffering humanity was expected to look elsewhere. The problem of course was that there was not really anywhere else to look. The situation in both Paris and the provinces darkened after 1845, as economic stagnation and growing hardship again tipped the country into revolution. As will now be seen, the charitable innovations implemented in the aftermath of 1848 were an interesting mixture of old and new. For hospices cases, however, the net effect of the tumultuous Second Republic was captured by the popular expression "the more things change, the more they stay the same."

# 10

## Caught between Initiative and Inertia

### Responses to the Incurably Ill from 1845 to 1905

During the second half of the nineteenth century, various private charitable initiatives began providing assistance to the incurably ill. For a start, they benefited from a growing number of focused charitable offerings. Of course, the therapeutic limitations of contemporary medicine meant that tremendous unmet needs remained. The elderly, infirm, and incurable were also still sorely neglected by the public welfare system. This slowly began to change after 1870, as political upheaval, humanitarian sentiment, and public health concerns progressively moved incurables closer to the top of the sociomedical agenda. Over time, modest and tentative steps were taken to deal with the strain they increasingly placed upon hospital services, though a decisive rejection of the charitable status quo only took place at the turn of the twentieth century. During this period, the bourgeoisie became increasingly concerned by rising working-class militancy. Coupled with a significant leftward political shift, this paved the way for the passage of landmark pension legislation on July 14, 1905. With this measure, incurables obtained both financial assistance and an important form of symbolic recognition.

This process of political and institutional reform had several noteworthy features. Perhaps most striking was its slow pace. As they had in the past, French decision makers remained reluctant to waste time and effort on hopeless cases. Humanitarian feelings and religious conviction, while important, simply weren't enough. Indeed, several ideological and political shifts had to gain traction before decisive action occurred. First, incurable illness had to be recast as more than an individual tragedy to be handled by female caregivers and religious virtuosos; it had to become a medical and political quandary. That this took place at the end of the nineteenth century reflected contemporary sociomedical imperatives and propitious political conditions. Quite simply, incurable consumption became an urgent issue because the right people became sufficiently concerned by the social effects of unassuaged suffering and the risks of contagion. Hospice reform, on the other hand, became politicized because the left, driven by egalitarian instincts and a genuine concern for the plight of the working class, made it a priority. For many radical republicans and socialists, however, hospice reform was particularly enticing because it allowed them to attack one of Catholicism's last remaining strongholds in French society.

## Incurables in the Aftermath of 1848; or, Opportunity Averted

The Revolution of 1848 was initially welcomed by a large segment of the population, including intellectuals, militant workers, and professional revolutionaries. Exceptionally, however, many Catholics and bourgeois also supported the fledgling Second Republic.[1] Unpopular decisions and economic crisis quickly took their toll, alienating rural voters in a largely rural country. In April 1848, the first free male vote since 1792, growing mistrust precipitated a conservative backlash. At the same time, material hardships increased revolutionaries' zeal for change. By June, street battles had broken out between Parisian rebels and government troops. The resulting civil war was brief but bloody and claimed over ten thousand lives, including Paris's archbishop. Widespread fears of another Terror paved the way for Louis Bonaparte's landslide victory in December's 1848 elections. The seasoned leaders of the newly formed Party of Order assumed that the president-elect would be putty in their hands. Stealing a page from his uncle, the future Napoleon III quickly and decisively turned the tables.

Shortly before the election that marked the end of the Second Republic, reformers hurriedly sought to transform civil society. Article 13 of the constitution, passed with great fanfare on November 4 1848, formalized the state's obligation to assist abandoned children, the infirm, and all elderly persons who could not be assisted by their families. In keeping with this spirit of generosity, Interior Minister Dufaure proposed a complete overhaul of the charitable system. The strict residency requirements that were previously required of beneficiaries would be eliminated. A new administrative entity, L'Assistance Publique, would oversee Parisian relief efforts. Finally, Dufaure presented an ambitious national plan on poverty that would centralize relief efforts. The national government would henceforth also heavily subsidize welfare bureaus in the country's poorest regions.

Unlike other proposals, the Assistance Publique was uncontroversial in that it involved overhauling rather than creating new services.[2] To be fair to the framers, modest improvements were made to Paris's home-care system.

The number of welfare bureau physicians increased substantially. Doctors were paid a modest salary for the first time. To entice doctors to the poorest neighborhoods, the wages there were significantly higher.

The law on hospitals and hospices, passed on August 7, 1851, was the last important health initiative of this era. It generously asserted that "when an individual without resources falls sick within a commune, no condition of domicile is required for his admission into the hospital." Yet despite its apparent liberality, the law was conservative in character. Although acutely ill indigents could expect to be cared for, the strict eligibility criteria for hospice relief remained unchanged. In addition, towns without an institution would henceforth have to pay a fee whenever residents were admitted to a neighboring commune. Importantly, the law left the establishment of intercommunal hospitalization agreements voluntary rather than mandatory. This left it toothless, as most communities didn't follow through on the matter. As in the past, most of the country's incurably ill, elderly, and infirm had nowhere to turn. Once again, they were hostages to the vicissitudes of private charity.

This legislation faithfully mirrored two features of contemporary French political economy. The first pertained to the contested issue of where responsibility for the unwanted started and ended. Since 1789, negotiations centered on one basic question: Whose problem was it? It was precedent that, in an emergency, one acted first and asked financial questions later. Hospice cases were another matter; if charity started at home, where did it end? Did responsibility stop at the extended family, the commune, the department, or did it include the entire nation?

Post-Revolutionary governments consciously rejected an open-ended view of social solidarity. This was exemplified by the passage of two critical and lasting pieces of legislation. The first was the law of 7th Fraimaire An V; in 1845, a Parisian administrator observed that "by creating the Charity Bureau at the communal level, [the law] transformed the old order of things and implicitly confirmed the salutary principle that the relief of the poor is a local burden."[3] The Civil Code played an equally decisive role; articles 205, 206, 207, and 212 outlined families' responsibilities toward elderly and dependent kin. Astride these precedents, the law of 1851 reiterated that hospice cases would remain a local matter. Regional and national initiatives were nonstarters; as with questions of public health, individual communities were responsible for their citizens.[4]

French charitable localism had deep and complex roots that included civic pride, moral conviction, and mistrust of distant authority.[5] That being said, these mid-century policy decisions were propelled less by regional politics than by concerns with Paris's stability. Unrest here, history had repeatedly confirmed, brought ruin upon all. A half-century of industrial and economic development had only increased the city's political and economic clout. Although most of France's 36 million inhabitants lived in small towns and hamlets, Paris was the major engine of growth. By 1850, its 1.2 million inhabitants controlled a quarter of the country's wealth.[6] In laying out a blueprint for charitable reform, the National Assembly was primarily preoccupied with protecting ratepayers and safeguarding the metropolis.

A beacon for both destitute and ambitious provincials, Paris also attracted ill people in search of a better life. Even before the Revolution of 1848, city authorities had expressed concern about growing demands for health services, particularly hospice care. Over the years, Paris' richly endowed medical institutions had become a favored destination of sick provincials and *banlieusards*. In 1845, a committee was hastily assembled to settle a dispute between Paris and surrounding municipalities. The latter claimed that their residents had the right to use Parisian hospitals and hospices, even though their local governments paid nothing in return. They reasoned that institutions such as Bicêtre and La Salpêtrière had inherited the broad mandate of the general hospitals of the ancien régime. They also claimed that the suburbs fueled Parisian prosperity, supplying it with labor, raw materials, and foodstuffs. This transfer of wealth, they insisted, justified the medical treatment of Parisian suburbanites.

Rejecting these claims, the committee declared that Paris's hospices belonged only to Parisians. The report implored all communes to build autonomous hospitals or reach some financial agreement with their neighbors. It was imperative, the committee insisted, to "confirm the true principle of public assistance: the burden is to be equally spread, *each commune will take care of its poor*."[7]

An 1855 circular by the head of the Assistance Publique indicated that the chronically ill were the administration's overriding concern. The preamble to the new admissions policy stressed how "the presence of outsiders (*étrangers*) in the hospitals every year means that the administration must refuse a hospital bed to Parisians, to whom it belongs before all others, or to multiply the number of hospital beds in contravention to all the laws of hygiene." If the connivance of neighboring communities was the root problem, incurables embodied it. Noting their newfound mobility, the policy asserted that "the inconveniences we signal tend to increase daily, either because of the increasing ease of movement offered by the railways or because of the just celebrity of its doctors. Those who have been judged incurable in the other departments, or those with tenacious afflictions very difficult to cure, come to Paris seeking the varied curative means that abound here."[8] Taking their cue from the 1845 commission, the framers of the law of 1851 hoped that Paris's problems would be solved if foreigners stopped cheating poor Parisians of that which was rightfully theirs.

If obviously mean-spirited, such arguments were not without merit in that most taxes were raised locally. Furthermore, if wealth and responsibility should go hand in hand, the status quo had an important distorting effect: it punished communities with hospitals and hospices and discouraged the creation of new ones. The most striking thing about mid-century charitable policies, however, was their fluid and self-serving understanding of citizenship. Mandatory conscription in times of war suggested that the basis of republican citizenship was the nation-state. And in the case of insanity, public safety trumped administrative boundaries. It was only when the duties and obligations were onerous and top-down that the upper class chose to frame "Frenchness" narrowly. The result was a form of administrative quarantine that sought to circumscribe the financial contagion. In a world of carefully erected boundaries, the government of all Frenchmen resembled the parish priest who exhorted his parishioners to do *something*. Given the limited interest in hospice cases, these case remained largely, though not totally, forgotten in the mad rush toward prosperity.

## Charitable Relief during the Second Empire: A Small Step Forward?

Few periods in French history have been viewed as ambivalently as the Second Empire, which has been called a "modernizing dictatorship."[9] Napoleon III's early political success reflected the premium that people placed on peace and order; as the Duc de Morny observed, "This country is so tired of revolutions that all it wants today is a good despotism."[10] Capitalizing on the family name, Napoleon III parlayed fears and aspirations into successive electoral landslides. A consummate populist and political outsider, he convinced conservatives that he would assiduously defend their interests. Mostly, he skillfully exploited Catholicism's political potential; by making it a focal point of national unity, he simultaneously weakened the left and the far right.[11] Defusing intra-elite tensions without alienating the population was a complex balancing act possible only in good economic times. Fortunately for Napoleon III, loose credit, railway construction, and the Haussmannization of Paris resulted in a decade-long boom.

Domestic and international events eventually unraveled Bonapartism. The collapse of the Crédit Mobilier (the French equivalent of Tea Pot Dome) and a free-trade agreement with Britain caused widespread discontent. Equally important, France's abandonment of the papacy during Italy's War of Unification led to a rupture between Altar and Empire. Yet as his original power base slipped away, Napoleon III chose to increase civil liberties rather than stifle dissent. He took a calculated risk, granting the right to strike and freedom of the press in 1864, and freedom of association in 1868. Unfortunately for him, this only fueled discontent. Strikingly, the period of semi-authoritarian rule engendered a livelier, more mature democratic culture.[12] The relative social peace of this period was illusory. Yet whether one loved the emperor or loathed him, the country's economic potential was productively harnessed under his rule.

As with his political legacy, Napoleon III's charitable record is viewed with ambivalence. The historian Timothy Smith has justly observed that no national assistance program was created, something he blames mostly on "the concerted opposition of the country's political and intellectual class, especially the liberals." Despite this political stalemate, he noted that progress was made at the local level "in the form of a gradual expansion of the bureaux de bienfaisance and mutual aid societies and the number of people annually assisted from 975,000 in 1850 to 1.35 million in 1870. But funding came from the communes, not the central state, and in any case all local efforts were the result of voluntary effort."[13] Strikingly, even a leftist contemporary acknowledged that Napoleon's government "did not stop founding orphanages, nurseries, asylums for children and for the elderly. . . . Amid constant expansion, various female religious orders were created to care for poor patients: the Auxiliatrices des Ames au Purgatoire, Auxiliatrices de l'Immaculée Conception, Petites-Soeurs de L'Assomption."[14] If more could have been done in a period of economic expansion, historians' tendency to minimize the importance of these activities partly reflects their own ideological commitments. During the era of Napoleon III, charities were administered by Royalists and staffed by female religious orders.[15] By downplaying their accomplishments, the actions of the "heroes of history"—left-wing reformers of the 1880s and 1890s—seem even more remarkable.

The rift between church and state presaged troubled times, as growing anticlericalism both fueled and fed off a burgeoning Catholic renaissance.[16] Generally hostile to Catholic efforts, secular historians have tended to emphasize the Church's desperate efforts to preserve its eroding power base. Yet we can acknowledge the Church's reactionary reflexes without denying that it provided an outlet for the commitments of believers. The historian Ruth Harris has grasped the challenges that this complexity poses. In elucidating the motives of Catholic women, she demonstrates that the Church encouraged their subordination but at the same time "offered them a world of opportunity and found a means of cultivating their loyalty and energies."[17]

The sick, elderly, and disabled were among the main beneficiaries of Catholic philanthropy. Les Petites Soeurs des Pauvres, who provided hospice care to the elderly, doubled in size during the Second Empire. A limited number of philanthropic efforts specifically targeted incurables. The most remarkable were hospices staffed by Les Dames du Calvaire, founded in Lyon in 1842 by a young Catholic widow named Jeanne Garnier. The organization expanded in Lyon and spread to five other French cities: Paris (1874),

Saint-Étienne (1874), Marseille (1881), Rouen, (1891), and Bordeaux (1909). Three foreign branches were also established: Brussels (1886), New York (1899), and Bethlehem (1920). These refuges harbored the undesirable and unwanted, patients with ulcerated cancers and skin conditions like *lupus devorans*. Widowed society ladies, assisted by a few paid auxiliaries, literally bandaged their wounds and tried to assuage their suffering. Catholicism was of course omnipresent, though past behavior and religious indifference reportedly weren't grounds for exclusion.

This initiative's considerable success reflected both its exclusivity and organizational suppleness. Other than an annual membership fee, each widow enjoyed complete autonomy. A handful of *dames résidentes* lived in the hospices and oversaw their functioning. Others' roles were more modest. The *veuves agrégés* came once or twice a week to change bandages, while the *veuves zélatrices* handled fund-raising. Drawing upon the devotion, wealth, and social connections of a core group of affluent widows, this association ministered to thousands of dying incurables. In the process, they perpetuated a venerable tradition wherein the Catholic elite performed physically repulsive tasks in a show of faith. Though the Dames did not take formal vows and retained worldly ties, their activities were structured around Catholic ritual and imagery. The high point of their day consisted of changing patients' bandages. This onerous duty was preceded by the following invocation: "My God, we offer up the dressing change we are about to perform, to honor the Passion and the Death of our Lord Jesus Christ; we offer it to you for the conversion of sinners, perseverance of the just, and the deliverance of the souls in purgatory."[18]

Through a series of gestures, dismal reality became cosmic drama, as those debased by illness became consubstantial with Jesus' suffering body. In a process that ritually reenacted the Passion, two vile phenomena—abject suffering and a nauseating nursing duty—served to collapse social distinctions. Struck by the fact that the list of Paris' *veuves agrégés* read like a who's who of elite royalist society, Maxim Du Camp observed in 1883 that

> the Dames du Calvaires who are the most sought out, the most desired, are those members of the upper aristocracy; it suffices to be a duchess or a princess to be sought out by all. The patient who was assisted by a grand lady could not suppress a smile of satisfaction. A cancer patient with literary pretensions and an elevated spirit readily exclaimed, "The duchess came in her fine English cab today; it is she who looked after me; she was so charming!" Who would have imagined that cancer had its vanities?[19]

Something analogous happened on a grander scale at Lourdes. Like most other charitable activities, these examples of exaggerated subordination remained a politically sanctioned outlet for female religious zeal even as they served as a compelling model of feminine authority and power.[20]

Harris and Thomas Kselman have justly emphasized the importance of healing shrines and Church rituals to millions of contemporaries.[21] Sacred ground fostered a sense of community and spiritual wholeness; even skeptics acknowledged that something remarkable happened at Lourdes. Invoking the elaborate consolatory rituals, Harris suggests that "the secular republic lacked the emotional and historical resources to challenge the power of this vision as effectively as it wished."[22]

During the second half of the century, private philanthropy had complex effects on the politics of illness. On the one hand, displays of Christian solidarity forced the Church's opponents to pay greater attention to problems that had previously gone ignored. At the same time, feminine devotion perpetuated a vision of incurable illness as an intricate physical and spiritual struggle rather than a social problem whose solution was political. Quite simply, if hospice care required a superhuman degree of devotion, mere mortals needn't apply. It also encouraged the view that devout women, not the state, were the natural protectors of the hopelessly ill. The greatest pitfall of contemporary healing rituals was thus that voluntarism reinforced political and gender hierarchies.[23] Religious virtuosity, like all forms of noblesse oblige, had a self-serving side. Spending a few hours at Calvaire or doing a week's service at Lourdes was far more edifying than aggressively combating the root causes of misery. In attacking private charity, radical republicans and socialists were adamant that occasional good deeds were no substitute for a tax-supported system of public assistance.

Even Catholic spokesmen recognized that private efforts only scratched the surface. In 1859, a liberal Catholic noted that eighty-four departments paid out 402,503 francs for deaf-mutes; only ten assisted incurables to the tune of 68,000 francs.[24] If some received hospital care, most were left to fend for themselves. Using the 1851 census, which showed that a large number of Frenchmen were disabled, August Cochin claimed that there were "at least 50–60,000 incurably infirm people in need of assistance."[25] Turned aside by both hospitals and hospices, they were "distressing exceptions who remain outside all rules, because their misery exceeds all usual bounds."[26] Like a growing number of notables after mid-century, he suggested that all levels of government contribute to their upkeep. Anticipating objections that such a plan was too "English," he insisted that such measures were desperately needed, long overdue, and addressed a social problem that private charity alone could not.[27]

Complacency proved quite entrenched, however; decades later, in January 1892, a leading reformer was still lamenting the fact that "almost everywhere in France, we witness the painful spectacle of many old people who are not taken in and incurables that suffer and die without receiving the least assistance."[28] It wasn't until 1905 that the state set up a universal assistance program for all hospice cases. This change reflected both pragmatism and idealism. In an atmosphere of sociomedical crisis and political agitation, the state began taking its obligations toward the incurably ill seriously.

## Social Crisis during the Early Third Republic

Many of those who complained about the perils of indiscriminate charity recognized that they had an interest in not neglecting the poor. It had long been understood that charity discouraged revolution and crime, that charitable relief was the velour glove that covered the state's iron fist.[29]

Yet prior to Koch's discovery of the tubercle bacillus in 1882, incurables were rarely regarded as dangerous per se. The social and medical strain they placed on others was a growing concern, however. Typical of an emerging mid-century literature, an aristocratic reformer indignantly denied that poverty-stricken families found suffering uplifting. Hinting that such discussions made a mockery of their experiences, the Countess de Gasparin insisted that the consequences of ignoring the plight of the ostracized ill were dire: "the family dissolves, the union subsists in the form of a heavy chain; criminal relations are established outside of marriage; habits of brutality and drunkenness are acquired; the rapport between father, mother, daughter and son are destroyed . . . this is a well established fact, that is frequently reproduced in Paris; increasingly miserable generations, more and more estranged from uplifting sentiments, are preparing our calamity and their ruin."[30] If prescient, the countess was no radical; like most of her ilk, she believed that care was best provided at home. Working-class families simply needed a bit of extra help and a whole lot of encouragement.

A well-known Catholic philanthropist, Albert de Melun, made a cleaner break with tradition. In a report to the legislative assembly in 1851, he noted that nothing devastated poor families as much as illness. He was also among the first to suggest that hospitals were a valuable safety valve, a source of social cohesion, not improvidence or neglect.[31] He was far ahead of his time, although the decades that followed witnessed a slow and uneven process of consciousness raising among the social elite. The process was greatly accelerated by the disastrous events of 1870–71, proving that few things rival street violence and revolution for getting the political class's attention.

As with every previous episode of upheaval, the "social question" was earnestly reopened in the early Third Republic. True to form, the government carried out a survey of the country's hospital and hospice services. The results, presented to the National Assembly in 1873, were predictably disheartening.[32] In Paris, where events had taken a savage turn, humanitarianism and self-interest led to a visible outpouring of concern. Interestingly, the admissions bureau was among the most prominent targets. In the mid-1870s, its raison d'être was forcefully questioned as part of a sharp critique of the hospital system.

Growing dissatisfaction led to calls for its closure at a meeting of the municipal council in 1875. The problem, critics insisted, were the legions of chronically ill patients whose local hospital told them "there are no beds, go to the admissions bureau." Upon their arrival, they were generally instructed to come back tomorrow. The result, predictably, wasn't pretty; as Maxim Du Camp observed, "one is barely able to calm them down and the majority leave cursing."[33] Two years after the idea of closing the bureau was first raised, a report from within the Assistance Publique came down on the side of the critics. It insisted that

> it is difficult to conjure up a clear idea of the mournful scenes and agonizing miseries that one witnesses at the admission bureau's consultations. You'd have to see, in the midst of this mass of miserable patients, the physician looking for those whose condition is most grave and to whom he can accord one of the few beds at his disposal. As for the great majority, the doctor cannot give in to their supplications; he has to send them away. . . . Thus we see those poor outcasts who have come from Belleville or Ternes, from the Porte du Trône or d'Italie, forced to come back three, four, five, and six days in a row. . . . And yet, these patients whom you force to drag themselves around, at the risk of collapsing on the way, across the four or five kilometers to the bureau, almost all live on the doorstep of one of the outlying hospitals where they should be received immediately. How can one explain such an anomalous, no, such a monstrous, state of affairs?[34]

Contemporaries increasingly believed that the configuration of the hospital system worsened people's misery. In a letter to the director of the Assistance Publique in 1875, a senior administrator insisted that hospitals needed to be more indulgent toward "uninteresting" patients. The results would be both immediate and palpable. The workload of the admissions bureau would decrease significantly. More importantly, fewer patients would undergo the ordeal of traveling downtown only to be admitted a few hours later to the same hospital that had refused them that morning.[35]

In response to the public outcry, two blue-ribbon panels were set up in 1877 to decide whether to close the admissions bureau. The Committee of the Medical Society of Hospital Doctors—which included many of the country's leading physicians[36]—defended the status quo. A modern hospital system, it insisted, needed a centralized triage system. Attending physicians' tendency to keep a few beds free "just in case" was also thoroughly defensible; it would be unconscionable to turn away acutely ill patients because the hospital was filled with incurables.[37] Rather than eliminating the bureau or overhauling the system, a bit of administrative fine-tuning would suffice. Complaints about doctors' callousness misrepresented the true problem, namely that *"there is not a single vacant bed in any hospital,* on the contrary, the wards are overflowing with patients; there are extra beds almost everywhere; in a word there is OVER-CROWDING."[38] A shortage of hospice beds and services meant that hospitals were filled with infirm and incurably ill patients who belonged elsewhere.[39] Rather than heartless, hospital doctors were overly indulgent. Faced with destitute people who had waited vainly for months to get into a hospice, they relented. This was a terrible mistake; in their words, "the hospital is thus gradually transformed, and becomes nothing but a branch of the hospice; and given that, for their part, the acutely ill don't stop coming, what is the result?" Rather than closing the bureau, the infirm and incurable need to be sent elsewhere, preferably to some modest purpose-built institution on the outskirts of the city.[40]

A report prepared by Paris's leading surgeons made many of the same observations and prescriptions, though it refined the traditional dichotomy between hospital patients and hospice cases. If hospitals should serve the acutely ill and injured while incurables belonged in hospices, the real problem were those who straddled these categories. Referring to chronically ill patients whose cases weren't altogether hopeless, the report noted, "When one goes through the hospice, the hospital, the convalescent hospitals, we everywhere see the chronic and the valetudinary. In the hospice where he has entered improperly, taking the place of the elderly and the infirm; in the hospital where he occupies the bed destined for true patients; in the convalescent hospitals were he again takes the place of the true patient, who should go there to complete his cure."[41] Like their medical colleagues, however, committee members were optimistic that "with temporary hospices, more economical, we would free up hospice beds, hospital beds, and space in the convalescent hospitals. The construction of new hospitals within Paris would be unnecessary, as hospitals that have rid themselves of those not requiring active treatment would suffice for the needs of all true patients."[42]

The fact that certain "chronics" benefited from hospitalization was inconvenient in that they couldn't simply be dismissed as hopeless. Yet at the same time, they were uninteresting professionally and offered an extremely modest return on the investment. It is little wonder that most physicians preferred to avoid them outright.[43]

In the end, professional expertise and bureaucratic inertia ensured that the admissions bureau survived until the turn of the century. The original outpouring of concern inaugurated a decades-long exercise in soul-searching, however. Ironically, efforts that were hurriedly put in place to deal with hospital overcrowding mostly confirmed that chronics and incurables were second-class citizens in a system disinclined to help.

One proposal involved the establishment of a new hospital for the chronically ill (Laënnec Hospital, founded 1878). Years later, critics noted that the project was rapidly sabotaged by physicians' distaste for chronic care. At the Third Conference on Tuberculosis in 1893, Dr. Clado insisted that attending physicians had consistently reserved a few beds for patients that they found "interesting." The net result, he noted, was that "slowly but surely Laënnec has become a hospital like all others, where consumptives occupy [only] 20–25 percent of the beds."[44] That same year, one of Paris's leading experts on the disease laconically observed that "Laënnec hospital, created for consumptives, has become a general hospital where, as in all the other Parisian general hospitals, they are gotten rid of as much as possible."[45]

In 1876, Parisian authorities also began offering a small pension to terminally ill consumptives who remained at home, modeled upon the long-standing entitlement program for cancer patients and epileptics. In keeping with tradition, however, the annual budget was modest and each stipend exceedingly small (8 francs per month). Years later, a respected and politically connected clinician observed that, to no one's surprise, the program had been a waste of money and a total flop. Without naming names, Joseph Grancher pointed out that even a high-ranked administrator agreed that the amounts offered were almost insulting. Both were cautiously optimistic that increasing the monthly pension fourfold to 30 francs per month might achieve the desired result, however.[46]

These failed endeavors confirm that, in the absence of the necessary professional and political will, guilty feelings don't solve anything. Incurables, meanwhile, continued to pay the price. In the 1890s, the admissions bureau was still admitting dying consumptives who had been "refused everywhere and shuttled back and forth between hospitals and the admissions bureau, often several days, *sometimes several weeks*."[47] The problem of bed scarcity worsened in the 1880s, despite the fact that hospital authorities had embraced the controversial solution of adding cots to existing wards. The net result was a fascinating paradox: even as hospitals were being transformed by new technologies, they struggled with the age-old problem of overcrowding. Doctors, for their part, alternated between blaming the system and blaming the patients; the only thing they knew for certain was "it was becoming urgent to send away the invading hordes of incurable consumptives."[48]

Things came to a head in the early 1890s because of concerns about the risk of contagion. At the height of the crisis, Dr. L. H. Petit invited Parisian hospital physicians to suggest ways of dealing with the problem.

Besieged and overwhelmed, their responses exposed their difficulty reconciling humanitarian feelings, utilitarian instincts, and distaste for futility. Given that incurable consumptives occupied up to a third of all beds, they steadfastly blamed them for hospital overcrowding.[49] Worse, the preference shown toward dying patients prevented them from admitting consumptives whose medium-term prognosis was less bleak.

While awaiting the construction of public sanatoria, they concurred that cutting-edge care should be reserved for those with early-stage disease, preferably in specially appointed isolation rooms. As for incurables, the solution was depressingly conventional: cavernous wards offering bare-bones palliative treatments. Though several physicians worried about the moral effects of segregating large numbers of hopeless cases, everyone's first priority was to stop squandering hospital resources.

At the level of daily routines, doctors' ambivalence played itself out in several ways. In extreme cases, they rejected consumptives outright. In a paradox whose irony wasn't lost on others, one senior hospital physician regretfully noted that many consultants treated consumptives as pariahs before acknowledging that he himself studiously avoided admitting them.[50] If no other respondent was that ruthless, others recognized that the fear of being overrun with incurables had perverse effects. Dr. Desnos confessed that he and others admitted mildly ill individuals who didn't need hospital care, merely to keep consumptives off their wards.[51] Even when they were admitted, late-stage patients tended to be systematically neglected.[52] They also risked expulsion. Joseph Grancher admitted that everyone felt a pang of remorse when the need to admit a more interesting case meant that "we find ourselves constrained, as we should, to chase the unhappy consumptives out of our wards to see them begin anew their peregrinations and efforts to gain admittance into another hospital? And this is not some chance event, it is a daily occurrence, and on the cobblestones of Paris there are several hundred consumptives condemned to this perpetual to and fro until their death."[53]

In some ways, the situation became even more complicated in 1893. The law on free medical assistance enacted that year was progressive in recognizing that certain categories of chronically ill patients, including early-stage consumptives, were officially "true patients." By May 1894, however, the Interior Ministry had sent out a corrective that stipulated, "The second condition required of those who are to receive free medical assistance is that they must be *patients*. The law of the 15 July 1893 thus leaves outside of its jurisdiction, the elderly and the incurably infirm. 'Patients' refer to those who could be received in a hospital, but not those received in hospices."[54] The moment a patient was judged incurable, the national government stopped paying their portion of hospital costs. If the patient's home commune refused to pay the going rate for hospice care, the patient was expected to leave.

In the resulting chaos, many incurables continued to lose out. In 1899, the acting director of the Assistance Publique noted that once a diagnosis of incurability was established the commune or department that had assisted them faced two options: break the rules and prolong their stay in hospital, or act immorally and send them out into the street. Examples of each, he observed, abounded.[55] Two decades of crisis had convinced everyone of the need for change. This hadn't provoked decisive action, however. The creation of an ambitious system of public assistance required the intervention of a national government determined to make the plight of incurables and other hospice cases, at long last, a priority.

## The Law of 1905: A Long and Winding Road

By 1888, the French state was regularly hectoring communes and departments to provide better home care. A year later, delegates at a high-profile conference at the Parisian World's Fair ambitiously declared that "public assistance must be made obligatory to assist those indigents who find themselves temporarily or permanently incapable of securing the material necessities of life."[56] The first manifestation of a new interventionist stance in France was the law on free medical assistance, passed with great fanfare on July 15, 1893. Bearing the imprint of physician-legislators and medical syndicates, it asserted that assistance was both a social duty and an individual right, political rhetoric rarely heard since the 1790s.[57] Concerned by the uneven scope of compulsory care, two members of the National Assembly suggested in February 1895 that hospice cases merited similar consideration.

This initiative gained momentum in December, when a legislative committee declared that hospice cases had a legal right to assistance. Soon after, the government asked the nation's highest legal authority, Le Conseil d'État, to draft legislation creating a national charitable system. They also set aside an annual sum of 500,000 francs to create a noncompulsory pension program for the elderly. The Conseil d'État finished its work in March 1898; using the law of 1893 as its model, it proposed a system of community-based assistance in which local governments bore nearly all of the costs.[58]

As with all contemporary social legislation, religious politics delayed its enactment.[59] Liberalism and regionalism stymied it more, ensuring that no further legislative action was taken until radical republicans' victory in the divisive election of 1902.[60] The newly constituted Bloc des gauches vigorously promoted Émile Combes's controversial agenda, including pension reform.[61] After speedy review in committee, two competing proposals were debated in the Assembly in May and June 1903. The government's opponents pointed out that certain departments had already established an effective hospice system without state prodding.[62] Proponents responded that existing services were, at best, patchy and inadequate.

In staking out their position, the government drew upon the work of a new breed of economists favorable to state intervention.[63] They also pointed to recent experience with the voluntary pension scheme. In the absence of sanctions, communes and departments had done little; only 5 percent of the 500,000 francs budgeted had been paid out during 1900 and 1901.[64] It was thus imperative to force the hand of local authorities more sensitive to the interests of ratepayers than to the plight of the abject.[65]

National and international events emboldened reform-minded politicians. The successful creation of a national pension system in 1889 by France's rival, Germany, proved that it could be done. Denmark and Belgium, which had also established universal assistance programs, gave a sense of the financial costs associated with different eligibility criteria.[66] Most importantly, working-class militancy and universal male suffrage imparted a sense of urgency to the question of social entitlements. Industrialization and democracy, in other words, made change hard to escape.[67] By 1894, even the mouthpiece for French industry admitted that "the best defense against socialism is social reform."[68]

In a poisonous political climate, the past was a source of both inspiration and consternation. Left-wing politicians insisted that the national government was finally taking up the noble agenda of the 1791 Poverty Committee; opponents invoked revolutionaries' catastrophic confiscation of Church property and nationalization of charity. Despite the differences that separated politicians, their lively reconsideration of history signaled the demise of laissez-faire liberalism and traditional charity ideology. If nothing else, the upper class had progressively come to understand that the state had a duty to assuage the elderly and chronically ill. Most decision makers also recognized that improvidence alone didn't explain working-class poverty. Low wages, involuntary unemployment, and ill health were also to blame.

In the final decades of the nineteenth century, intellectuals and politicians began to embrace the newly minted concept of "solidarism." Its main tenet was that publicly funded charity was both desirable and republican; its proponents drew on biology and sociology in an effort to defend its scientific credibility. Under its aegis, programs were established to encourage working-class property ownership, the expansion of savings plans, and the creation of workplace cooperatives in which employees shared in company profits.[69] Solidarists also promoted public health measures, wrapped in the republican rallying cry of "equal protection against disease."[70] Employers were, of course, largely concerned with limiting costs while preserving the country's human capital. Yet in using the language of equality and fraternity, mandatory, tax-funded assistance programs were successfully framed as a quintessentially French solution to the ills engendered by modern capitalism.[71]

Despite the growing currency of these ideas, older views about illness and charity continued to permeate political debates. Decision makers, for example, contested the root causes of tuberculosis. Socialists implicated misery, malnutrition, and long hours even as they called for higher wages and a shorter work week; conservative opponents, on the other hand, blamed alcoholism, debauchery, and syphilis for its spread.[72] A few die-hard traditionalists also worried that publicly funded pensions sent the wrong message. They risked undermining social cohesion, one senator argued, because they'd encourage workers to expect even more outlandish entitlements.[73]

For the first time, the French state also proclaimed that assistance wouldn't be arbitrarily capped but proportionate to the needs of the poor. This was both reasonable and desirable, they averred, for traditional charity was self-serving, inadequate, and humiliating.[74] As the acclaimed French socialist Jean Jaurès declared, "What is the idea behind this law? It is to substitute the certitude of law for the arbitrariness of donations. . . . It is to give to those who are to be assisted not only a degree of well-being, but a little more dignity, more independence."[75] Making it a birthright, in other words, spared people the humiliation of begging.[76]

If political rhetoric is any indication, nearly all of French society had accepted the urgency and morality of hospice reform. Even those who worried about the organizational challenges and the financial costs voiced support for its merits.[77] Times had changed; one deputy who originally voted against the measure admitted to his adversaries that "the Assembly did not share my views. If I had only had your friends against me, so be it; but the clergy, the king, and the emperor were all against me!"[78] So confident of this plan's popular appeal, the government dared the opposition to oppose it.[79] A few notables tried to rally opposition, but to no avail.[80] The Assembly passed the bill on June 15, 1903, 552 votes to 3.[81] Two years later, the French Senate unanimously approved a modified version.[82] The Assembly quickly followed suit.[83]

Such apparent unanimity and consensus did not erase traditional concerns, particularly those that turned on religion and money. From the start, lawmakers were confronted with two widely divergent estimates of the projected costs. A 1901 study by the commerce department estimated that 600,000 persons would apply for benefits, including 225,000 incurables. It calculated the cost of care to be 165 million francs, which didn't include hospice construction and refurbishment that the government ambitiously envisaged. To quell the expected panic, the Interior Ministry commissioned its own study, which concluded that fewer people would apply at a fraction of the costs. Once outlays for existing relief programs had been accounted for, the total new tax burden would only be 17.4 million francs.[84] Opponents responded with howls of derision; even the government's friends admitted that no one knew the exact price tag.[85]

By the time the law made it to the Senate in 1905, the opposition had settled on 100 million francs, far more than society could afford.[86] Two branches of the government, on the other hand, presented somewhat more reassuring figures.[87] In the end, the costs incurred during the first year were not quite 49 million francs.[88] This was an extraordinarily expensive entitlement program by French standards, however. A few years earlier, the total cost of free medical assistance for indigents was only 8.7 million francs.[89]

While the debate focused mostly on the program's affordability, politicians also sparred over how to divide up the costs. Eager to redistribute wealth from richer to poorer regions, the government nonetheless insisted that local governments should bear the brunt of the cost.[90] This was partly because most taxes were levied locally; giving officials other people's money to spend also increased the likelihood of administrative abuse. Driven by fears that communes and departments would politically sabotage the program, the Senate forced the government to increase its contribution. It proposed a new formula for apportioning costs, turning the relative financial commitments upside down. The French state would now pay over half the cost (37 out of 66.7 million). Local ratepayers benefited most from this new arrangement; their contribution plunged from 31 to 18 million.[91] This vital concession, approved by 270 out of 271 senators, allowed the draft law to be passed. Beyond decreasing constituents' financial burden, the opposition had cleverly calculated that radical republicans would be left facing unpalatable political choices: reduce spending elsewhere or levy new taxes.

When the Assembly was poised to pass the initial version of the bill, an opponent provided the critical subtext to these debates when he insisted that he was the adversary of all forms of socialism.[92] Every conservative politician hoped that this show of support would allow them to postpone an even costlier program—state-subsidized insurance for retired workers—indefinitely.[93] For the far left, the law of July 14, 1905, was simply a small step forward. As socialist leader Édouard Vaillant proclaimed, it inaugurated a political order in which "just as assistance has replaced charity, insurance will come to replace assistance, constituting an intermediate step for the working class until it has completed the conquest of all of its rights, and completed its emancipation."[94]

The government's harshest critic also saw this as an important step on the road to godless socialism, almost as bad as recently passed legislation separating church and state.[95] Edouard Aynard's invocation of state-sponsored anticlericalism wasn't gratuitous. This legislation did, in fact, target one of Catholicism's last remaining strongholds, its charitable apparatus. For as several left-wing politicians noted, charity was often used as an inducement to encourage Church membership.[96] The law's passage, following the incendiary separation of church and state, marked the culmination of long-standing efforts to decrease Catholicism's political influence. The laicization of welfare bureaus, hospitals, and education was one to two decades old; hospice assistance remained the Church's last vestige of influence. Radical republicans did their best to make up for lost time. Rather than building upon existing initiatives as the Conseil d'État had suggested, they demanded a public system that excluded the Church.

Several aspects of the proposed legislation were particularly contentious. Beyond creating publicly funded, nondenominational hospices alongside existing confessional ones, the government sought to force all pensioners, even committed Catholics, to use public facilities. The state would pay for private care only if a public hospice was at too great a distance.[97] Ironically, legislators invoked the protections of religious freedom to defend their actions; in a democracy, no organization or church could monopolize the provision of care.[98] Catholic organizations would also be denied a role in screening applicants. And unlike socialist-dominated mutual-aid societies, Catholic representatives were barred from the cantonal commission entrusted to review appeals. Despite forceful requests, the government brushed aside calls for more Catholic involvement.[99]

Critics also criticized the government's plans to appropriate revenue from existing hospice programs. Even individual bequests, most of which had come from devout Catholics, were to be appropriated by the state unless the donor had left specific instructions regarding their use.[100] Finally, the Senate commission added a new measure, ostensibly to reduce costs. Unlike interest income from personal saving or stipends from mutual-aid societies that triggered a modest reduction in benefits, funds from private (that is, Catholic) donations would result in a significantly larger claw-back.[101] The government claimed that individual savings merited greater consideration than alms; critics, rightly enough, read this as another thinly veiled attack on religion.

The government's opponents charged that taxpayers were being asked to bankroll its ideological excesses. It was inefficient, they pointed out, to build a new hospice alongside a preexisting one. They also cautioned that a souring of relations between private and public charities would hurt the interests of the poor. Hospice donations would immediately dry up, they warned, as had happened to welfare bureaus after their de-Christianization in the 1890s.[102] Despite this credible threat, Combes's militantly anticlerical administration was determined to make the most of its legislative majority.[103] Henri Monod spoke for all when he asserted that "a public service does not live off donations."[104]

The government did make a few conciliatory gestures. For a start, private gifts were treated like other forms of income.[105] Private hospices were also given a reprieve; provided they passed regular inspections, they were eligible for public funds. Plans to build new hospices were also scaled back. These decisions were more pragmatic than principled, however. Radical Republicans basically wanted to secularize hospice care without completely alienating those serving on the front lines. To get what it wanted, the government declared a truce on one front and claimed the larger battle.

Though they supported the new measure, moderate republicans and liberals again found themselves in an awkward position, squeezed between Catholics and militant anticlericals.[106] Like the freethinking doctors who resisted closing Lourdes, most appreciated the importance of religion in the lives of many elderly, infirm, and incurable individuals. In 1883, just as state-sponsored anticlericalism was gaining the upper hand, one committed republican found himself singing the praises of private charity. Though agnostic, Maxim Du Camp wondered, "Is clericalism really the enemy? I am too mediocre a cleric to decide the question, but I affirm that, for nations as for man, spiritualism is life-giving and materialism equals death."[107] He could only praise those who spent their lives serving others; in a city such as Paris they were "like a beacon over an abyss."[108] Unlike those who wanted to sever all ties between hospices and the Church, he and other moderates appreciated the contributions, however partial, that Catholics had historically provided to France's neglected and neediest citizens. In their mind, religious conviction inspired a selflessness that secular values would never match.

# Conclusion

Today we speak of chronic and/or degenerative diseases, and sufferers previously classified as incurable are now considered disabled, chronic, or terminally ill. There are no longer any Homes for Incurables in Boston, Philadelphia, and Brooklyn; "reputedly incurable" is also a forgotten notion. Yet despite changes in vocabulary, the related issues of prognosis and disease trajectory are as significant today as they were a century and a half ago. Importantly, many of the developments that make "being incurable" what it is today trace their origins to the nineteenth century.

During that period, physicians wielded new forms of knowledge, new technologies, and new skills that allowed them to diagnose and, in some cases, treat illnesses more effectively. Thanks to these and other developments, physicians came to enjoy a newfound measure of prestige and authority. This process gained momentum in the twentieth century, as various breakthroughs dramatically improved medicine's ability to cure and to transform disease, mostly for the better. Indeed, one needs look no further than the discovery of antibiotics for tuberculosis to appreciate scientific medicine's dramatic impact on human health and experience. Yet the emergence of AIDS and drug-resistant tuberculosis vividly demonstrates that both disease ecology and (in)curability remain nearly as contingent and unstable today as they were in the past. Health outcomes are not random events. Just as in the nineteenth century, the incidence and prognosis of chronic disease is profoundly affected by socioeconomic and geopolitical factors. For millions in the developing world, AIDS remains incurable because of "how the world works." For various reasons, life-saving drugs don't reach the people that need them, cruelly exposing the limits of transnational justice and global solidarity. Of course even in affluent countries, many of the same issues play a role. Race, poverty, and access to care are not only important social determinants of health; they profoundly affect the evolution and prognosis of chronic disease. In the end, though biology and bad luck are important, (in)curability is also driven by income and education, as well as by the decisions that policy makers take on our behalf.

The progressive secularization and professionalization of end-of-life care is another important historical development. Since the mid-nineteenth century, physicians, nurses, and other paid caregivers have assumed many of the roles previously filled by pastors, priests, nuns, and families. In the case of incurable illness, this process has been both uneven and problematic. Critics, both past and present, have used these disorders to draw attention to the therapeutic limits of modern medicine and to highlight the importance of adequately addressing patients' emotional, existential, and spiritual concerns.

Finally, new forms of sociopolitical activism came to the fore during the late nineteenth century, initiatives that culminated in the creation of the modern welfare state. In both France and elsewhere, state-sponsored programs progressively replaced private, religiously inspired efforts at assuaging incurables. Despite their cost and apparent wastefulness, such activities were no longer simply a moral or religious duty but a social and professional challenge that more agreed was worth the effort.

Together, these developments contributed to the politicization and partial medicalization of incurable illness. By the early twentieth century, doctors and other decision makers viewed the treatment of chronic disease with a newfound optimism. Therapeutic innovations such as radiotherapy and hypodermic morphine allowed them to palliate suffering more effectively. At the same time, physicians and society at large increasingly recognized that many incurables required a level of care only available in institutions. In fact, as time went on, incurables from all social classes progressively turned to hospitals en masse. Twentieth-century medicine's growing ambition and optimism also had an important spillover effect; incurables came to be seen as appropriate, eventually even desirable, subjects of scientific research.

The magnitude of this medical and cultural shift is apparent if one considers the case of a leading incurable illness, cancer. In the first decades of the twentieth century, doctors and social reformers exuberantly launched campaigns across Europe and North America to improve its diagnosis and treatment. Joseph Recamier's 1911 address to an international conference vividly illustrated an important aspect of this ambitious new ethos: "for patients afflicted with inoperable cancer, especially when it is ulcerated and necessitates dressing changes, relief during the last months is only possible through hospitalization. This hospitalization must differ from ordinary hospital services in that the rules must be less severe, the alimentation easier to vary, visits allowed and encouraged. For such charitable efforts to fulfill their full goals, one must make it a center for scientific study, and annex the asylum for incurables to an active service and to a laboratory, the only means to avoid a general sense of discouragement."[1]

Even before the country emerged as a scientific juggernaut, the United States had taken the lead in the struggle against cancer and other chronic diseases. A critical early step in this crusade involved questioning the scientific validity and social consequences of the term *incurable*. This was a headline issue, for example, in Ernest Boas and Nicholas Michelson's landmark 1929 treatise, *The Challenges of Chronic Disease*. Based on their work at the Montefiore Hospital for Chronic Diseases in New York City, Boas and Michelson concluded that the treatment of chronic disease had been hindered by two important misconceptions: their presumed association with old age and the mistaken belief that they were incurable. In their words, this label was unconscionably harsh because "to the sick it signifies lost hope and permanent invalidism; to the physician it spells defeat and ignorance; to society it means human wastage and added economic burdens; to all it carries the sadness of a wrecked or crippled life." The term also encouraged the belief that society's sole obligation was to provide them with food and shelter. Citing the uncertainties of clinical medicine and devastating effects of therapeutic nihilism, they insisted that "not infrequently, an incurable can be restored to comparative health and economic usefulness, and, in many instances, properly directed efforts will serve to prolong life and relieve pain and discomfort."[2] The key to transforming perceptions, they and others believed, was to reframe the study of chronic disease as a fascinating, even gratifying, medicoscientific project.

Subsequent decades were marked by growing concern with these disorders' far-reaching consequences. Public health surveys, the nascent insurance industry, the mass screening of military conscripts, and government commissions served as catalysts in a process that accelerated at mid-century.[3] In 1952, the blue-ribbon Magnuson Report presented a compelling analysis of the economic and human costs of chronic disease in the United States. In calling for aggressive action, its authors noted that interest in these disorders had increased dramatically in the past decade, in part because of the successful rehabilitation of injured soldiers. A few years later, the appearance of the first issue of the *Journal of Chronic Diseases* (January 1955) confirmed that attitudes had changed. Describing itself as a "new venture in medical literature," its introductory article noted that it "finds its stimulus and reason for being in an awakening medical and public interest in the increasing importance of chronic illness."[4] Beyond confirming that problems officially exist only when enough powerful people choose to notice them, these events also indicated that opinion leaders' views were converging. It was imperative, they concurred, to encourage research and improve existing screening, treatment, and rehabilitation programs. Fragmentation of care, indifference, and neglect were unacceptable; only state-of-the-art, "total care," and a broad-based prevention strategy could prevent unnecessary suffering and waste.[5] Since then, of course, chronic disease has progressively become a major, arguably the leading, public health concern.[6]

The immediate postwar period also marked the beginning of an exciting new era as growing numbers of clinicians and social scientists devoted their professional lives to issues that had previously remained in the shadows. In tandem with the chronically ill, they have explored existing realities and forged new ones. During the last half century, interest in both fields (chronic disease and terminal illness) has exploded, mobilizing a broad array of social actors.

A central focus of twentieth-century efforts against chronic disease has been to transform prognostic perceptions and disease outcomes. Efforts at circumscribing and limiting incurability fell into two broad categories, curative and temporizing. One can better understand the distinction between the two by considering the case of cancer. During the twentieth century, the disease has increasingly become the object of high-profile efforts to encourage early detection and aggressive treatment. Considerable resources—emotional, human, and financial—were deployed to disseminate a reassuring message: surgery can cure cancer. Social commentators and social scientists have drawn attention to both the strengths and the limitations of these sociomedical campaigns. One thing, however, is clear and unequivocal: the focus was curative, to cut off the flow of incurables at the source.

Two other treatment modalities, radiotherapy and chemotherapy, became staples of cancer treatment.[7] And though each can occasionally be curative, these treatments typically only push back the boundaries of incurability and temporarily allay the threat of death. In the last few decades, the proliferation of such treatments has resulted in the creation of a new form/new phase of malignant disease: the so-called chronic phase. Together, these interventions have helped limit the number of incurable individuals for whom "nothing" could be done. They have also helped to diminish the length of time that patients spend in the final phase of their disease when the focus becomes the palliation of suffering and preparation for death.

As was the case in the nineteenth century, the acts of curing, temporizing, and palliating still overlap to a significant degree; all anticancer treatments can potentially serve all three purposes. Importantly, each of them carries risks and is associated with significant side effects. Yet despite their shortcomings, these innovations have had an enormous practical and social impact. Historically, they have acted as a counterweight to hopelessness, encouraging doctors and patients to "keep up the fight."

Notwithstanding these advancements, the majority of twentieth-century cancer patients still died from their diseases. For these and other "hopeless cases," life remained an arduous struggle to secure care and keep up their morale.[8] Perhaps predictably, nineteenth-century biases against incurables hadn't magically disappeared.[9] Frustration and despair often found expression in anger and accusation: the perception that a loved one had been dismissed as hopeless was a prominent feature of American antimedical rhetoric during the 1950s.[10] Even critiques leveled by late twentieth-century terminal care reformers leave one with an uneasy sense of déjà vu.

Troubled by the ongoing problem of therapeutic neglect, a small but vocal community of practitioners and theorists began to draw attention to the unmet needs of incurables. A series of six short articles in the *Nursing Times* by a then-unknown physician named Cicely Saunders signaled her debut in a field she came to both define and dominate: modern hospice care.[11] The sources of this movement's success were multiple and varied. Partly, it reflected the fact that reformers successfully identified and assuaged many unmet physical and emotional needs. Leading spokespeople also put forward a reassuring vision of cancer's terminal phase as a time of personal and spiritual growth, drawing on many of the same cultural resources that inspired nineteenth-century representations of consumption.

At the same time, the hospice movement attacked both the methods and the priorities of the medical establishment. Over time, a growing number of critics suggested that doctors' need and desire to sustain an illusion of omnipotence led to grave lapses in patient care. Hiding behind a wall of deceit was only the tip of the iceberg. Equally disturbing was that the inherent bias of the system was to either abandon the dying or do "too much," technologically prolonging death at the expense of more meaningful contact between patients and their loved ones. Especially since the late 1960s, technology was indicted by the hospice movement for at least two reasons: technology got it wrong, misapprehending the value of a natural death to patients and families. Technological medicine was also depicted as costly and futile, an argument that has preoccupied governments and lawmakers since.

In retrospect, technology's role in the setting of incurable illness is more complicated. Many critics of medical reductionism nonetheless welcomed the benefits of new, sophisticated (and often aggressive) palliative technologies. Equally importantly, the "cure-at-all-costs" mentality of the twentieth century was probably prerequisite to the emergence of a compelling alternative discourse as its limits and downside became apparent.[12] In other words, if twentieth-century cancer care is marked by many regrettable excesses, it has also stimulated scrutiny of existing practices and of the boundaries between curable and incurable, ameliorable and hopeless, salvageable and truly terminal.

The various continuities in the history of incurability indicate why a better understanding of the past is so important. Facilitated by advances in technology and broad socioeconomic trends, the late twentieth century witnessed a single-minded assault on the suffering of the terminally ill. Compassionate care of the dying came to be seen not only as a moral imperative (which it always was, at least in theory) but an urgent collective priority. Therein lies the unique and ultimately greater merit of those who fought hard to improve the system. But I think it also says something about the potential fragility of their accomplishments. If it is true that the modern hospice movement is a singular achievement that reflects the scientific, economic, social, and political atmosphere of the 1960s and 1970s, it is an accomplishment that will require nurturing lest changing circumstances cause us to revert to patterns of behavior and thinking that were typical not of the "good old days" but rather of the bad old ones.

"Good deaths," even in the limited sense of death with dignity, may well be rare and elusive nowadays.[13] Acknowledging this may not be a bad thing. Rather than look to the past for rarefied behavioral ideals, we should critically scrutinize it in order to map out our own priorities, both as individuals and as a collective. This may be more pressing than ever in that industrialized societies have to find ways of coping with growing numbers of chronically ill, disabled, and dying citizens.

# NOTES

## INTRODUCTION

1. A recent book on the history of cancer asserts that "indeed in many ways it is a quintessentially 'modern' affliction: although previous generations endured the ravages of cancer, they more often succumbed to contagious than neoplastic diseases." Barbara Clow, *Negotiating Disease: Power and Cancer Care, 1900–1950* (Montreal: McGill-Queen's University Press, 2001), xi. See also James T. Patterson, *The Dread Disease: Cancer and Modern American Culture* (Cambridge, MA: Harvard University Press, 1987), viii.

2. François-Joseph-Victor Broussais, *Histoire des phlegmasies ou inflammations chroniques*, 2nd ed. (Paris: Gabon, 1816), xii.

3. Anonymous, *Process verbal de l'assemblée générale du bureau de bienfaisance, 6e arrondissement, compte moral et administratif de l'exercice 1835—Rapport médical* (Paris, 1836), 26.

4. Eugene Weber, *Peasants into Frenchmen: The Modernization of Rural France* (Stanford, CA: Stanford University Press, 1976), 150–51.

5. These included scrofula, pulmonary phthisis, cancers, aneurysms, dropsy, gangrene, rickets, concretions (*concrétions*), chlorosis, and scurvy. Henri Meding, *Paris médical. Vade-mecum des médecins étrangers. Renseignements historiques, statistiques, administratifs et scientifiques sur les hôpitaux et hospices civils et militaires, l'enseignement de la médecine, les académies et sociétés savantes. Précédés d'une topographie médicale de Paris et suivis d'un précis de bibliographie médicale française et des adresses de tous les médecins de Paris* (Paris: Baillière, 1852), I: 154–55.

6. This category included tuberculosis, scrofula, syphilis, gout, rheumatism, rickets, hydrocephalus, and mesenteric tabes. Tuberculosis and cancer alone accounted for 94.9 percent of these deaths (9,893 of 10,428). Léon Vacher, *Étude médicale et statistique sur la mortalité à Paris, à Londres, à Vienne, et à New York* (Paris: Savy, 1866), 162.

7. Ibid., 117. Not only was the proportion of deaths from acute causes dramatically inflated by cholera that year, but the stigma of cancer and the difficulty establishing a diagnosis undoubtedly led to underreporting. Mortality figures also only give an incomplete sense of the cancer burden; not everyone with the disease would have died within a year after it was first detected.

8. J.F.K. Hecker, "Discours sur les diathèses morbides qui ont successivement affectées les peuples de l'Europe, traduit par M. Martin," *Revue médicale française et étrangère* I (1838): 12–23.

9. Jules Rengade, *Les grands maux et les grands remèdes. Traité complet des maladies qui frappent le genre humain avec l'exposition détaillée de leurs causes, de leurs symptômes, des troubles et des lésions qu'elles produisent dans l'organisme et des moyens les plus rationnels de les prévenir et de les combattre* (Paris: Librairie Illustrée, 1879), 35.

10. Erwin H. Ackerknecht, "Diathesis: The Word and the Concept in Medical History," *Bulletin of the History of Medicine* 56 (1982): 317–25.

11. Certain important nineteenth-century diagnostic categories have essentially disappeared. Mark S. Micale, "On the Disappearance of Hysteria: A Study in the Clinical Deconstruction of a Diagnosis," *Isis* 84, no. 3 (September 1993): 496–526.

12. Gerald Grob, *The Deadly Truth: A History of Disease in America* (Cambridge, MA: Harvard University Press, 2002), 217–42.

13. Charles E. Rosenberg, "Disease and Social Order in America: Perceptions and Expectations," *Milbank Quarterly* 64, suppl. 1 (1986): 34–55.

14. Charles E. Rosenberg, *The Cholera Years: The United States in 1832, 1849, and 1866* (Chicago: University of Chicago Press, 1962).

15. Andrew Cunningham, "Transforming Plague: The Laboratory and the Identity of Infectious Disease," in *The Laboratory Revolution in Medicine*, ed. Andrew Cunningham and Perry Williams (Cambridge: Cambridge University Press, 1992), 209–44.

16. Selman A. Waksman, *The Conquest of Tuberculosis* (Berkeley: University of California Press, 1964).

17. The disorder's fate in the hands of historical demographers such as Thomas McKeown and his successors has inadvertently contributed to this bias. In his famous analysis of population mortality since the eighteenth century, McKeown included tuberculosis in the category of infectious diseases, along with scarlet fever, diarrheal illnesses, typhoid fever, and smallpox. Thomas McKeown, *The Modern Rise of Population* (London: Edward Arnold, 1976).

18. Charles E. Rosenberg, *The Care of Strangers: The Rise of America's Hospital System* (New York: Basic Books, 1987).

19. Herman Feifel, epilogue to *New Meanings of Death*, ed. Herman Feifel (New York: McGraw-Hill, 1977), 355.

20. Sheila M. Rothman, *Living in the Shadow of Death: Tuberculosis and the Social Experience of Illness in American History* (New York: Basic Books, 1994); Emily K. Abel, *Suffering in the Land of Sunshine: A Los Angeles Illness Narrative* (New Brunswick, NJ: Rutgers University Press, 2007).

21. Robert Aronowitz, *Unnatural History: Breast Cancer and American Society* (Cambridge: Cambridge University Press, 2007).

22. David S. Barnes, *The Making of a Social Disease: Tuberculosis in Nineteenth-Century France* (Berkeley: University of California Press, 1995); Pierre Guillaume, *Du désespoir au salut:le tuberculeux aux XIXe et XXe siècles* (Paris: Aubier, 1986).

23. Ruth Harris, *Lourdes: Body and Spirit in the Secular Age* (London: Allen Lane, 1999).

24. Anonymous, *Compte moral et administratif du bureau de bienfaisance du 5e arrondissement de Paris, présenté par M. Vée, adjoint au maire, à l'assemblée générale tenue le 13 juillet 1843*, 17.

25. Administrators in her affluent *arrondissement* had recently earmarked funds for the terminally ill, one of the only such relief efforts in the country at that time.

26. Alexis Lefebvre, *La science de bien mourir, 2e partie. Annales de l'Association de la Bonne Mort . . . rédigées et mises en ordre par le R. P. Alexis Lefebvre*, 3 vols. (Paris: Cretté, 1865–1870).

27. The phenomenology and history of pain and pain medicine have been carefully scrutinized. Certain anthropologists have also explored suffering's personal consequences and sociopolitical dimensions. See Elaine Scarry, *The Body in Pain: The Making and Unmaking of the World* (Oxford: Oxford University Press, 1985); Roselyn Rey, *The History of Pain*, trans. Louise Elliot Wallace, J. A. Cadden, and S. W. Cadden (Cambridge, MA: Harvard University Press, 1995); Isabelle Baszanger, *Inventing Pain Medicine: From the Laboratory to the Clinic* (New Brunswick, NJ: Rutgers University Press, 1998); Arthur Kleinman, *The Illness Narratives: Suffering, Healing, and the Human Condition* (New York: Basic Books, 1988); Arthur Kleinman, Veena Das, and Margaret Lock, eds., *Social Suffering* (Berkeley: University of California Press, 1997); Paul Farmer, *Pathologies of Power: Health, Human Rights, and the New War on the Poor* (Berkeley: University of California Press, 2003).

28. Barbara Bates, *Bargaining for Life: A Social History of Tuberculosis, 1876–1938* (Philadelphia: University of Pennsylvania Press, 1992).

29. Dr. A. Jaumes, *Des maladies réputées incurables; des causes qui paraissent établir leur incurabilité; de la conduite du médecin dans le traitement de ces maladies* (Thèse de Concours, Montpellier, 1848), 127.

30. Charles E. Rosenberg, "The Bitter Fruit: Heredity, Disease and Social Thought," in *No Other Gods: On Science and American Social Thought*, 2nd ed. (Baltimore: Johns Hopkins University Press, 1997), 25–53; Charles E. Rosenberg, "Banishing Risk: Continuity and Change in the Moral Management of Disease," in *Morality and Health*, ed. Allan M. Brandt and Paul Rozin (London: Routledge, 1997), 35–51.

31. *Nouveau dictionnaire de médecine et de chirurgie pratique*, 1875, s.v. "Maladie," 468.

32. For but two examples, see Rosenberg, *The Cholera Years*, 15; Barnes, *The Making*, 138–73, 215–46.

33. Alexandre Brierre de Boismont, *Du suicide et de la folie suicidaire*, 2nd ed. (Paris: Baillière, 1865), 199–211.

34. John Harley Warner, *Against the Spirit of System: The French Impulse in Nineteenth-Century American Medicine* (Princeton, NJ: Princeton University Press, 1998).

35. Thomas A. Kselman, *Miracles and Prophecies in Nineteenth-Century France* (New Brunswick, NJ: Rutgers University Press, 1983).

## CHAPTER 1  "WHAT ARE HIS CHANCES, DOCTOR?": THE SEMANTICS OF INCURABILITY IN THE NINETEENTH CENTURY

1. This analysis builds on George Weisz's analysis of medical reasoning at the French Academy of Medicine. Weisz, *The Medical Mandarins: The French Academy of Medicine in the Nineteenth and Early Twentieth Centuries* (New York: Oxford University Press, 1995), 159–88.

2. Nineteenth-century contagionist/anti-contagionist debates, Margaret Pelling convincingly suggests, weren't as cut and dry as such mutually exclusive labels would suggest. Echoing Charles Rosenberg's observation about cholera in America, most British physicians adopted a position she calls "contingent contagionism." Borrowing from their nomenclature, one can reasonably say that most physicians viewed chronic progressive diseases as contingently (in)curable. Rosenberg, *The*

*Cholera Years*, 78; Margaret Pelling, *Cholera, Fever, and English Medicine, 1825–1865* (Oxford: Oxford University Press, 1978).

3. Jaumes, "Des maladies," 138.

4. Louis Fleury, *Traité pratique et raisonné d'hydrothérapie: recherches cliniques sur l'application de cette médication au traitement des congestions chroniques* (Paris: Labé, 1856), 347.

5. This reconstruction is based upon a reading of the leading French- and English-language monographs on tuberculosis and cancer. Several hundred works examining the (in)curability of chronic disease were also published in France during this period. Finally, I consulted most French medical theses that dealt with the treatment or prognosis of chronic disease between 1800 and 1910.

6. Anonymous, *Manuel des commissaires et dames de charité* (Paris: Mme Huzard, 1830), 13–14. The list of disorders granting access to Lyon's Hospice for Incurables included "paralysis, continuous tremors, incontinence, internal aneurysms, cancers, blindness, deformity, the loss of a member, mutilations, ulcers, grave and complete hernias." Olivier Faure, *Genèse de l'hôpital moderne: Les Hospices Civils de Lyon de 1802 à 1845* (Lyon: Presses Universitaires de Lyon, 1982), 242.

7. The best available definition (albeit from a slightly later period) stated that "an incurable illness is a slowly progressive chronic affliction caused by an organic lesion that we cannot hope to cure." Eugène Ravon, *Guide du médecin examinateur de l'assistance aux vieillards, infirmes, et incurables et du médecin inspecteur des enfants protégés et assistés et des écoles* (Paris: Berger-Levrault, 1911), 313. See also François-Joseph-Victor Broussais, *Cours de pathologie et de thérapeutique générales/professé à la Faculté de médecine de Paris par F.-J.V. Broussais; sténographié par M. Tasset; rédigé par P.-M. Gaubert, et revue par l'auteur* (Paris: Baillière, 1834), I: 155; Jaumes, "Des maladies," 7.

8. Fleury, *Traité pratique*, 86–87.

9. Joseph Marie Alfred Beni-Barde, *Traité théorique et pratique d'hydrothérapie comprenant les applications de la méthode hydrothérapeutique au traitement des maladies nerveuses et des maladies chroniques* (Paris: Masson, 1874), 293.

10. Jaumes, "Des maladies," 9, 12.

11. In 1803, Henri Michel Hounaud's official title was "Chef de clinique interne, et chef de clinique de perfectionnement pour les maladies réputées incurables" (c.f. endnote 62). In letters to the famous French actress Rachel, a former notary and a former traveling salesman both referred to tuberculosis as "reputedly incurable." Dr. Tampier, *Dernières heures de Rachel : Lettres qui lui ont été adressées sur sa maladie; examen des diverses médications préconisées contre la phthisie pulmonaire* (Paris: Labé, 1858), 31, 35.

12. Jaumes, *Des maladies*, 15–72.

13. Ibid., 53.

14. "A well-established agonizing state is the highest form of incurability and also the easiest to recognize." Jaumes, *Des maladies*, 81.

15. Marie-Joseph Pinel de Goville, for example, singled out four "incurable illnesses": phthisis, cancer, scrofula, and nervous diseases (chorea, epilepsy, and hysteria). Marie-Joseph Pinel de Goville, *Remarques sur les maladies réputées incurables et sur les moyens d'en obtenir la guérison* (Paris: Aniéré, 1862), 10–13. Psychiatrist Paul Moreau de Tours singled out five: cancer, tuberculosis, scrofula, epilepsy, and general

paresis. Paul Moreau de Tours, *Des pseudo-guérisons dans les maladies incurables* (Paris: Parent, 1877).

16. L. F. Gaillard, "Histoire générale des sept diathèses," *Gazette médicale de Paris* 1 (1846): 264.

17. A. Coural, "Comparer les affections diathésiques avec les maladies chroniques non diathésiques" (thèse de concours, Montpellier, 1872), 19–20.

18. Alfred Castan, *Traité élémentaire des diathèses* (Paris: Delahaye, 1867), 48.

19. Ibid., 186–87.

20. Gaillard, "Histoire général," 264.

21. By mid-century, cancer was deemed "more incurable" than tuberculosis, which was no longer judged inherently incurable. M. Barth, "Du diagnostic et de la curabilité du cancer, Séance du 3 octobre 1854," *Bulletin de l'académie impériale de médecine* 20 (1854–55): 12.

22. Jacalyn Duffin, *To See with a Better Eye: A Life of R.T.H. Laënnec* (Princeton, NJ: Princeton University Press, 1998), 67.

23. The term "heteromorphic" reflected the fact that these tissues had no equivalent in the normal human body.

24. René Théophile Hyacinthe Laënnec, *De l'auscultation médiate, ou, traité du diagnostic des maladies des poumons et du cœur: fondé principalement sur ce nouveau moyen d'exploration* (Paris: Brosson et Chaudé, 1819), 1: 59.

25. Hermann Lebert, *Traité pratique des maladies cancéreuses et des affections curables confondues avec le cancer* (Paris: Baillière, 1851), 4.

26. Dr. C. Rogée, "Essai sur la curabilité de la phthisie pulmonaire, ou recherches anatomico-pathologiques sur la transformation des tubercules et la cicatrisation des excavations tuberculeuses des poumons," *Archives générales de médecine, journal complémentaire des sciences médicales* 5 (1839): 191–209, 289–307, 460–76 (quote is from p. 191).

27. James Turnbull, *An Inquiry How Far Consumption Is Curable with Observations on the Treatment and on the Use of Cod-Liver Oil and Other Remedies, with Cases*, 2nd ed. (London: Churchill, 1850), 3.

28. "No one is unaware that we have just passed through a systematizing era [*une époque systématique*] where the prognosis of phthisis was resolutely declared fatal, always fatal; and this epoch coincides, it must be noted, with the era of so-called anatomico-pathological medicine." Jean Sales-Giron, "La curabilité de la phthisie," *La revue médicale française et étrangère* (1854): 129.

29. Aleksander Zurkowski, "Du degré d'utilité des exutoires permanents dans le traitement des maladies chroniques," *Mémoires de l'Académie impériale de médecine* 22 (1858): 501.

30. Augustin Grisolle, *Traité élémentaire et pratique de pathologie interne* (Paris: Fortin, 1844), 2: 483.

31. Louis-Auguste Rougier, *Rapport fait à la société de médecine de Lyon, le 15 juin 1835, au nom d'une commission chargée d'examiner les mémoires envoyés au concours pour les prix de l'année 1835* (Lyon, 1835), 7, 47.

32. Gaspard-Laurent Bayle, *Recherches sur la phthisie pulmonaire* (Paris: Gabon, 1810), 416.

33. *Dictionnaire des sciences médicales, par une société de médecins et chirurgiens*, s.v. "Cancer," 671.

34. Ibid., 673.

35. Duffin, *To See*, 268.

36. Elisabeth Williams, *A Cultural History of Medical Vitalism in Enlightenment Montpellier* (Aldershot: Ashgate, 2003).

37. *Dictionnaire des sciences médicales*, s.v. "Cancer," 672.

38. "When these illnesses are not hereditary, one does not find in their etiology this fatal rapport of cause and effect which characterizes [acute] illnesses." Coural, "Comparer," 23.

39. Ibid., 33.

40. Castan, *Traité élémentaire*, 30.

41. François Saint-Léger, "Essai sur la phthisie pulmonaire" (MD thesis, Paris, 1833), 14.

42. Broussais, *Histoire des phlégmasies*, 633.

43. Erwin H. Ackerknecht, *La médecine hospitalière à Paris*, translated from English by Françoise Blateau (Paris: Payot, 1986), 90, 102–4.

44. Broussais believed that he had recovered from tuberculosis. At his autopsy (which he requested), there was evidence of scarring in the right lung, apparently confirming his suspicion. Rogée, "Essai," 472.

45. John Pickstone, "Bureaucracy, Liberalism, and the Body in Post-Revolutionary France: Bichat's Physiology and the Paris School of Medicine," *History of Science* 19 (1981): 115–42. Jacques Léonard, *La médecine entre les pouvoirs et savoirs: Histoire intellectuelle et politique de la médecine française au XIXe siècle* (Paris: Aubier Montaigne, 1981), 118. Jean-François Braunstein, *Broussais et le matérialisme: Médecine et philosophie au XIXe siècle* (Paris: Méridiens Klincksieck, 1986), 192–95.

46. Braunstein, *Broussais*, 14–15.

47. Ibid., 186–200.

48. Duffin, *To See*, 82–90, 108, 240–45, 251–55.

49. Paul Broca, who believed that there existed an incurable cancerous diathesis, was a republican and a freethinker. For details on his life and work, see Francis Schiller, *Paul Broca: Founder of French Anthropology, Explorer of the Brain* (Berkeley: University of California Press, 1979).

50. Ibid., 4.

51. Pierre Jérôme Sébastien Téallier, *Du cancer de la matrice: De ses causes, de son diagnostic et de son traitement* (Paris: Baillière), 33–34.

52. René Théophile Hyacinthe Laënnec, *Traité de l'auscultation médiate et des maladies des poumons et du cœur*, 2nd ed. (Paris: J.-S. Chaudé, 1826), I: xxi.

53. Frédéric Duparcque, *Réfutation de la doctrine d'inévitabilité et d'incurabilité du cancer* (Paris: Le Normant, 1837), 5.

54. Horace de Montègre, *Notice historique sur la vie, les travaux, les opinions médicales et philosophiques de F.-J.-V. Broussais précédé de sa profession de foi, et suivie des discours prononcés sur sa tombe* (Paris: Baillière, 1839), 128. The quote is from Broussais, *Histoire des phlégmasies*, 2nd ed., I: xiii.

55. Broussais, *Histoires des phlégmasies*, I: 458.

56. Broussais, *Cours de pathologie*, 4: 401.

57. Ibid., 1: 68.

58. Michel Joseph Maire Richard, "Dissertation sur les erreurs populaires relatives à la médecine, et leurs dangers" (MD thesis, Paris, 1833), 6.

59. Tampier, Dernières heures, 12.

60. Léonard, La médicine, 24.

61. Charles-Louis Dumas, Doctrine des maladies chroniques, pour servir de fondement à la connaissance théorique et pratique de ces maladies (Paris: Déterville, 1812).

62. Henry-Michel Hounau, "Quelques recherches sur les principales sources des maladies chroniques" (MD thesis, Montpellier, 1807), 20.

63. Broussais, Cours de pathologie, 2: 619.

64. René Laënnec, Traité de l'auscultation mediate, et des maladies des poumons et du cœur, 4th ed. (Paris: J.-S. Chaudé, 1837), 2: 258.

65. At a large medical conference, one orator called Laënnec "a fervent believer in the curability of tuberculosis." Dr. Gourdin, "Sur la curabilité de la pthisie pulmonaire,"Congrès médical de France, 2e session tenue à Lyons de 26 septembre au 1er octobre (Paris: Baillière, 1864), 122.

66. Laënnec, Traité de l'auscultation, 2nd ed., 1: 704–5.

67. Ibid, 123–24.

68. Duffin, To See, 235–39.

69. Broussais, Cours de pathologie, 4: 401.

70. Laënnec, Traité de l'auscultation, 2nd ed., 1: 703–4.

71. Ibid., 704. See also Dictionnaire universel de matière médicale et de thérapeutique générale, s.v. "Anti-phthisiques," 328.

72. Laënnec, Traité de l'auscultation, 2nd ed., 1: 707.

73. François Saint-Léger, "Essai sur la phthisie pulmonaire" (MD thesis, Paris, 1833), 32.

74. Terence D. Murphy, "Medical Knowledge and Statistical Methods in Early Nineteenth-Century France," Medical History 25 (1981): 310, 315.

75. J. Rosser Matthews, Quantification and the Quest for Medical Certainty (Princeton, NJ: Princeton University Press, 1995), 31–32.

76. Murphy, "Medical Knowledge," 318.

77. Matthews, Quantification, 5, 70–85.

78. Ibid., 21–22, 26–29, 37, 67–68.

79. Matthews, Quantification, 66; Weisz, The Medical Mandarins, 159–88.

80. Pierre Charles Alexandre Louis, Recherches anatomiques, pathologiques et thérapeutiques sur la phthisie, 2nd ed. (Paris: Baillière, 1843), 651.

81. Alfred Velpeau, Traité des maladies des seins et de la région mammaire (Paris: Masson, 1854), 550.

82. Broussais, Cours de pathologie, 4: 400.

83. Stanislaus Tanchou, Recherches sur le traitement médical des tumeurs cancéreuses du sein, ouvrage pratique basé sur trois cents observations (extraites d'un grand nombre d'auteurs), avec . . . une statistique sur la fréquence de ces maladies (Paris: Baillière, 1844).

84. Velpeau, Traité des maladies, 563–64.

85. Grisolle, Traité élémentaire, 2: 484–85.

86. *Dictionnaire des sciences médicales*, s.v. "Cancer," 565, 576–77.

87. Weisz, *Medical Mandarins*, xiii.

88. Jean Cruveilhier, "Mémoire sur les corps fibreux de la mamelle. Séance du 9 janvier 1844," *Bulletin de l'académie royale de médecine* 9 (1843–44): 336–38; Roux, "Suite de la discussion du Mémoire de M. Cruveilhier relatif aux tumeurs des mamelles. Séance du 30 janvier 1844," *Bulletin de l'académie royale de médecine* 9 (1843–44): 380, 385.

89. Cruveilhier, "Mémoire de M. Cruveilhier concernant les tumeurs des mamelles, Séance du 23 janvier 1844," *Bulletin de l'académie royale de médecine* 9 (1843–44): 367; Moreau, "Mémoire de M. Cruveilhier concernant les tumeurs des mamelles. Séance du 16 janvier 1844," *Bulletin de l'académie royale de médecine* 9 (1843–44): 367–68; Blandin, "Suite de la discussion du Mémoire de M. Cruveilhier relatif aux tumeurs des mamelles. Séance du 5 mars 1844," *Bulletin de l'académie royale de médecine* 9 (1843–44): 511.

90. *Bulletin de l'académie royale de médecine* 9 (1843–44): 359, 388–89, 391, 495–96, 606.

91. J. Z. Amussat, "Suite de la discussion du Mémoire de M. Cruveilhier concernant les tumeurs de la mamelle. Séance du 13 février 1844," *Bulletin de l'académie royale de médecine* 9 (1843–44): 438.

92. "Those of my honorable colleagues who believed that I was bringing an accusation against surgeons who had adopted the doctrine of removing all tumors of the mamma that were not susceptible to resolution have sorely misunderstood my words. I accuse the inadequacies of science, and that's all; as to the practitioners, I respect them, I honor them. I may believe them to be in error, under an illusion, but I never believed in the ill faith of a physician or surgeon penetrated with the dignity of our profession." Cruveilhier, "Suite de la discussion du Mémoire de M. Cruveilhier concernant les tumeurs de la mamelle. Séance du 27 février 1844," *Bulletin de l'académie royale de médecine* 9 (1843–44): 497.

93. Roux, "Suite de la discussion du Mémoire de M. Cruveilhier concernant les tumeurs des mamelles. Séance du 26 mars 1844," *Bulletin de l'académie royale de médecine* 9 (1843–44): 589.

94. Velpeau, "Suite de la discussion du Mémoire de M. Cruveilhier concernant les tumeurs des mamelles. Séance du 26 mars 1844," *Bulletin de l'académie royale de médecine* 9 (1843–44): 647.

95. Desportes, "Suite de la Discussion du Mémoire de M. Cruveilhier concernant les tumeurs des mamelles. Séance du 26 mars 1844," *Bulletin de l'académie royale de médecine* 9 (1843–44): 613.

96. Roux, "Suite de la discussion du Mémoire de M. Cruveilhier relatif aux tumeurs des mamelles. Séance du 30 janvier 1844," *Bulletin de l'académie royale de médecine* 9 (1843–44): 377.

97. These debates were covered in both the French and international medical press, and authors' opinions mirrored those of the principal protagonists. It even made it into local medical presses. See, for instance, Anonymous, "Discussion on the Diagnosis of Cancer in the French Academy of Medicine," *Buffalo Medical Journal* 13 (1857–58): 73–90.

98. *Nouveau dictionnaire de médecine et de chirurgie pratiques*, s.v. "Cancer," 131.

99. Roux noted that even statistical evidence couldn't settle the matter as partisans on both sides would only record favorable cases. Roux, "Suite de la Discussion du

mémoire de M. Cruveilhier relatif aux tumeurs de la mamelle. Séance du 30 janvier 1844," *Bulletin de l'académie royale de médecine* 9 (1843–44): 404–5.

100. Velpeau, "Du diagnostic et de la curabilité du cancer. Séance du 7 septembre 1854," *Bulletin de l'académie impériale de médecine* 20 (1854–55): 184.

101. Robert, "Du diagnostic et de la curabilité du cancer. Séance du 10 octobre 1854," *Bulletin de l'académie impériale de médecine* 20 (1854–55): 21–25.

102. Velpeau, "Suite de la Discussion du mémoire de M. Cruveilhier relatif aux tumeurs des mamelles. Seance du 23 janvier 1844," *Bulletin de l'académie royale de médecine* 9 (1843–44): 363.

103. The idea that there exists "thought styles within communities," first proposed by Ludwig Fleck and sharpened by subsequent generations of medical sociologists and historians, posits that the community in which one is trained and continues to work decisively influences one's perception of reality.

104. Velpeau, "Du diagnostic et de la curabilité du cancer. Séance du 16 janvier 1855," *Bulletin de l'académie impériale de médecine* 20 (1854–55): 443–44.

105. For a compelling account of patient decision making, see Susan Garfinkel, "This Trial Was Sent in Love and Mercy for My Refinement": A Quaker Woman's Experience of Breast Cancer Surgery in 1814," in *Women and Health in America*, ed. Judith Walzer Leavitt, 2nd ed. (Madison: University of Wisconsin Press, 1999), 68–90; Susan Emlen's case is also examined in Robert A. Aronowitz, *Unnatural History: Breast Cancer and American Society* (Cambridge: Cambridge University Press, 2007), 21–50.

106. Velpeau, *Traité des maladies*, 656.

107. *Dictionnaire encyclopédique des sciences médicales*, s.v. "Carcinome," 407.

108. An early twentieth-century observer insisted that Velpeau had "preached in vain." René Ledoux-Lebard, *La lutte contre le cancer* (M.D. thesis, Paris, 1906), 28.

109. Dr. Denis de Saint-Pierre, *Petit manuel des prétendus incurables* (Paris: A. Appert, 1866), 8–9.

110. Dr. Després, "Récidive, un squirrhe du sein neuf ans seulement après la première opération," *Mémoires et Bulletins de la société de chirurgie de Paris* 7 (1881): 532–33.

111. "Marjolin and Boyer, and most of our masters, came to sanction it (the surgical incurability of cancer) in their mature years." Robert, "Du diagnostic et de la curabilité du cancer," *Bulletin de l'académie impériale de médecine* 20 (1854–55): 370.

112. E. Garreau, "Considérations pratiques sur le cancer," *Revue médicale française et étrangère* 3 (1846): 26.

113. J. Benoit, "Principes de traitement des tumeurs cancéreuses," *Montpellier médical* 7 (July–December 1861): 317.

114. Jean-Baptiste Fonssagrives, *Thérapeutique de la phtisie pulmonaire basée sur les indications, 2e édition révisée avec soin et précédée d'une introduction sur la doctrine de Laënnec en regard des travaux récents sur la phthisie pulmonaire* (Paris: Baillière, 1880), vii–viii.

115. Broussias's fall from grace, it was noted, "cannot but carry along all the discouraged souls and lead them to embrace a skepticism that reason and morality together condemn." Maximillien Simon, *Déontologie médicale ou des devoirs et des droits des médecins dans l'état actuel de la civilisation* (Paris: Baillière, 1845), 112–13.

116. Augustin Grisolle, *Traité de pathologie interne*, 9th ed. (Paris: Masson, 1869), 2: 552.

117. Raoul Le Roy, *Guérit-on la phthisie? Par quels moyens?* (Paris: Masson, 1875), 57.

118. Hermann Pidoux, *Études générales et pratiques sur la phthisie* (Paris: Asselin, 1873), 508–9.

119. For one example, see J. Cossy, "Mémoire sur le traitement par les préparations alcalines, jointes à une température élevée et chargées de vapeurs amoniacales," *Archives générales de médecine, journal complémentaire des sciences médicales* 6 (1844): 431–54.

120. Fonssagrives, *Thérapeutique*, 74–75.

121. Dr. E. Quintard, "Forces morales médicatrices" (MD thesis, Paris, 1875), 30.

122. Léon Vallée (et un bibliophile ami), *La Sarabande ou choix d'anecdotes, bons mots, chansons, gauloiseries, épigrammes, réflexions et pièces en vers des français depuis le XVe siècle jusqu'à nos jours* (Paris: H. Welter, 1903), 301.

123. After the tubercle bacillus was identified, physicians began searching for and supposedly discovering the micro-organism that caused cancer. Eugène Louis Doyen, *Étiologie et le traitement du cancer* (Paris: Maloine, 1904).

124. Pidoux, *Études générales*, 243.

125. Ibid., 140.

126. Most commentators agreed that, contingencies aside, "true incurability is that which, in the present state of science, resists even the most competent care." Jaumes, *Des maladies*, 63.

127. Rogée, "Essai," 191–92.

128. "This word *reputedly* expresses more than doubt. It is a type of *fiction* provisionally admitted for the needs of the moment." Jaumes, "Des maladies," 12–14 (emphasis in original).

## CHAPTER 2    REINVENTING HOPE IN THE LATE NINETEENTH CENTURY

1. Dr. J. Benoit approvingly noted that this question "almost entirely abandoned as fatally resolved in favour of death, reappears virginal and attractive in the eyes of practitioners." Benoit, "Principes du traitement," 326.

2. A. Jaumes, "Des maladies," 57.

3. Fonssagrives, *Thérapeutique*, 12–13.

4. Lion Murard and Patrick Zylberman, *L'hygiène dans la République: La santé publique ou l'utopie contrariée 1870–1918* (Paris: Fayard, 1996), 498–500.

5. For a brief but cogent discussion of medical "essentialism" (i.e., that consumption was part of a person's essence), see Barnes, *The Making*, 26–30. The importance of medical constitutionalism and the diatheses within American medicine have been explored by several authors. So too has their professional and sociopolitical valence (which differed along sectional lines). Rosenberg, *No Other Gods*, 25–53; Georgina D. Feldberg, *Disease and Class: Tuberculosis and the Shaping of Modern North American Society* (New Brunswick, NJ: Rutgers University Press, 1995), 11–35; Katherine Ott, *Fevered Lives: Tuberculosis in American Culture since 1870* (Cambridge, MA: Harvard University Press, 1996), 6–19.

6. Coural, "Comparer," 9.

7. Maxime Durand-Fardel, *Leçon d'ouverture du cours sur les eaux minérales et les maladies chroniques, professée à l'École Pratique* (Paris: O. Douin, 1888), 12–13.

8. *Nouveau dictionnaire de médecine et de chirurgie pratiques*, s.v. "Diathèse," 446.

9. Victor Trinquier, "Des diathèses; l'état actuel des sciences médicales est-il favorable ou défavorable à leur admission?" (thèse de concours, Montpellier, 1836), 43.

10. John Harley Warner, *The Therapeutic Perspective: Medical Practice, Knowledge, and Identity in America, 1820–1885* (Cambridge, MA: Harvard University Press, 1986), 235–57.

11. *Nouveau dictionnaire de médecine et de chirurgie pratiques*, s.v. "Maladie," 474.

12. Ibid., 412.

13. Jean-Jacques Yvorel, *Les poisons de l'esprit: Drogues et drogués au 19e siècle* (Paris: Quai Voltaire, 1992), 76.

14. Jaumes, *Des maladies*, 58–59.

15. Laënnec accorded heredity a significant though secondary role, mostly because it didn't satisfy his exacting criteria for determining causality. Duffin, *To See*, 162.

16. Téallier, *Du cancer de la matrice*, 40–41.

17. François Saint-Léger, "Essai sur la phthisie pulmonaire" (MD thesis, Paris, 1833), 14.

18. Coural, "Comparer," 41–42.

19. Daniel Pick, *Faces of Degeneration: A European Disorder, circa 1848–1918* (Cambridge: Cambridge University Press, 1993).

20. Apollinaire Bourchardat, "De l'étiologie et de la prophylaxie de la tuberculisation pulmonaire," *Supplément à l'Annuaire de thérapeutique* 21 (1861).

21. Pidoux, *Études*, 519.

22. René-Marie Briau, *Sur quelques difficultés de diagnostic dans les maladies chroniques des organes pulmonaires: Mémoire lue à la société d'hydrologie médicale de Paris dans la séance du 7 mars 1859* (Paris: Masson, 1859).

23. "We might think that physicians, like hydrologists, who partly provide care to the privileged classes, and who, besides that, have at their disposal a therapeutic agent whose action, which acts upon the entire organism, should seemingly be so powerful against as formally a diathesic an illness as phthisis, should be converts to the doctrine of curability. This is not the case, however, and I could point to unbelievers among my most distinguished colleagues." Dr Desnos, "De la curabilité de la phthisie pulmonaire," *Congres médico-chirurgical de France 1e session tenue à Rouen du 30 septembre au 3 octobre 1863* (Paris: Baillière, 1863), 255.

24. In the 1830s, some argued that the diatheses offered an alluring therapeutic target. Maximillien Simon, "L'admission des différentes diathèses des anciens est d'une grande valeur en thérapeutique," *Bulletin général de thérapeutique* 10 (1836): 105–10.

25. Douglas Peter Mackaman, *Leisure Settings: Bourgeois Culture, Medicine, and the Spa in Modern France* (Chicago: University of Chicago Press, 1998), 44–46, 86–96, 99–101, 121.

26. Tampier, *Dernières heures de Rachel*, 96.

27. Sigismond Jaccoud, *Leçons de clinique médicale faites à l'hôpital de la Charité* (Paris: Delahaye, 1867), 153.

28. Le Roy, *Guérit-on la phthisie?*, 3.

29. Castan, *Traité élémentaire*, 124.

30. "One must never abandon the struggle, one must always rouse oneself to hope, even in those cases which appear most discouraging." Noel Gueneau de Mussy, *Leçons cliniques sur les causes et le traitement de la tuberculisation pulmonaire* (Paris: Delahaye, 1860), 53. See also Zurkowski, "Du degré d'utilité," 496.

31. Prosper de Pietra Santa, *Traitement rationnel de la phtisie pulmonaire* (Paris: O. Doin, 1875), 1–2.

32. Michael Worboys, *Spreading Germs: Disease Theories and Medical Practice in Britain 1865–1900* (New York: Cambridge University Press, 2000), 200.

33. "Does it not seem, sirs, that we are far from Laënnec and Virchow? We affirm the natural curability of the tubercle; we affirm that instead of being a miserable neoplasm incapable of organisation, the tubercle tends naturally to fibrous organisation." Joseph Grancher, *Maladies de l'appareil respiratoire. Tuberculose et auscultation* (Paris: Octave Doin, 1890), 245.

34. Grisolle, *Traité de pathologie interne*, 9th ed., 2: 539–40.

35. "If personally I cannot yet be certain to have seen phthisis cured, I am no less convinced of the doctrine of curability." Desnos, "De la curabilité," 256.

36. "Not only can phthisis be cured, gentlemen, but it can be cured in all of its degrees. It would be easy for me, by consulting my memory, to find numerous facts to support this proposition." Gueneau de Mussy, *Leçons cliniques*, 56. A few years later, Dr. Hugues presented ten cures from his practice and that of several other hydro-therapists, before describing the evidence as "imposing." Dr. Hugues, "Guérison de la phtisie," *Congres médico-chirurgical de France, 2e session tenue à Lyon de 26 septembre au 1er octobre 1864* (Paris: Baillière, 1865), 133–47.

37. Georges Daremberg, *Traitement de la phtisie pulmonaire* (Paris J. Rueff, 1892), 10–11.

38. Rothman, *Living in the Shadow of Death*, 148–60.

39. Le Roy, *Guérit-on la phtisie?* 19–20, 33.

40. Castan, *Traité élémentaire*, 124.

41. Sigismond Jaccoud, *Curabilité et traitement de la phthisie pulmonaire: Leçons cliniques faites à la Faculté de médecine* (Paris: Delahaye et Lecrosnier, 1881), 16.

42. M. le Professeur Boudant, "Du traitement de la phtisie par les eaux minérales," *Congres médico-chirurgical de France, 2e session tenue à Lyon du 26 septembre au 1er octobre 1864* (Paris: Baillière, 1865), 199.

43. Fonssagrives, *Thérapeutique*, xxii.

44. Desnos, "De la curabilité," 258–59.

45. Describing his "curative" treatment, Piorry noted that "of one hundred *pneumophymiques* submitted to the treatment indicated in this paper, there were perhaps eighty where the improvement was very marked, in whom life was prolonged from a few weeks to a few years." Pierre Adolphe Piorry, *Mémoire sur la curabilité et le traitement de la phthisie pulmonaire et des tubercules* (Paris: Baillière, 1859), 14–15.

46. Jaccoud, *Curabilité*, 178.

47. Ibid., 39–40.

48. Pidoux, *Études*, 391.

49. "To conclude as to the arrest of the tuberculous process, a period of calm does not suffice; it is necessary that a long time, two or three years at least, pass without the

slightest recrudescence, in an excellent general state of health, in which the local state [of the lung] is progressively improving." Grancher, *Maladies*, 471.

50. Daremberg, *Traitement*, 21–22.

51. Benjamin Verdo, *Le charlatanisme et les charlatans en médecine: Étude psychologique* (Paris: Baillière, 1867), 37–41.

52. Pidoux, *Études*, 347.

53. Grancher, *Maladies*, 246.

54. Pierre Charles Alexandre Louis, *Recherches anatomiques, pathologiques et thérapeutiques sur la phthisie*, 2nd ed. (Paris: Baillière, 1843), 574, 656 (quote is from p. 574).

55. Gueneau de Mussy, *Leçons*, 29–32.

56. Pidoux, *Études*, 364–68. Like many of those who spoke up, Pidoux was a practicing hydrotherapist. Although there were pockets of incredulity within elite medicine, hydrotherapy was not part of the lunatic fringe. Various practitioners, including Pidoux, were members of the Academy of Medicine. This body also took the field seriously; it established a permanent commission on mineral waters in 1823. A chair in hydrotherapy was also established at the Paris Medical School. Importantly, there were no significant differences of opinion between spa physicians and the medical, or surgical, mainstream when it came to either tuberculosis or cancer. For an overview of medical hydrology, see Weisz, *Medical Mandarins*, 137–58.

57. Jaccoud, *Curabilité*, 35, 108–9 (quote is from pp. 108–9).

58. Grancher, *Maladies*, 144–69 (quote is from p. 169; emphasis is in the original).

59. Ibid., 315–16, 369–71.

60. Ibid., 367–68.

61. Maurice Letulle, "Preface," in Éliseé Ribard, *La tuberculose est curable, moyens de la reconnaître et de la guérir. Instructions pratiques à l'usage des familles* (Paris: G. Carée et C. Naud, 1900), vi.

62. Ibid., 93–94, 98–99 (quote is from pp. 93–94).

63. Grancher, *Maladies*, 367.

64. Georges Daremberg, *Les différentes formes cliniques et sociales de la tuberculose pulmonaire: Pronostic, diagnostic, traitement* (Paris: Masson, 1905), 66.

65. Thomas Mann, *The Magic Mountain: A Novel* (New York: Knopf, 1996).

66. Joseph Castri, "Du traitement palliatif du cancer du col ulcéré de l'utérus et en particulier de l'emploi d'une préparation spéciale d'iodoforme" (MD thesis, Paris, 1883), 6.

67. Verneuil, *Gazette Hebdomadaire de médecine et de chirurgie* 39, no. 11 (March 12, 1892): 148–49.

68. Ornealla Moscucci, *The Science of Woman: Gynaecology and Gender in England, 1800–1929* (Cambridge: Cambridge University Press, 1990), 137, 143–44, 152–60.

69. Wendy Mitchinson, "Gynecological Operations on Insane Women: London, Ontario, 1895–1901," *Journal of Social History* 15 (2001): 467–84; Barbara Ehrenreich and Deirdre English, *For Her Own Good: 150 Years of the Experts' Advice to Women* (Garden City, NY: Anchor Books, 1978); Andrea Tone, *Devices and Desires: A History of Contraception in America* (New York: Hill and Wang, 2001); Emily Martin, *The Woman in the Body: A Cultural Analysis of Reproduction* (Boston: Beacon Press, 1987); Ann Douglas Wood, "The Fashionable Diseases: Women's Complaints and Their Treatment in Nineteenth-Century America," *Journal of Interdisciplinary History* 4, no. 1 (Summer 1973): 25–52.

70. James Murphy, "The Influence of Surgery on Gynaecology," *Provincial Medical Journal* 10 (1891): 404.

71. Émile Forgue, "Cancer du col," in *Nouveau traité de chirurgie*, vol. 34 *Gynécologie*, ed. Auguste Le Dentu and Pierre Delbet (Paris: Bailliere, 1916), 353.

72. Professeur Koberlé (de Strasbourg), "Traitements des cancers de la matrice par l'hystérotomie," *Gazette hebdomadaire de médecine et de chirurgie* 23, no. 9 (26 February 1886): 140.

73. Després, "Discussion," *Bulletins et mémoires de la société de chirurgie de Paris* 14 (1887): 747–49.

74. Dr. A. Reeves Jackson, "The Modern Treatment of Cancer of the Uterus," in *Transactions of the International Medical Conference, Ninth Session*, ed. John B. Hamilton, 799–800 (Washington, DC: Fell, 1887). His views circulated in France. See Adrien Pozzi, "Le traitement du cancer de l'utérus (en dehors de la grossesse)" (MD thesis, Paris, 1888), 59.

75. M. Bouilly, "Suite de la discussion sur l'hystérectomie vaginale contre le cancer utérin," *Bulletins et mémoires de la société de chirurgie de Paris* 17 (1891): 711; Joseph Auclair, "De l'hystérectomie abdominale totale dans le traitement du cancer de l'utérus" (MD thesis, Paris, 1899), 79.

76. Jackson, "The Modern Treatment," 798.

77. Félix Terrier, "Discussion sur l'hystérectomie vaginale contre le cancer utérin," *Bulletins et mémoires de la société de chirurgie de Paris* 17 (1891): 666.

78. Renée C. Fox and Judith P. Swazey, *The Courage to Fail: A Social View of Organ Transplants and Dialysis* (Chicago: University of Chicago Press, 1974).

79. Gynecologists fell into one of three camps: conservatives, moderates, and radicals. Regina Morantz-Sanchez, *Conduct Unbecoming a Woman: Medicine on Trial in Turn-of-the-Century Brooklyn* (New York: Oxford University Press, 1999), 105–11, 129, 196, 201–3.

80. Louis-Gustave Richelot, "Suite de la discussion sur l'hystérectomie vaginale contre le cancer utérin," *Bulletins et mémoires de la société de chirurgie de Paris* 17 (1891): 714.

81. Charles Émile Lairé, "Des résultats éloignés de l'hystérectomie vaginale totale dans le cancer de l'utérus" (MD thesis, Paris, 1896), 166–67.

82. Léon Le Fort, "Sur le concours pour le Prix de l'Académie en 1887. Séance du 29 novembre," *Bulletin de l'Académie de Médecine* (1887): 663–64. See also Morantz-Sanchez, *Conduct*, 106.

83. Morantz-Sanchez, *Conduct*, 72–78, 80, 152–53, 161–62, 185, 201, 209–210.

84. Richelot, "Hystérectomie vaginale suivie de mort," *Bulletins et mémoires de l'Académie de Chirurgie de Paris* 12 (1885): 746–50.

85. Richelot, "Note sur l'hystérectomie vaginale," *Bulletins et mémoires de la société de chirurgie de Paris* 14 (1887): 151.

86. Fox and Swazey, *The Courage to Fail*, 2nd ed., 1978, especially 71–73, 81–82, 108–34.

87. Alfred Henri Marchand, "Note sur la valeur thérapeutique de l'hystérectomie vaginale dans le traitement du cancer utérin," *Bulletins et mémoires de la société de chirurgie de Paris* 18 (1892): 67.

88. Richelot, "L'hystérectomie vaginale contre le cancer utérin," *Bulletins et mémoires de la société de chirurgie de Paris* 17 (1891): 629.

89. Lairé, "Des résultats," 27.

90. Aronowitz, *Unnatural History*, 90–92, 95–96.

91. Richelot, "L'hystérectomie vaginale contre le cancer utérin," *Bulletins et mémoires de la société de chirurgie de Paris* (28 October 1891): 623.

92. Richelot, "Suite de la discussion sur l'hystérectomie vaginale contre le cancer utérin," *Bulletins et mémoires de la société de chirurgie de Paris* 17 (1891): 713–14.

93. Charles Monod, "Enseignement complémentaire et éducation du public," *Travail de la 2e conférence internationale pour l'étude du cancer tenue à Paris du 1er au 5 octobre 1910* (Paris: Alcan, 1911), 26.

94. Gueneau de Mussy, *Leçons*, 2.

95. Jaccoud, *Curabilité*, 69. Grancher, *Maladies*, 469–70.

96. Pidoux, *Études*, 512–14.

97. Ribard, *La tuberculose*, 11.

98. Daremberg, *Traitement*, 4–5

99. Jean Baptiste François Étienne Lefevre, "Quelques idées sur la médecine en général tendant à prouver son utilité" (MD thesis, Paris, 1833), 22–23.

100. John Christopher Feutdner, *Bittersweet: Diabetes, Insulin, and the Transformation of Illness* (Chapel Hill: University of North Carolina Press, 2003).

101. Georges Dujardin-Beaumetz, "Sur la prophylaxie de la tuberculose. Séance du 6 août 1889," *Bulletin de l'Académie de Médecine* 22 (1889): 126. "One must combat to the bitter end the opinion of people, still too numerous, that one cannot cure pulmonary phthisis." Daremberg, *Les différentes formes*, 249.

102. Physicians apparently rarely found evidence of healing in autopsies of hospital patients, something Daremberg ascribed to rampant alcoholism. Daremberg, *Les différentes formes*, 300–301.

103. Charles E. Rosenberg, "The Therapeutic Revolution: Medicine, Meaning, and Social Change in Nineteenth-Century America," *Perspectives in Biology and Medicine* 20 (1977): 3–25.

104. Paul Farmer, "Social Scientists and the New Tuberculosis," *Social Sciences of Medicine* 44, no. 3 (February 1997): 347–58. Explaining treatment failure has also been a key issue with AIDS. S. Grabar et al., "Factors Associated with Clinical and Virological Failure in Patients Receiving a Triple Therapy Including a Protease Inhibitor," *AIDS* 14, no. 2 (January 28, 2000): 141–49.

105. Ravon, *Guide du médecin*, 309–10.

106. Anonymous, "Communication du Président," *Bulletin de la société médicale des médecins des bureaux de bienfaisance de Paris* 55 (March 1907): 69.

107. Ravon, *Guide du médecin*, 302, 358, 385. Compensated chronic endocarditis could be scored anywhere from of 10–50 percent; a stomach ulcer, 5–75 percent; deafness 15–25 percent; varicose veins 20–33 percent. Doctors could also consider secondary diagnoses (i.e., varicose veins) in the final tally. The entire scoring system can be found in Ravon, *Guide du médecin*, 415–19.

## CHAPTER 3 "I TOLD YOU SO":
## THE RHYME AND REASON OF CHRONIC DISEASE

1. "Every being is endowed with a divine direction or instinct, which is, is a manner, interwoven with its proper essence, whereby it removes those ills from itself. And this is manifest in the natural termination of many *acute diseases* (which

generally proceed from God, as chronic ones do from ourselves)." John Swan, *The entire works of FDr. Thomas Sydenham, newly made English from the originals: . . . To which are added, explanatory and practical notes, from the best medicinal writers; with others by the translator. . . . The fifth edition, with all the notes inserted in the proper places* (London: F. Newbury, 1769), 385–86. Sydenham's ideas were approvingly cited in Coural, "Comparer," 46–47, and Pidoux, *Études*, 538.

2. James Paget, *Lectures on Tumours, Delivered at the Royal College of Surgeons of England* (London: Longman, Brown, and Green, 1853), 2: 618–19.

3. Rosenberg, "Banishing Risk," 35–51.

4. Paul-Louis Gastou, *Hygiène sociale, contribution à la lutte contre la causes de la dégénérescence de l'espèce humaine et les maladies qui la provoquent (alcoolisme, cancer, syphilis, tuberculose* (Le Havre: Imprimerie du commerce, 1900), II.

5. Hounau, "Quelques recherches," i–iii.

6. M. Léraillé, "Discours pour l'inauguration de l'Hôpital des Incurables d'Amiens, prononcé à l'Église Cathédrale" (Amiens: Imprimerie de Caron-Vitet, 1829), 9–10.

7. Rosenberg, *No Other Gods*, 38–39.

8. Castan, *Traité*, 15–16.

9. Hubert Lauvergne, *De l'agonie et de la mort dans toutes les classes de la société, sous le rapport humanitaire, physiologique, et religieux* (Paris: Baillière, 1842), 2: 430.

10. Charles E. Rosenberg, "Pathologies of Progress: The Idea of Civilization as Risk," *Bulletin of the History of Medicine* 72 (1998): 714–30.

II. Jean-Louis-Marie Alibert, *Clinique de l'hôpital Saint-Louis ou traité complet des maladies de la peau, contenant la description et leurs meilleurs modes de traitement* (Paris: Cormon et Blanc, 1833), 193, 204.

12. Tanchou, *Recherches sur le traitement médical*, iii.

13. Robert N. Proctor, *Cancer Wars: How Politics Shapes What We Know and Don't Know about Cancer* (New York: Basic Books, 1995), 16–34.

14. Bertillon, "Documents relatifs à l'anthropologie de l'Afrique australe (Extraits du voyage du docteur Livingstone)," *Bulletin de la société d'anthropologie de Paris* I, no. I (1859–60): 221–49; M. Berchon, "Documents sur le Sénégal," *Bulletin de la société d'anthropologie de Paris* I, no. I (1859–60): 519–34; Dr. Landry, "Document sur le Canada," *Bulletin de la société d'anthropologie de Paris* 2, no. I (1861): 12–18. In a survey of recent gynecological literature from 1879, it was noted that "cancerous affections are rare in female negroes," *Bulletin de la société d'anthropologie de Paris* 2 (1879): 615.

15. Patterson, *The Dread Disease*, 79, 185, 271–72.

16. Hermann Lebert, *Traité clinique et pratique de la phthisie pulmonaire et des maladies tuberculeuses des divers organes* (Paris: V. Adrien Delahaye, 1879), 28.

17. Broussais, *Cours de pathologie*, 2: 568, 4: 398–99 (quote is from pp. 4: 398–99).

18. Peter, *Leçons*, 2: 383.

19. This has been carefully documented by a large number of historians. See, for example, Guillaume, *"Du désespoir au salut*, 155–69; Barnes, *The Making*, 141–48; Feldberg, *Disease and Class*, 29–33.

20. Paul Laignel-Lavastine, "La psychologie des tuberculeux," *Revue de médecine* 27 (1907): 244.

21. Aimé Hubert Gouget, "Du malade ou de l'importance de son étude" (MD thesis, Paris, 1833), 14–15.

22. Tampier, *Dernières heures de Rachel*, 49.

23. J. Andrew Mendelsohn, "Medicine and the Making of Bodily Inequality in Twentieth-Century Europe," in *Heredity and Infection: The History of Disease Transmission*, ed. Jean-Paul Gaudillière and Ilana Löwy (London: Routledge, 2001), 21–79.

24. Gueneau de Mussy, *Leçons*, 7–8.

25. J. G. de Bonqueval, *Traité théorique et pratique de l'électro-homéopathie. Système Sauter ou nouvelles thérapeutique guérissant d'après des principes certains les maladies chroniques et aiguës et même celle réputées incurables* (Paris: Jacques Lecavalier, Paris, 1885), 131.

26. Rosenberg, "Bitter Fruit," 42.

27. Rosenberg, "Banishing Risk," 37–39, 44.

28. Lauvergne, *De l'agonie*, 2: 110–14.

29. Roy Porter and G. S. Rousseau, *Gout: The Patrician Malady* (New Haven: Yale University Press, 1998).

30. Pidoux, *Études*, 533.

31. Peter, *Leçons*, 2: 406.

32. Allan Brandt, *No Magic Bullet: A Social History of Venereal Disease in the United States since 1880* (New York: Oxford University Press, 1985).

33. Barnes, *The Making*, 138–73.

34. Alain Corbin, *Women for Hire: Prostitution and Sexuality in France after 1850* (Cambridge, MA: Harvard University Press, 1990).

35. Antoine Portal, *Considérations sur la nature et le traitement de quelques maladies héréditaires ou de famille* (Paris: Baudouin, 1808), 36–43.

36. Jean-Louis-Marie Alibert, *Précis théorique sur les maladies de la peau* (Paris: Caille et Ravier, 1818), 2: 305–6, 360.

37. Seventy percent of chronically ill patients admitted that they, their parents, or ancestors were afflicted with syphilis. Lauvergne, *De l'agonie de la mort*, 2: 431.

38. Dr. Denis de Saint-Pierre, *Petit manuel des prétendus incurables* (Paris: A. Allpert, n.d. [c. 1835]), 1.

39. Barnes, *The Making*, 30.

40. Rosenberg, "The Bitter Fruit," 40.

41. Louis, *Recherches anatomiques*, 333–34.

42. Guillaume, *Du désespoir au salut*, 293–94. For a contemporary viewpoint, see Daremberg, *Les différentes formes*, 136.

43. Alibert, *Clinique de l'hôpital Saint-Louis*, 204–5.

44. Frédéric Duparcque, *Réfutation de la doctrine d'inévitabilité et d'incurabilité du cancer* (Paris: Le Normant, 1837), 24–25.

45. A. Jaumes, "Des maladies," 130.

46. Dr. E. Salmon, *Le nouveau médecin des villes et des campagnes ou recueil de conseils pour la conservation de la santé, suivi de l'exposé des soins relatifs à la première enfance ou code de la jeune mère, et de réflexions sur les maladies invétérées dites incurables, terminé par une monographie du cancer, des tumeurs externes, etc.* (Cherbourg: Bedel Fontaine et Syffert, 1864), 11–12.

47. Daniel Pick, *Faces of Degeneration: A European Disorder, circa 1848–1918* (Cambridge: Cambridge University Press, 1993).

48. Ruth Harris, *Murders and Madness: Medicine, Law, and Society in the Fin de Siècle* (Oxford: Clarendon Press, 1989), 51–56.

49. Benedict-Augustin Morel, *Traité des dégénérescences physiques, intellectuelles et morales de l'espèce humaine* (Paris: Baillière, 1857), 1: 679.

50. Robert Nye, *Crime, Madness, and Politics in Modern France: The Medical Concept of National Decline* (Princeton, NJ: Princeton University Press, 1984).

51. Harris, *Murders and Madness*, 78.

52. Antoine Petit, *Essai sur les maladies héréditaires, considérées sous les rapports de leur nature, de leur origine, des moyens d'en prévenir la transmission, d'en empêcher le développement, du traitement qu'elles réclament, une fois qu'elles sont développées* (Paris: Gabon, 1817).

53. François-Joseph-Victor Broussais, *Traité de physiologie appliquée à la pathologie* (Paris, Baillière, 1834), 2: 568.

54. *Dictionnaire des sciences médicales, par une société de médecins et de chirurgiens*, s.v. "Mariage," 32.

55. Barnes, *The Making*, 141–48.

56. Thomas H. Huxley, "On the Reception of the Origin of Species," in *Life and Letters of Charles Darwin*, ed. Francis Darwin (New York: D. Appleton, 1925), 1: 539. For a cogent discussion of this issue, see Robert E. Stebbins, "France," in *The Comparative Reception of Darwinism*, ed. Thomas F. Glick (Austin: University of Texas Press, 1972), 122, 146–49.

57. Stebins, "France," 117–21.

58. Constantin James, *Du Darwinisme, ou l'Homme-singe* (Paris: Plon, 1877).

59. For an overview of the process by which the Church gradually reconciled itself to Darwinism, see Harry W. Paul, *The Edge of Contingency: French Catholic Reaction to Scientific Change from Darwin to Duhem* (Gainesville: University Presses of Florida, 1979), 64–107.

60. Mark B. Adams, "Eugenics in the History of Science," in *The Wellborn Science: Eugenics in Germany, France, Brazil, and Russia*, ed. Mark B. Adams (New York: Oxford University Press, 1990), 5.

61. Clémence Royer, cited in William H. Schneider, "The Eugenics Movement in France 1890–1940," in *The Wellborn Science: Eugenics in Germany, France, Brazil, and Russia*, ed. Mark B. Adams (New York: Oxford University Press, 1990), 71.

62. Schneider, "The Eugenics Movement," 69–109. One of the best general histories remains Daniel J. Kevles, *In the Name of Eugenics: Genetics and the Uses of Human Heredity* (New York: Knopf, 1985).

63. Gueneau de Mussy, *Leçons*, 6.

64. Pidoux, *Études*, 152, 163, 167, 528, 536–37.

65. Frédéric Morin, *Les diathèses et les cachexies aux eaux de la Bourboule: Scofule, tubercule, goutte et rhumatisme, diabète-sucré, dartres et syphilis* (Clermont-Ferrand: A. Vigot, 1879), 20–21.

66. Peter, *Leçons*, 2: 147–48.

67. *Dictionnaire encyclopédique des sciences médicales*, s.v. "Dégénérescence (biologie anthropologique)," 214.

68. *Nouveau dictionnaire de médecine et de chirurgie pratiques*, s.v. "Diathèse," 437.

69. *Dictionnaire de médecine et de chirurgie pratiques*, s.v. "Hérédité," 457; Jules Rengade, *Les grands maux*, 4.

70. Paul Moreau de Tours, *Des pseudo-guérisons*; Benjamin Ball, "Phthisise et folie, leçon professé à la Clinique des maladies mentales, à l'Asile Sainte-Anne," *Encéphale: Journal des maladies mentales et nerveuses* 1 (1881): 177.

71. J. Edward Chamberlin and Sander L. Gilman, *Degeneration: The Dark Side of Progress* (New York: Columbia University Press, 1985).

72. Sander L. Gilman, *Disease and Representation: Images of Illness from Madness to AIDS* (Ithaca, NY: Cornell University Press, 1988).

73. Alain Corbin, "Hereditary Syphilis or the Impossible Redemption: A Contribution to the History of Morbid Heredity," *Time, Desire, and Horror: Towards a History of the Senses*, trans. Jean Birrell (Oxford: Polity Press, 1995), 119.

74. "We never cease to have recourse to the most gratuitous suppositions to explain that which, in the end, we cannot explain." Hermann Lebert, *Traité pratique des maladies cancéreuses et des affections curables confondues avec le cancer* (Paris: Baillière, 1851), 60. See also Ball, "Phthisise et folie," 178.

75. "It has even been said that it [tuberculosis] was always hereditary and that when a consumptive denied its existence, he was accused of wanting to hide phthisis as a stain on the family." *Dictionnaire populaire de médecine usuelle d'hygiène publique et privée*, s.v. "Phtisie," 2: 726. See also *Dictionnaire de médecine et de chirurgie pratiques*, s.v. "Hérédité," 467.

76. Gustave-Simon Lagneau, "Rapport sur la coopération des médecins traitants à la détermination des causes de décès," *Bulletin de l'Académie de médecine* 7 (1879): 609.

77. Daremberg, *Les différentes formes*, 138.

78. Linda Bryder, *Below the Magic Mountain: A Social History of Tuberculosis in Twentieth-Century Britain* (Oxford: Oxford University Press, 1988), 200–214.

79. Barnes, *The Making*, 30.

## CHAPTER 4   DEATH, DECAY, AND THE GENESIS OF SHAME

1. One of the classics in a crowded genre is John Donne, *Devotions upon Emergent Occasions and Several Steps in My Sickness, etc.* (London: Thomas Iones, 1624). See also Alexis Lefebvre, *La science de bien mourir, manuel de l'Association de la Bonne Mort* (Paris: Putoit-Cretté, 1864), 51–52, 169–70.

2. John McManners, *Death and the Enlightenment: Changing Attitudes to Death among Christians and Unbelievers in Eighteenth-Century France* (Oxford: Oxford University Press, 1981), 255–57.

3. Susan Sontag, *Illness as Metaphor* (New York: Random House, 1979).

4. Clark Lawlor and Akihito Suzuki, "The Disease of the Self: Representing Consumption, 1700–1830," *Bulletin of the History of Medicine* 74, no. 2 (2000): 458–94, quote is on pp. 461–62.

5. "Separate system of honor" was originally used to refer to stigmatized ethnic minorities who celebrated, even made an ostentatious display of, their deviance. Erving Goffman, *Stigma: Notes on the Management of Spoiled Identity* (Englewood Cliffs, NJ: Prentice-Hall, 1963), 6–7. A recent study of Somali immigrants to Canada

insists that they reject the stigma of race and often engage in "stigma reversal." Abdi M. Kusow, "Contesting Stigma: On Goffmann's Assumptions of Normative Order," *Symbolic Interaction* 27, no. 2 (2004): 179–97.

6. Henri Peyre, *Qu'est ce que le Romantisme?* (Paris: Presses Universitaires de France, 1971), 5–49.

7. The fact that "Romantic" is a noun and an adjective (both upper and lower case) compounds the problem. Understandably, most commentators are far more comfortable speaking in terms of Romanticism(s).

8. Isaiah Berlin, *The Roots of Romanticism* (Princeton, NJ: Princeton University Press, 1999), 88, 94–95 (quote is from p. 88).

9. Jerome J. McGann, *The Romantic Ideology: A Critical Investigation* (Chicago: University of Chicago Press, 1983), 71.

10. From the diary of Pauline de La Ferronays, cited in Philippe Ariès, *The Hour of Our Death*, trans. Helen Weaver (New York: Knopf, 1981), 423.

11. Lawlor and Suzuki, "The Disease of the Self," 466–68.

12. Lauvergne, *De l'agonie*, 2: 435.

13. Ibid., 433–34.

14. Lebert, *Traité clinique*, 141.

15. Claudine Herzlich and Janine Pierret, *Illness and Self in Society*, trans. Elborg Forster (Baltimore: Johns Hopkins University Press, 1987), 32–37 (quote is from pp. 32–33).

16. Marc-Antoine Petit, *Essai sur la médecine du cœur; auquel on a joint les principaux discours prononcés à l'ouverture des Cours d'Anatomie, d'Opérations et de Chirurgie clinique, de l'Hôtel-Dieu de Lyon; savoir: 1e Sur l'influence de la Révolution sur la santé publique; 2e Sur la manière d'exercer la bienfaisance dans les hôpitaux; 3e Sur la Douleur; 4e Sur les Maladies observées dans l'Hôtel-Dieu de Lyon pendant neuf années; 5e L'Éloge de Desault* (Lyon: Garnier, 1806), 71 (emphasis in the original).

17. Émile Tardieu, "Psychologie du malade," *Revue philosophique*, Paris, 45 (June 1898): 568.

18. Herzlich and Perret, *Illness and Self*, 35–37.

19. McManners, *Death*, 255.

20. Guillaume, *Du désespoir au salut*, 24.

21. Simon, *Déontologie médicale*, 1.

22. Jean-Louis-Marie Alibert, *Précis théorique sur les maladies de la peau* (Paris: Caille et Ravier, 1818), 2: 302–4, 311–12; *Nouveau dictionnaire de médecine et de chirurgie pratiques*, s.v. "Diathèse," 449.

23. For an interesting American example, see Abel, *Suffering in the Land of Sunshine*, 122–27.

24. De Bonqueval, *Traité théorique*, v.

25. Peter, *Leçons*, 2: 504.

26. Guillaume, *Du désespoir au salut*, 35–36; quote is from p. 36.

27. Barnes, *The Making*, 61–63, 165–73.

28. Lawlor and Suzuki are essentially silent about other available narratives. Lawlor and Suzuki, "The Disease of the Self," 478.

29. Alibert, *Précis théorique*, 1: 334.

30. The one comparably ennobling trait that the affluent (and their doctors) frequently invoked was ambition, at school or in world of business.

31. Lawlor and Suzuki, "The Disease of the Self," 463.

32. An early-century authority described scrofula as an infirmity "as shameful as it is disgusting, that turns one into the scum of our fellow men; it leads to dread over conjugal union, it is transmitted to our descendants and strikes the infant in the arms of its mother. It transforms the best years of life into ones of sorrow and suffering." Alibert, *Précis théorique*, 2: 307.

33. The best analyses of the therapeutic practices and the disciplinary structures of modern sanatoria can be found in Bryder, *Below the Magic Mountain* and Barron Lerner, *Contagion and Confinement: Controlling Tuberculosis along the Skid Row* (Baltimore: Johns Hopkins University Press, 1998).

34. *Dictionnaire des sciences médicales, par une société de médecins et de chirurgiens*, s.v. "Mariage," 35.

35. Hezlich and Perret, *Illness and Self*, 25. See also Joseph-Claude-Anselme Récamier, *Recherches sur le traitement du cancer par la compression méthodique simple ou combinée, et sur l'histoire générale de la même maladie, suivies de notes sur les forces et la dynamétrie vitale, sur l'inflammation et l'état fébrile* (Paris: Gabon, 1829), 1: xviii.

36. Fodéré, *Marriage*, 44.

37. Warren Richey, "Boycott Groups: Klein Ads Carry Scent of Heroin Chic," *Christian Science Monitor*, 25 October 1996.

38. At the low point of the AIDS epidemic in the West, one Hollywood studio used a Romantic storyline to attack homophobia and the stigmatization of AIDS patients. The movie *Philadelphia* earned Tom Hanks an Academy Award for best actor. *Philadelphia*, written by Ron Nyswaner, directed by Jonathan Demme, 1993, Tri-Star Pictures.

39. Jonathan Larson's rock musical *Rent* has been running continuously on Broadway for over ten years. In 2005, Sony Pictures released a full-length movie version produced and directed by Chris Columbus.

40. McGann, *The Romantic Ideology*, 132.

41. Howard Becker, *Outsiders: Studies in the Sociology of Deviance* (New York: Free Press, 1963).

42. Erving Goffman, *The Presentation of Self in Everyday Life* (Garden City, NY: Doubleday, 1959); Goffman, *Asylums: Essays on the Social Situation of Mental Patients and Other Inmates* (Chicago: Aldine, 1961).

43. Goffman, *Stigma*, 41–104.

44. Ibid., 127–28, 131–33, 137–38.

45. Eliot Freidson, *Profession of Medicine: A Study of the Sociology of Applied Knowledge* (New York: Dodd, Mead, 1974), 203–77.

46. Anselm Strauss, *Chronic Illness and the Quality of Life* (St. Louis: Mosby, 1975); Anselm Strauss and Juliet Corbin et al., *Chronic Illness and the Quality of Life*, 2nd ed. (St. Louis: Mosby, 1984).

47. Michael Bury, "Chronic Illness as Disruption," *Sociology of Health and Illness* 4, no. 2 (1982): 167–82.

48. Graham Scambler and Anthony Hopkins, "Being Epileptic: Coming to Terms with Stigma," *Sociology of Health and Illness* 8, no. 1 (1986): 26–43.

49. Kathy Charmaz, "Experiencing Chronic Illness," in *Handbook of Social Studies in Health and Medicine*, ed. G. Albrecht, R. Fitzpatrick, and S. Scrimshaw (London: Sage, 2000), 285.

50. Social class and education help diminish the stigma associated with predicaments such as childlessness. Catherine Riessman, "Stigma and Everyday Resistance Practices: Childless Women in South India," *Gender and Society* 14 (2000): 111–35.

51. Bruce G. Link and Jo C. Phelan, "Conceptualizing Stigma," *Annual Review of Sociology* 27 (2001): 375.

52. Colin Jones, "Plague and Its Metaphors in Early Modern France," *Representations* 53 (1996): 97–127; Rosenberg, *The Cholera Years*.

53. Alan M. Kraut, *Silent Travelers: Germs, Genes, and the Immigrant Menace* (Baltimore: Johns Hopkins University Press, 1994), 50–78.

54. Rosenberg, "Banishing Risk."

55. Lauvergne, *De l'agonie*, 2: 460, 462.

56. Simon, *Déontologie médicale*, 354.

57. Brierre de Boismont, *Du suicide*, 208.

58. Suzanne Kaufman, "Miracles, Medicine, and the Spectacle of Lourdes" (PhD thesis, Rutgers University, 1996), 312–15.

59. Simon, *Déontologie médicale*, 310–15.

60. Brierre de Boismont, *Du suicide*, 200.

61. Tardieu, "Psychologie du malade," 583–84.

62. Louis Chevalier, *Laboring Classes and Dangerous Classes in Paris during the First Half of the Nineteenth Century*, trans. Frank Jellinek (New York: Howard Fertig, 1973), 359–60.

63. Pidoux, *Études*, 566.

64. Rengade, *Les grands maux*, 12.

65. Tardieu, "Psychologie," 573.

66. Anonymous, "Reine Beaubis, veuve Bodier," *Les Prix de Vertu fondés par M. de Montyon. Discours prononcés à l'Académie Française. Réunis et publiés avec une notice sur M. De Montyon par Frédéric Lock et J. Couly D'Aragon*, vol. 1, 1819–1838 (Paris: Garnier Frères, 1858), 163–64.

67. Tardieu, "Psychologie du malade," 572.

68. De Saint-Pierre, *Petit manuel des prétendus incurables*, 1–2.

69. Bouillaud, "Discussion du diagnostic et de la curabilité du cancer," séance du 5 décembre 1854, *Bulletin de l'Académie impériale de médecine* 20, 19e année (1854–55): 310.

70. Salmon, *Le nouveau médecin des villes et des campagnes*, 12–13; Tardieu, "Psychologie du malade," 565–66.

71. Dr. Gourdin, "Sur la curabilité de la pthisie pulmonaire," *Congrès médical de France, 2e session tenue à Lyons du 26 septembre au 1er octobre*, 126 (Paris: Baillière, 1864).

72. Rosenberg, *No Other Gods*, 25–53.

73. Simon, *Déontologie médicale*, 223; emphasis added.

74. Cited in Tampier, *Dernières heures de Rachel*, 48.

75. Salmon, *Le nouveau médecin*, 52.

76. Kathy Charmaz, "Identity Dilemmas of Chronically Ill Men," *Sociological Quarterly* 35, no. 2 (May 1994): 269–88.

77. This analysis specifically excludes syphilis because its stigmatization was over-determined by the fact that it's sexually transmitted.

78. Sontag, *Illness as Metaphor*, 8.

79. *Dictionnaire de médecine usuelle*, s.v. "Cachexies."

80. Morin, *Les diathèses et les cachexies*, 11.

81. Moral contagion was traditionally associated with mental illness or undesirable behaviors that spread via imitation, such as "outbreaks" of hysteria or epilepsy. The use of the term here similarly assumes that patients could have such a dramatic effect on others that they too fell ill.

82. Guillaume, *Du désespoir au salut*, 38.

83. Laënnec, *Traité de l'auscultation médiate*, 4th ed., 2: 179–80.

84. "Without precisely believing in the contagiousness of phthisis, two distinguished professors, Laënnec and Andral, recommend as a prudent measure to those habit-ually living with phthisics to take certain precautions, especially at an advanced state of their affliction, and to avoid that an individual should sleep in the same bed as the patient, or constantly live with them in the same atmosphere. These are good pieces of advice to follow, given that the miasmas that phthisics' bodies exude can only be harmful to health; but we believe that there is no foundation to the fear of contagion, at least in the climate in which we live." Grisolle, *Traité élémentaire*, 2: 580.

85. Pidoux, *Études*, 220.

86. Bernard Peyrilhe, *A Dissertation on Cancerous Diseases*, translated from the Latin with notes (London: Wilkie, 1777).

87. Velpeau, *Traité des maladies du sein*, 545–46.

88. Alain Corbin, *The Foul and the Fragrant: Odor and the French Imagination* (Cambridge, MA: Harvard University Press, 1986).

89. Alibert, *Précis théorique*, 2: 315–16.

90. Pidoux, *Études*, 222.

91. Joseph Castri, "Du traitement palliatif du cancer ulcéré du col de l'utérus et en particulier de l'emploi d'une préparation spéciale d'iodoforme" (MD thesis, Paris, 1883), 11–12.

92. Pidoux, *Études*, 235. Jean-Paul Gaudrillière and Ilana Löwy, eds., *Heredity and Infection: The History of Disease Transmission* (London: Routledge, 2001).

93. Rengade, *Les grands maux*, 130.

94. Everett C. Hughes, "Dilemmas and Contradictions of Status," *American Journal of Sociology* 50 (1945): 353–59; Becker, *Outsiders*; Charmaz, "Identity Dilemmas," 277.

95. Tera W. Hunter, *To Joy My Freedom: Southern Black Women's Lives and Labors after the Civil War* (Cambridge, MA: Harvard University Press, 1997), 187–218.

96. Lion Murard and Patrick Zylberman, *L'hygiène dans la République*, 443–46, 459–68, 52–523; Bruno Latour, *The Pasteurization of France*, trans. Alan Sheridan and John Law (Cambridge, MA: Harvard University Press, 1988); Nancy Tomes, *The Gospel of Germs: Men, Women, and the Microbe in American Life* (Cambridge, MA: Harvard University Press, 1998); Kraut, *Silent Travelers*.

97. A. Haviland, "Cancer Houses," *Lancet* 145, no. 3739 (April 1895): 1049–50. Paul Juillerat, "Les maisons à cancer de Paris," *Bulletin de l'Association Française pour l'étude du cancer* 3 (1910): 61–66.

98. Mendelsohn, "Medicine and the Making of Bodily Inequality," 21–79.

99. Daremberg, *Les différentes formes*, 191.

100. Petit, *Essai sur la medicine du coeur*, 181–82. The issue of moral contagion was regularly cited to justify the separation of incurable and potentially curable consumptives.

101. Lupus was the most severe manifestation of the so-called dartrous diathesis. See Jean-Louis-Marie Alibert, *Clinique de l'hôpital Saint-Louis* (Paris: Cormon et Blanc, 1833), 191.

102. Ibid., 191.

103. Émile Guillaumin, *The Life of a Simple Man*, revised translation by Margaret Crosland (Hanover, NH: University Press of New England, 1983), 183–84. The original version is *La vie d'un simple: Mémoires d'un métayer* (Paris: Stock, 1904).

104. Charles Richet, "Essai sur les causes du dégoût," *Revue des deux mondes*, 33e année, Troisième période, Tome 22e, Paris (1877): 662, 671.

105. Alibert, *Précis théorique*, 2: 332.

106. André Moussous, "De la mort chez les phtisiques" (thèse de concours, Paris, 1886), 14–15. He borrowed this description from the well-known German physician Felix Von Niemeyer.

107. Lefebvre, *La science de bien mourir, 2e partie*, 3: 117–20 (quote is from pp. 118–19).

108. The cancerous cachexia was "the cachexia of the cachexias, it is dissolution, death magnified." De Bonqueval, *Traité théorique*, 347.

109. Récamier, *Recherches*, 2: 135–36.

110. Simon, *Déontologie médicale*, 54–55.

111. Simon, *Déontologie médicale*, 205–6; Jack D. Ellis, *The Physicians-Legislators of France: Medicine and Politics in the Early Third Republic* (Cambridge: Cambridge University Press, 1990), 107–8.

112. Barnes, *The Making*, 48–73.

113. Like many others, Lauvergne equated aberrancy and wasting: "the erotic form of hysteria leads to marasmus, suicide, and insanity." Lauvergne, *De l'agonie*, 1: 369.

114. Simon, *Déontologie médicale*, 96.

115. Herzlich and Pierret, *Illness and Self*, 73.

116. "In the nineteenth century the epidemics were in regression, and with them a certain immediate apprehension of bodily ill faded away or changed its meaning. Yet, paradoxically, the horror of the sick body was expressed more and more frequently in literary works." Herzlich and Pierret, *Illness and Self*, 78.

117. Georges Bataille, *Eroticism: Death and Sensuality*, trans. Mary Dalwood (San Francisco: City Light Books, 1986), 45–47.

118. Susan E. Lederer, "Dark Victory: Cancer and Popular Hollywood Film," *Bulletin of the History of Medicine* 81, no. 1 (2007): 94–115.

119. Julia Kristeva, "Holbein's Dead Christ," in *Fragments of a Human Body*, ed. Michel Fehr (New York: Zone, 1989), 238–69.

120. Ariès, *The Hour of Our Death*, 110–29, 569.

121. Ibid., 368.

122. Lebert, *Traité pratique des maladies cancéreuses*, 118.

CHAPTER 5   MEDICAL ATTITUDES TOWARD THE CARE OF INCURABLES

1. Lefebvre, *La science de bien mourir, 2e partie*, 2: 267–71.

2. Pierre-Jean-Corneille Debreyne, *Thérapeutique appliquée, ou traitements spéciaux de la plupart des maladies chroniques* (Paris: Baillière, 1841), 4.

3. J.L.A. Delacoux Désroseau, "Simples réflexions sur les devoirs du médecin considéré comme homme" (MD thesis, Paris, 1835), 9.

4. Simon, *Déontologie médicale*, 273.

5. I would like to thank Alex Dracobly for bringing nine of the most important reviews to my attention.

6. Anonymous, *Journal de médecine et de chirurgie* 4 (1846): 285–87. Dr. H. Thirial, *Journal des connaissances médico-chirurgicales* 13 (March 1846): 110–11.

7. Louis Delasiauve, *Revue médicale française et étrangère. Journal des progrès de la médecine hippocratique*, nouvelle série, 2 (1846): 241.

8. Ibid., 247.

9. Charles-Polydore Forget, *Des devoirs du médecin* (Strasbourg: Derivaux and Paris: Baillière, 1849), 6.

10. Tampier, *Dernières heures de Rachel*, 68.

11. "It often happens that, at the beginning of their career, physicians are forced to make themselves stand out and draw attention to themselves, to have recourse to certain maneuvers and to make a certain splash that constitutes a form of honest charlatanism that I cannot resolve myself to blame." Benjamin Verdo, *Le Charlatanisme et les charlatans en médecine, étude psychologique* (Paris: Baillière, 1867), 37–38.

12. Adrien Coriveaud, "Le médecin en face des maladies incurables: Son rôle et ses devoirs. Discours prononcé à l'assemblée de l'Association des Médecins de la Gironde tenue à Bourg le dimanche 31 mai 1885" (Bordeaux: G. Gounouilhou, 1885), 12.

13. Joseph-Marie Audin-Rouvière, *La médecine sans médecin, ou un manuel de santé, ouvrage destiné à soulager les infirmités, à prévenir les maladies aiguës, à guérir les maladies chroniques, sans le secours d'une main étrangère*, 2nd ed. (Paris: Chez l'auteur, 1824), 468–69.

14. Matthew Ramsey, "Academic Medicine and Medical Industrialism: The Regulation of Secret Remedies in Nineteenth-Century France," in *French Medical Culture in the Nineteenth Century*, ed. Ann La Berge and Mordechai Feingold (Amsterdam: Rodopi, 1994), 29.

15. Tampier, "Dernières heures de Rachel," 36.

16. Dr. Desparquets, *Des maladies chroniques réputées incurables: Maladies de poitrine; affections nerveuses, goutteuses, rhumatismales, lymphatiques, scrofuleuses, scorbutiques, cancéreuses, syphilitiques; maladies de la peau; maladies des yeux; paralysies, affections de vessie, et matrice; etc., etc., et de leur traitement rationnel par l'hygiène et le régime alimentaire associés à une médication spéciale. Suivis d'une appréciation des méthodes médicales régnantes* (Paris: l'auteur, 1855), 5.

17. "It is often when the mission of [medical] artist ends that the mission of the man of charity begins." Simon, *Déontologie médicale*, 351–52.

18. Paul S. Mueller, "William Osler's Study of the Act of Dying: An Analysis of the Original Data," *Journal of Medical Biography* 15, supp. 1 (2007): 59; R. L. Golden, "Sir William Osler: Humanist Thanatologist," *OMEGA: Journal of Death and Dying* 36 (1997–98): 241–58.

19. Théodore Tuffier, "Traitement du cancer utérin inopérable," *L'Œuvre médico-chirurgical* 63 (February 1911): 2710.

20. Weisz, *The Medical Mandarins*, 215–36. Jacques Léonard, *La médicine entre les pouvoirs et les savoirs* (Paris: Aubier, 1981), 327.

21. Daremberg, *Les différentes formes*, III.

22. Coural, "Comparer," 4.

23. The obvious physical signs of organic illness were a key marker for pioneering anatomico-pathologists out to establish the legitimacy of their method for diagnosing illness.

24. Grancher, *Maladies*, 206.

25. Charles Monod and Felix Jayle, *Cancer du sein* (Paris: Rueff, 1894), 60–61.

26. Joseph Récamier, *Traitement du cancer utérin inopérable* (Paris: G. Steinheil, 1905), 1–2.

27. *Dictionnaire de sciences médicales, par une société de médecins et de chirurgiens*, s.v. "Guérison," 554–55.

28. Desparquets, *Des maladies*, 4.

29. Jules Rengade, *Les grands maux*, 42.

30. Gerald L. Geison, *The Private Life of Louis Pasteur* (Princeton, NJ: Princeton University Press, 1995), 145–47; Bert Hansen, "America's First Medical Breakthrough: How Popular Excitement about a French Rabies Cure in 1885 Raised New Expectations for Medical Progress," *American Historical Review* 103, no. 2 (April 1998), 373–418.

31. Jaumes, *Des maladies*, 138.

32. Ibid., 138.

33. Jules-Zulema Amussat, "Discussion. Du diagnostic et de la curabilité du cancer," séance du 21 novembre 1854, *Bulletin de l'Académie impériale de médecine* 20, 19e Année (1854–1855): 234.

34. Barrier, *Traitement des maladies scrofuleuses*, 195.

35. Simon, *Déontologie médicale*, 146–48, 151, 383.

36. Coriveaud, *Le médecin*, 5.

37. Tuffier, "Traitement du cancer inopérable," 2709–10.

38. Edouard Auber, *Philosophie de la médecine* (Paris: Baillière, 1865), 160.

39. Joseph Bullar, "On the Use of Small Doses of Opium in the Act of Dying from Phthisis," *Associated Medical Journal of London* (April 1856): 268–69. He ended his article by stating, "I have the less hesitation in making this communication, though it may have no novelty; for we often need to be reminded of what is old, as well as to be taught what is new; and the very purpose of our JOURNAL is to communicate amongst ourselves those minor matters which we often make the subject of medical talk when we meet."

40. Oswald Browne, *On the Care of the Dying: A Lecture to Nurses* (London: George Allan, 1894), 29.

41. Daremberg, *Les différentes formes*, 304.

42. Salmon, *Le nouveau médecin des villes*, 5.

43. Hermann Pidoux, "De la superstition médicale et de l'hypochondrie dans la médecine des maladies chroniques, discours prononcé à l'ouverture de la société d'hydrologie médicale de Paris, le 10 novembre 1862," *Annales de la Société d'hydrologie médicale de Paris*, 9 (1862–63): 437.

44. Forget, *Des devoirs*, 21.

45. Léonard, *La médecine entre les pouvoirs et les savoirs*, 15, 68.

46. Louis Peisse, *La médecine et les médecins. Philosophie, doctrines, institutions, critiques mœurs, et biographies médicales* (Paris: Baillière, 1857), 449.

47. Tampier, *Les dernières heures de Rachel*, 32.

48. Desparquets, *Des maladies chroniques réputées incurables*, 18–19.

49. Audin-Rouvière, *La médecine sans médecin*, 482–84.

50. Jacques Léonard, *La vie quotidienne du médecin de province au XIXe siècle* (Paris: Hachette, 1977), 173–76.

51. Léonard, *La médecine entre les pouvoirs et les savoirs*, 175.

52. Léonard, *La médecine entre les pouvoirs et les savoirs*, 203–8, 224–26; Duffin, *To See*, 245.

53. E. Faneau-Delacour, "Considérations et observations sur la nature et le traitement du cancer," *Journal Universel des sciences médicales*, Paris 42 (1826): 9.

54. Forget, *Des devoirs* , 29–30.

55. Jaumes, *Des maladies* , 89.

56. Coriveaud, *Le médecin*, 10–11.

57. Auguste François Chomel, "De l'importance des moyens pour soutenir le moral des malades," *Gazette des hôpitaux* 8 (1846): 498.

58. Delacoux Desroseau, "Simples réflexions," 12.

59. Tirat de Malemort, *Des maladies chroniques, spécialement de la phthisie pulmonaire et des affections qui la produisent le plus souvent, les darteres, les scrofules, le rhumatisme et la goutte, le gastrite, le cattarrhe, l'asthme, l'aménorrhée (maladies des femmes) considérées dans leurs causes, dans leurs effets et dans leur traitement curatif et préservatif* (Paris: Baillière, 1845), 126.

60. Tampier, *Dernières heures de Rachel*, 27–28.

61. Ibid., 30.

62. Simon, *Déontologie médicale*, 330–31.

63. H. F. Ragonneau, "Considérations sur l'agonie" (MD thesis, Paris, 1817), 23, 25 (quote is on p. 25).

64. Ibid., 23–24.

65. François-Joseph-Victor Broussais, *Histoire des phlégmasies ou inflammations chroniques*, 5th ed. (Paris: Mequinon-Marvis, 1838), 330.

66. Jaumes, "Des maladies," 141.

67. Ibid., 97.

68. *Dictionnaire de médecine usuelle à l'usage des gens du monde des chefs de famille et de grands établissements, des administrateurs, des magistrats et des officiers de police judiciaire, enfin pouvant servir à tous ceux qui se dévouent au soulagement des malades*, s.v. "Agonie," 58–59.

69. Tardieu, "Psychologie du malade," 591.

70. "Without a doubt, one must make inquiries of interested parties, to know whether the affairs of the patient are in order or not and to act in consequence. One is even authorized in certain grave instances to prolong the dying state, to delay death by a few minutes with the help of more or less violent forms of stimulation (a hammer submerged in boiling water and applied to the skin, cauterisation, etc)." *Dictionnaire populaire de médecine usuelle d'hygiène publique et privée*, s.v. "Agonie," 59–60. Administering tonics and cordials as well as force-feeding late-stage cancer and tuberculosis patients remained socially acceptable throughout the nineteenth century.

71. Pierre Adolphe Piorry, *Mémoire sur l'agonie sur les causes matérielles de la mort et sur les soins à donner aux mourants* (Paris: E. Martinet, 1875), 6–7.

72. Keith Thomas has suggested that guilty feelings played a decisive role in prompting witchcraft accusations against poverty-stricken widows who begged too aggressively. Thomas, *Religion and the Decline of Magic* (New York: Scribner, 1971).

73. Louis, *Recherches anatomiques*, 676.

74. Coriveaud, *Le médecin*, 6–7.

75. Simon, *Déontologie médicale*, 85.

76. Ibid., 2.

77. Auclair, "De l'hystérectomie abdominale totale," 81. He claims to have taken the quote from Labadie-Lagrave et Legueu, *Traité médico-chirurgical de gynécologie* (Paris, 1898), page not specified.

78. Daremberg, *Les différentes formes*, 7–8, 57 (quote pp.7–8).

79. Tardieu, "Psychologie du malade," 572–73.

80. Lefevre, "Quelques idées," 19.

81. Brierre de Boismont, *Du suicide*, 200.

82. Velpeau, *Traité des maladies du sein*, 602.

83. Barrier, *Traitement des maladies scrofuleuses*, 72.

84. Simon, *Déontologie médicale*, 1–2.

85. Tardieu, "Psychologie du malade," 575–76.

86. Austin Flint, *Medical Ethics and Etiquette*, the code of ethics adopted by the American Medical Association, with commentaries (New York: D. Appleton, 1883), 25; Jaumes, "Des maladies," 138–39.

87. Desparquets, *Des maladies chroniques réputées incurables*, 4–6.

88. Tirat de Malemort, *Des maladies chroniques*, 94.

89. Ibid., 121.

90. The vicomtesse de Chappedelaine similarly praised him for having cured her godchild, a sickly young girl who "had been abandoned as incurable." Tirat de Malemort, *Des maladies chroniques*, 98, 120.

91. Ibid., 348.

92. Tampier, *Dernières heures de Rachel*, 21.

93. Ibid., 35.

94. Chambeouf, *Principes de médecine naturelle*, 5.

95. Ibid., 139.

96. *Dictionnaire annuelle des progrès des sciences et institutions médicales: suite et complément de tous les dictionnaires*, s.v. "Cancer," 79.

97. *Dictionnaire de médecine et de thérapeutique médicale et chirurgicale comprenant le résumé de toute la chirurgie, les indications thérapeutiques de chaque maladie, la médecine opératoire, les accouchements, l'oculistique, l'odontechnie, l'électrisation, la matière médicale, les eaux minérales*, s.v. "Cancer," 234.

98. Tuffier, "Traitement du cancer inopérable," 2690.

99. *Dictionnaire de médecine usuelle à l'usage des gens du monde, des chefs de famille et de grands établissements, des administrateurs, des magistrats et des officiers de police judiciaire, enfin pouvant servir à tous ceux qui se dévouent au soulagement des malades*, s.v. "Phthisie," 651.

100. Maurice Letulle, "Prophylaxie et traitement de la tuberculose pulmonaire dans la classe pauvre," *Presse médicale*, VIIe année, 20 (1899): 95.

101. Récamier, *Traitement du cancer*, 200–201.

102. Tardieu, "Psychologie du malade," 591.

103. Coriveaud, *Le médecin*, 8.

104. Petit, *Essai sur la médecine du cœur*, 69–70, 189 (quote pp. 69–70).

105. *Arrêts et Circulaires de l'Assistance publique*, "Les médecins ne doivent pas négliger de visiter à domicile les malades dont l'état est reconnu par eux incurable [Circulaire du 16 août 1856 aux Maires de Paris]."

106. Henri Napias, *Annales d'Hygiène publique et de médecine légale* (1879): 62.

107. François-Louis-Isidore Valleix, "Coup d'œil général sur l'hydrothérapie; détermination des cas auxquels, d'après l'observation, elle est utilement applicable, et appréciation de sa valeur thérapeutique," *Bulletin général de thérapeutique* 35 (15 August 1848): 103–4.

108. Simon, *Déontologie médicale*, 310–11.

109. Coriveaud, *Le médecin*, 8–9.

110. Ball, "Phthisie et folie," 172–73.

111. J.-B.-C. Garoz, "Considérations générales sur les qualités morales du médecin, suivies du traitement moral dans les maladies" (MD thesis, Paris, 1835), 11; P.-M.-A. Ouelley, "De l'indispensable utilité des nécropsies dans la pratique particulière, dans l'intérêt des familles, du médecin et de la science en général, par rapport aux maladies héréditaires" (MD thesis, Paris, 1833), 45–46.

112. Petit, *Essai sur la médecine du coeur*, 34–35.

113. Garoz, "Considérations générales," 10, 12. See also Léonard, *La médecine*, 80–83.

114. Léonard, *La vie quotidienne*, 17.

115. Ibid., 35.

116. Casper "Durée probable de la vie des médecins," *Annales d'hygiène et de médecine légale*, 11 (1834): 375–84.

117. Simon, *Déontologie médicale*, 377.

118. Forget, *Des devoirs du médecin*, 20, 28.

119. Daremberg, *Les différentes formes*, 101.

## CHAPTER 6 MEDICAL STRATEGIES, SOCIAL CONVENTIONS, AND PALLIATIVE MEDICINE

1. This influential notion was first articulated by the sociologists Anselm L. Strauss and Barney G. Glaser in *Anguish: A Case History of a Dying Trajectory* (Mill Valley, CA: Sociology Press, 1970). For an early twentieth-century appraisal of incurability's effects on behavioral norms, see Daremberg, *Les différentes formes*, 260.

2. Simon, *Déontologie médicale*, 313–14.

3. Chomel, "De l'importance," 499.

4. Rothman, *Living in the Shadow of Death*, 110.

5. Michel de Montaigne, cited in E. Quintard, "Forces morales médicatrices" (MD thesis, Paris, 1875), 31.

6. Chomel, "De l'importance," 502.

7. Peter, *Leçons*, 2: 567.

8. Chomel, "De l'importance," 498.

9. Delacoux Désroseau, "Simples réflexions," 11.

10. *Nouveau dictionnaire de médecine et de chirurgie pratiques* (supplement), s.v. "Secret médical," 453.

11. Flint, *Medical Ethics*, 25.

12. Chomel, "De l'importance," 503.

13. Charles Bosk, *Forgive and Remember: Managing Medical Failure* (Chicago: University of Chicago Press, 1979), 33, 103–10.

14. Ibid., 503.

15. Garoz, "Considérations générales," 13.

16. Nicholas Christakis, *Death Foretold: Prophecy and Prognosis in Medical Care* (Chicago: University of Chicago Press, 1999) 128, 131–34.

17. Chomel, "De l'importance," 503.

18. Worthington Hooker, *Physician and Patient; or, A Practical View of the Mutual Duties, Relations, and Interests of the Medical Profession and the Community* (New York: Baker and Scribner, 1849), 382.

19. Charles Auguste Chevreuse, "Influence de l'imagination sur les maladies" (MD thesis, Paris, 1833), 34.

20. Lauvergne, *De l'agonie*, 2: 438.

21. Barrier, *Traitement des maladies scrofuleuses*, 289.

22. *Dictionnaire populaire de médecine usuelle d'hygiène publique et privée*, s.v. "Pthisie," 730.

23. Tampier, *Dernières heures de Rachel*, 1858, 87.

24. Garoz, *Considérations générales*, 19.

25. The English physician Thomas Percival's work on medical ethics (1803) was the standard reference for generations of Anglo-American doctors. While eschewing "absolutism," Percival recommended being forthright with the entourage and inscrutable to a fault with desperately ill patients. Percival, *Medical Ethics; or, a Code of Institutes and Precepts, Adapted to the Professional Conduct of Physicians and Surgeons, I. In Hospital Practice. II. In Private, or General Practice. III. In Relation to Apothecaries. IV. In Cases Which May Require a Knowledge of Law* (Manchester: S. Russell, 1803), 31–32.

26. William Munk, *Euthanasia; or, Medical Treatment in Aid of an Easy Death* (London: Longmans, Green, 1887). Here the term euthanasia referred to easing, not hastening death. See also Oswald Browne, *On the Care of the Dying*, 22–25.

27. *Dictionnaire populaire de médecine usuelle d'hygiène publique et privée*, s.v. "Agonie," 59.

28. Many doctors still believe that hope, no matter how contrived, prolongs the lives of terminally ill patients and that excessive forthrightness shortens it. These beliefs have been likened to a form of modern medical folklore. Christakis, *Death Foretold*, 137–52.

29. Broussais, *Traité de physiologie*, 171.

30. Martha Noel Evans, *Fits and Starts: A Genealogy of Hysteria in Modern France* (Ithaca, NY: Cornell University Press, 1991), 57–65.

31. A. L. Coural, "Des influences psychiques dans l'étiologie des états morbides" (MD thesis, Bordeaux, 1889), 24.

32. "In certain circumstances *emotional pain* is no less advantageous: thus we have seen it cure the most resistant catarrhal afflictions, lead to the disappearance of muteness, paralysis of the limbs, and the atrocious pains of rheumatism or of gout" (emphasis in the original). Jean Baptiste Felix Descuret, *La médecine des passions, ou les passions considérées dans leurs rapports avec les maladies, des lois et la religion* (Paris: Labé, 1844), 238. See also Barrier, *Traitement*, 81–82.

33. Petit, *Essai sur la médecine du cœur*, 67.

34. This is one of the major "stories" of mind-body medicine explored in Anne Harrington, *The Cure Within: A History of Mind-Body Medicine* (New York: Norton, 2008), 103–38.

35. Descuret, *La médecine*, 236–37.

36. Dr. A. Bertrand, *Phthisie pulmonaire et maladies de l'appareil respiratoire réputées incurables: Traitement physique- guérison* (Paris: A. Dutemple, 1875), 30.

37. Christopher C. Goetz, Michel Bonduelle, Toby Gelfand, *Charcot: Constructing Neurology* (New York: Oxford University Press, 1995), 205–8. This view was eventually supplanted by one that insisted that hysterical stigmata did not reflect material changes in brain but were, rather, the expression of psychological processes. Evans, *Fit and Starts*, 51–76.

38. Jean-Martin Charcot, "Faith Cure," *New Review* II (1892): 244–62.

39. Harris, *Lourdes*, 288–319.

40. In letters dripping with irony, Catholic doctors pointed out that two leading anti-clerical professors (Charcot and Larbode) and France's most famous Jewish one (Hippolyte Bernheim) regularly sent patients to Lourdes. Eugène Vincent, *Doit-on fermer Lourdes au nom de l'hygiène? Réponse des médecins qui ne font pas de politique: Non* (Lyon: Paquet, 1906), 35, 62.

41. Étienne Martin, *Précis de déontologie et de médecine professionelle* (Paris: Masson, 1914), 55.

42. Forget, *Des devoirs du médecin*, 18.

43. Braunstein, *Broussais*, 175–79, 227–30. For a sense of what this meant in practice, see Lefebvre, *La science de bien mourir, 2e partie*, 2: 272–74.

44. Vincent, *Doit-on fermer Lourdes?* 31.

45. Ibid., 176.

46. Harris, *Lourdes*, 320–56.

47. Matthew Ramsey, "Alternative Medicine in Modern France," *Medical History* 43 (1999): 304.

48. Mark S. Micale and Paul Lerner, eds., *Traumatic Pasts: History, Psychiatry, and Trauma in the Modern Age, 1870–1930* (Cambridge: Cambridge University Press, 2001).

49. Quintard, "Forces morales médicatrices," 56–57 (emphasis in the original).

50. J.-B. Fonnsagrives characterized late-stage tuberculosis as the time when the doctor "reached the end of his resources and was reduced to employing inadequate palliatives." Fonnsagrives, *Thérapeutique*, 516.

51. Coriveaud, "Le médecin," 13.

52. Selim Cosmao-Dumenez, *Sur un nouveau matelas d'eau employé à la Maison municipale de santé de Paris, pour prévenir la gangrène par compression dans les maladies chroniques* (Paris: H. Galante, 1862), 5–6.

53. L. H. Petit, "Des opérations palliatives chez les cancéreux," *Bulletin générale de thérapie* 45 (1878): 298–311.

54. Tuffier, "Traitement du cancer," 2708.

55. Colostomies were obviously extremely messy in the era before plastics.

56. Broussais, *Cours de pathologie*, 1: 276.

57. Peter, *Leçons*, 2: 597.

58. Ibid., 591.

59. Jaumes, "Des maladies," 95–96 (quote is from p. 96).

60. *Dictionnaire de la santé et des maladies, ou la médecine domestique par alphabet*, s.v. "Palliatif," 511.

61. *Nouveau dictionnaire de médecine et de chirurgie pratiques*, s.v. "Diathèse," 461.

62. Fleury, *Traité pratique et raisonné d'hydrothérapie*, 531–32.

63. Tardieu, "Psychologie du malade," 591.

64. Fleury, *Traité pratique et raisonné d'hydrothérapie*, 593–94.

65. Philibert Patissier, "Quelques considérations générales sur les diathèses à manifestations chroniques et sur leur traitement par les eaux minérales naturelles," *Revue médicale française et étrangère* 1 (1857): 601.

66. Lefebvre, *La science de bien mourir, 2e partie*, 1: 184–85.

67. For a compelling portrait of spa culture and socialization, see Mackaman, *Leisure Settings*.

68. Durand-Fardel, *Les eaux minérales et les maladies chroniques*, 127.

69. Mackaman, *Leisure Settings*, 43.

70. Morin, *Les diathèses et les cachexies*, 9–10.

71. Louis, *Recherches anatomiques*, 654–55.

72. Forget, *Des devoirs du médecin*, 28.

73. Lefebvre, *La science de bien mourir, 2e partie*, 3: 99–100.

74. Chevreuse, "Influence de l'imagination," 33–34.

75. Jaumes, "Des maladies," 123–24.

76. *Dictionnaire encyclopédique des sciences médicales*, s.v. "Carcinome (Partie clinique)," 408.

77. Chevreuse, "Influence de l'imagination," 33–34.

78. Ramsey, "Alternative Medicine," 286–90.

79. Jacques Léonard, La médecine, 72–73, 84. Also Léonard, Médecins, malades, et société dans la France du XIXe siècle (Paris: Sciences en situation, 1992), 71.

80. The turf battles cut both ways, as some physicians had the right (and generated much of their income) from preparing and selling prescription medication.

81. Léonard, Médecins, malades, et société, 70.

82. Ibid., 36.

83. Ibid., 33–61.

84. Léonard, La médicine, 77, 292.

85. Léonard, Médecins, malades, et société, 33–82; Jacques Léonard, La vie quotidienne du médecin de province au XIXe siècle (Paris: Hachette, 1977), 154–64.

86. Jacques Léonard, "Les guérisseurs en France au XIXe siècle," Revue d'histoire moderne et contemporaine 27 (1980): 501–3; Léonard, La médicine entre les pouvoirs et les savoirs, 69–70.

87. Léonard, Médecins, maladies, et société, 51.

88. Matthew Ramsey has aptly described the country as "authoritarian but non-interventionist." Ramsey, "Academic Medicine and Medical Industrialism: The Regulation of Secret Remedies in Nineteenth-Century France," in French Medical Culture in the Nineteenth Century, ed. Anna La Berge and Mordechai Feingold (Amsterdam: Rodopi, 1994), 29, 55, 61, 64.

89. Ibid., 42–51.

90. Léonard, Médecins, malades, et société, 51.

91. Ramsey, "Alternative Medicine," 300.

92. Verdo, Le charlatanisme, 9–10.

93. Theodor Billroth, General surgical pathology and therapeutics, in fifty-one lectures; a text-book for students and physicians; translated from the 4th German edition, with the special permission of the author and revised from the 8th edition, 3rd American ed. (New York: Appleton, 1879), 712.

94. Dictionnaire de médecine, de chirurgie, de pharmacie, de l'art vétérinaire et des sciences qui s'y rapportent, s.v. "Palliatifs," 1134.

95. Dictionnaire des sciences médicales, par une société de médecins et chirurgiens, s.v. "Palliatifs," 121.

96. Dictionnaire des sciences médicales, par une société de médecine et de chirurgiens, s.v. "Cancer," 668.

97. "The use of cabalistic signs and foreign languages in the writing of prescriptions can be justified only by a genuine need to dissimulate a remedy, in the interest of the patient and not because of a so-called professional dignity, dignity that can never be based upon fraud and charlatanism." Forget, Des devoirs du médecin, 28. See also Simon, Déontologie médicale, 286–87.

98. Verdo, Le charlatanisme, 37–41.

99. Petit, Essai, 33–34.

100. Theodore Zeldin, France 1848–1945 (Oxford: Clarendon Press, 1973) I: 26–28.

101. Dr. Charles Fauvel, La Vraie vérité sur M. Vries, dit le Docteur noir (Paris: Delahaye, 1859).

102. Jan Hendrick Vries (dit le Docteur noir), *Ordre de Dieu d'ériger le temple du royaume du Christ prophétisé par Salomom . . . décrit par Ézéchiel . . . manifesté en vision à Vries . . . Réforme universelle par la civilisation et l'union des nations. Érection à Paris d'un temple symbolique en albâtre réunissant et confondant en un culte unique le protestantisme, le catholicisme et le judaïsme, auxquels viennent se joindre toutes les religions professées dans l'univers. Paris, centre du monde, devient le soleil dont les rayons répandent partout l'amour, l'union et la civilisation des peuples* (Paris: De Dubuison, 1856); see also Anonymous, *La vérité sur le docteur noir* (Paris: Librairie Nouvelle, 1859), 25.

103. Fauvel, *La Vraie vérité*, 42–43. For another version of these events, see *La verité sur le docteur noir*, 27–30.

104. Anonymous, *La vérité sur le docteur noir*, 1859, 5. Philippe Ricord was the attending physician. He consulted Alfred Velpeau regarding the possibility of surgery. For details, see *Grand dictionnaire universel du XIXe siècle: Français, historique, géographique, mythologique, bibliographique, littéraire, artistique, scientifique, etc., etc*, 1867 edition, s.v. "Cancer," 254.

105. Anonymous, *La vérité*, 31–32.

106. Ibid., 254.

107. Ibid., 254.

108. "Le docteur noir-Vriès: Exercise illegal de la medicine," *Chroniques Judiciaires*, 3e brochure (Jan. 1860): 22.

109. Though it is unclear whether it occurred in this case, physicians sometimes received kickbacks from successful "outsiders."

110. Anonymous, "Expériences sur le traitement du cancer institué par le sieur Vriès à l'hôpital de la Charité, sous la surveillance de MM. Manec et Velpeau. Compte rendu par M. Velpeau. Séance du 28 mars 1859," *Bulletin de l'Académie Impériale de Médecine* 24 (1858–59): 658.

111. Velpeau's "generous spirit took offence at the idea of injustice and charlatanism; whatever the source, it was offensive, odious to him . . . But the triumph of truth is often a costly one, and few are aware of the bitterness that one of his last battles, that with the famous *Docteur noir*, brought down upon him." Éloge de M. Richet in "Obsèques de M. Velpeau," *Gazette des hôpitaux* (29 August 1867): 399.

112. Vries's strange and outlandish persona may have increased some people's faith in his healing powers.

113. Fauvel, *La vraie vérité*, 14–15.

114. Gueneau de Mussy, *Leçons*, 67–68.

115. Paul Broca, *Traité des tumeurs* (Paris: Asselin, 1866), 398.

116. For an interesting discussion of this issue in mid twentieth-century America, see David Cantor, "Cancer, Quackery, and the Vernacular Meanings of Hope in 1950s America," *Journal of the History of Medicine and Allied Sciences* 61, no. 3 (July 2006): 324–68.

117. Lebert, *Traité clinique et pratique*, 464.

118. Rengade, *Les grands maux*, 27–28.

119. A. Moussous, "De la mort chez les phtisiques" (MD thesis, Paris, 1886), 29.

120. Rengade, *Les grands maux*, 27–28.

121. *Dictionnaire populaire de médecine usuelle d'hygiène publique et privée*, s.v. "Agonie," 59–60.

122. Chomel, "De l'importance," 502.

123. Forget, *Des devoirs du médecin*, 18–19.

124. Simon, *Déontologie médicale*, 312.

125. Alphonse Goix, *Note sur les devoirs du médecin chrétien auprès de mourants* (Lille: Bureau du Journal des sciences médicales, 1889), 6.

126. Percival, *Medical Ethics*, 31; Hooker, *Doctor and Patient*, 352–53; Flint, *Medical Ethics*, 25.

127. Ragonneau, "Considérations sur l'agonie," 19.

128. Thomas Kselman, *Death and the Afterlife in Modern France* (Princeton, NJ: Princeton University Press, 1993), 90.

129. Ibid., 99–102.

130. Lefebvre, *La science de bien mourir, manuel de l'Association de la Bonne Mort*, 226–27.

131. Amédée Dechambre, *Le Médecin: devoirs privés et publics, leurs rapports avec la jurisprudence* (Paris: Masson, 1883), 217.

132. Goix, *Note sur les devoirs*, 5.

133. Pierre Jean Corneille Debreyne, *La Théologie morale et les sciences médicales*, 6th ed. (Paris: Poussielgue, 1884), 229. Cited in Kselman, *Death and the Afterlife*, 98.

134. Lefebvre, *La science de bien mourir, 2e partie*, 2: 47–48.

135. Ivan Waddington, "The Role of the Hospital in the Development in Modern Medicine: A Sociological Analysis," *Sociology* 72 (May 1973): 211–24.

136. Zurkowski, "Du degré d'utilité," 517.

137. E. Garreau, "Considérations pratiques sur le cancer," *Revue médicale française et étrangère* 3(1846): 51.

138. Ibid., 54.

139. "An almost constant effect of chronic illness is to make the person worried, somber, egotistical, and irascible." Descuret, *La médecine*, 70.

140. Lebert, *Traité clinique*, 464.

141. Daremberg, *Les différentes formes*, 319.

142. Lebert, *Traité pratique des maladies cancéreuses*, 365.

143. Ibid., 287–88.

144. Daremberg, *Les différentes formes*, 89–90.

## CHAPTER 7  *ECCE HOMO*: OPIATES, SUFFERING, AND THE ART OF PALLIATION

1. David F. Musto, *The American Disease: Origins of Narcotic Control* (New Haven: Yale University Press, 1973). Virginia Berridge, *Opium and the People: Opiate Use and Drug Control Policy in Nineteenth and Early Twentieth Century England*, 2nd ed. (London: Free Association Books, 1999). David T. Coutwright, *Dark Paradise: A History of Opiate Addiction in America* (Cambridge, MA: Harvard University Press, 2001).

2. Yvorel, *Les poisons de l'esprit*.

3. Ibid., 114–15.

4. There were four sources of morphine addiction during the same period in U.S. history (iatrogenic, the Civil War, self-dosage, and nontherapeutic). Chronic disease (or at least chronic complaints) played a critical role in the first of these.

Yet notwithstanding a decline in the absolute numbers of addicts, the shift from medicinal use (primarily among relatively affluent women) to self-use (primarily among lower-class men) drove perceptions that addiction was "dirty" and that the drug posed a growing threat. This transformation, in turn, played a decisive role in encouraging the subsequent enactment of heavy-handed legislation. Courtwright, *Dark Paradise*, 2–3, 9–60, 110–44.

5. B. Cyprien Hontang, "Essai sur l'opium, son importance et son emploi thérapeutique" (MD thesis, Paris, 1833), 44–55.

6. Démetrius Zambaco, "De la Morphéomanie," *Encéphale: Journal des maladies mentales et nerveuses* 2 (1882): 637–38.

7. Berridge, *Opium*, 136–38.

8. It was an equally pressing issue in Britain. For details, see Berridge, *Opium*, xxx, 21–22, 62, 87–93.

9. *Dictionnaire des sciences médicales, par une société de médecins et chirurgiens*, s.v. "Opium," 470.

10. MM. Ollivier (D'Angers), Labarraque et Gaultier de Claubry, "Rapport sur divers opiums livrés au commerce et suspectés de falsification," *Annales d'hygiène publique et de médecine légale* 22 (1839): 374.

11. Ibid., 390, 393.

12. Lebert, *Traité pratique des maladies cancéreuses*, 282.

13. Berridige, *Opium*, 88–89.

14. Hector Aubergier, "De la culture du pavot en France pour la récolte de l'opium," *Mémoires de l'académie impériale de médecine* 19 (1855): 53. Despite the inhospitable climate, small-scale poppy farming was also attempted in England in the early nineteenth century. Berridge, *Opium*, 11–17.

15. Ibid., 80.

16. *Nouveau dictionnaire de médecine et de chirurgie*, s.v. "Opium," 633.

17. Yvorel, *Les poisons de l'esprit*, 49–51; Berridge, *Opium*, 97–105.

18. Berridge, *Opium*, 79–80; Foxcroft, 89–91.

19. *Dictionnaire des sciences médicales, par une société de médecins et chirurgiens*, s.v. "Opium," 492.

20. Berridge, *Opium*, 21–61.

21. Yvorel, *Les poisons de l'esprit*, 104–5.

22. Charles Polydore Forget, "Clinique de l'opium," *Bulletin général de thérapeutique* 49 (August 1855): 154.

23. Lebert, *Traité pratique des maladies cancéreuses*, 540.

24. Ragonneau, "Considérations sur l'agonie" (MD thesis, Paris, 1817), 20.

25. Simon, *Déontologie médicale*, 385.

26. Dechambre, *Le Médecin*, 218.

27. *Dictionnaire des sciences médicales, par une société de médecins et chirurgiens*, s.v. "Opium," 482.

28. Louis, *Recherches anatomiques*, 669.

29. Armand Trousseau and Hermann Pidoux, *Traité de thérapeutique et de matière médicale*, 9th ed. (Paris: Asselin, 1877), 2: 156–57. Subcutaneous administration results in brisk and near-complete systemic absorption mimicking hypodermic injection.

Berridge has aptly called these innovations "curtain raisers for the true hypodermic method," Berridge, *Opium*, 138–39.

30. Léonard, *La médecine*, 73.

31. *Dictionnaire des sciences médicales, par une société de médecins et chirurgiens*, s.v. "Morphine," 304–5.

32. Debreyne, *Thérapeutique appliquée*, 173.

33. "The humble folk, who are exposed to morphine only in the hospital, do not have the financial means to continue its usage, once they get out." Édouard Levinstein, *La morphinomanie: Basée sur des observations personnelles*, 2nd ed. (Paris: Masson, 1880), 6. In a thesis on the palliative treatment of uterine cancer (1886), one doctor spoke of a forty-year-old woman whose horrible pain was relieved only by cocaine. The high cost of the drug forced the doctor to stop prescribing it after only a few days. Gaches Sarraute, "Du traitement palliatif du cancer utérin inopérable" (MD thesis, Paris, 1886), 12.

34. Lebert, *Traité pratique des maladies cancéreuses*, 118.

35. Lefebvre, *La science de bien mourir, 2e partie*, 1: 34–36, 76–77.

36. Ibid., 1: 287, 3: 81–82.

37. Forget, "Clinique de l'opium," 148.

38. Foxcroft, *The Making of Addiction*, 151.

39. Jules Rochard, *Questions d'hygiène sociale* (Paris: Hachette, 1891), 238.

40. Berridge, *Opium*, 139–40.

41. Georges Cochet, "Contributions à l'étude des injections hypodermiques" (MD thesis, Paris, 1883), 7.

42. Alfred-Joseph de Lebeaupin, *La méthode de Jennings pour le traitement de l'intoxication par l'opium et la morphine et la cure de Vichy* (Paris: Masson, 1906), 4.

43. Maxim Du Camp, "La charité privée à Paris. II. Les Dames du Calvaire," *Revue des deux mondes* 3, no. 57 (1883): 294.

44. The work was translated by Alfred de Mussy in 1827 and was very influential in French literary circles. See Yvorel, *Les poisons de l'esprit*, 37.

45. Morel, *Traité des dégénérescences physiques*, 394–413.

46. Forget, "Clinique de l'opium," 156.

47. Clifford Albutt, "On the Abuse of Hypodermic Injections of Morphia," *Practitioner* 5 (1870): 327–31.

48. Levinstein, *La morphinomanie*, 3.

49. Ibid., 5.

50. Benjamin Ball, *La morphinomanie: Les frontières de la folie, le dualisme cérébral, les rêves prolongés, la folie gémellaire ou aliénation mentale chez les jumeaux* (Paris: Asselin et Houzeau, 1885), 23.

51. Ibid., 25.

52. "Most often we are deceived by patients and often by their families. There reigns in this case a singular complicity between the morphine maniac and his entourage; the mother, the wife, the sister, the friends, seek to cast a veil over the vice that they should denounce to the physician in the interest of the patient." Ball, *La morphinomanie*, 50–51.

53. *Nouveau dictionnaire de médecine et de chirurgie*, s.v. "Opium," 650.

54. Benjamin Ball, *La morphinomanie. De la responsabilité partielle des aliénés. Les frontières de la folie. Les rêves prolongés. Opuscules divers,* 2nd ed. (Paris: Lefrançois, 1888), 75.

55. Howard I. Kushner, "Taking Biology Seriously: The Next Task for Historians of Addiction?" *Bulletin of the History of Medicine* 80, no. 2 (2006): 115–43.

56. Barbara Hodgson, *In the Arms of Morpheus: The Tragic History of Laudanum, Morphine, and Patent Medicine* (Vancouver, BC: Greystone Books, 2001), 85.

57. Estimates from the 1880s placed the number of Parisian addicts between 40,000 and 100,000. Yvorel, *Les poisons de l'esprit,* 107, 109, 124, 126, 131, 216.

58. Ruth Harris, *Murders and Madness: Medicine, Law, and Society in the Fin de Siècle* (Oxford: Clarendon Press, 1989), 312–20.

59. Yvorel, *Les poisons de l'esprit,* 140–41, 170–75.

60. Ibid., 73–77, 173–74.

61. Alcohol abuse was the leading public health problem in France during this period (alongside syphilis and tuberculosis). Partly this reflects the magnitude of the problem. Yet its association with working-class "excess" also decisively affected perceptions.

62. Berridge, *Opium,* 192, 198.

63. Regnard, 313.

64. Yvorel, *Les poisons de l'esprit,* 90, 121, 173–74, 207.

65. Ibid., 113–14, 135; Foxcroft, *The Making of Addiction,* 130–31.

66. Yvorel, *Les poisons de l'esprit,* 199.

67. Paul Regnard, *Sorcellerie, magnétisme, morphinisme, délire des grandeurs* (Paris: Plon, 1887), 322–23.

68. Levinstein, *la morphinomanie,* 7–8. Yvorel estimates that physicians were overrepresented by a factor of over one hundred; Yvorel, *Les poisons de l'esprit,* 125–28. A startling number of (male) American physicians also apparently had a problem with addiction at the turn of the twentieth century. Coutwright, *Dark Paradise,* 41.

69. Regnard, *Sorcellerie,* 326.

70. Ibid., 301.

71. Yvorel, *Les poisons de l'esprit,* 185–88.

72. Berridge, *Opium,* 173–75.

73. Yvorel, *Les poisons de l'esprit,* 165–67.

74. *Nouveau dictionnaire de médecine et de chirurgie,* s.v. "Opium," 650.

75. Peter, *Leçons,* 2: 537.

76. Narcotics are one of several medications where tolerance readily develops with prolonged usage.

77. Jules Rochard, *Questions d'hygiène sociale* (Paris: Hachette, 1891), 261–62.

78. Levinstein, *La morphinomanie,* 8.

79. Léopold Calvet, "Essai sur le morphinisme aigu et chronique: Étude expérimentale et clinique sur l'action physiologique de la morphine" (MD thesis, Paris, 1876), 68–75.

80. Ibid., 71.

81. Ibid., 71, 73.

82. *Nouveau dictionnaire de médecine et de chirurgie*, s.v. "Opium," 665.

83. Regnard expressed sympathy for those who became addicted because of a painful chronic illness while heaping scorn on those who were overly sensitive or lacking moral fiber. Regnard, *Sorcellerie*, 313.

84. Yvorel, *Les Poisons de l'esprit*, 199

85. Levinstein, *La morphinomanie*, 68.

86. Ibid., 75–80.

87. Paul Brouardel, "Opium, morphine et cocaïne: intoxication aiguë par l'opium, mangeurs et fumeurs d'opium, morphinomanes et cocaïnomanes," *Cours de médecine légale de la Faculté de médecine de Paris* (Paris: Baillière, 1906), 12: 141–42.

88. Ball, *La morphinomanie* (1885), 70.

89. Bullar, "On the Use of Small Doses of Opium," 268–69.

90. Pierre Guillaume, *Médecins, église et foi XIXe–XXe siècles* (Paris: Aubier, 1990), 117.

91. Snow believed that the nervous system played a critical role in the development of cancer and argued that pain caused the disease to progress and spread.

92. Herbert Snow, *The Palliative Treatment of Incurable Cancer: With an Appendix on the Use of the Opium-Pipe. Being a lecture delivered at the cancer hospital, March 7th, 1890* (London: Churchill, 1890), 47.

93. Joseph Récamier, "Traitement des malades inopérables et questions d'assistance," *Travaux de la 2e conférence internationale pour l'étude du cancer 1910* (Paris: Alcan, 1911), 187.

94. Courtwright, *Dark Paradise*, 52–53, 121, 81–104.

95. Regnard, *Sorcellerie*, 337.

96. Tuffier, "Traitement du cancer inopérable," 2713–14.

97. Daniel Critzman, *Le cancer* (Paris: Masson, 1894), 154–55. This work was also published in *Encyclopédie scientifique des aide-mémoire* (Paris: Gauthier-Villers et Fils, 1892–1913).

98. Récamier, *Traitement du cancer*, 187.

99. Ibid., 187–88.

100. Tuffier, "Traitement du cancer inopérable," 2713–14.

101. Ball, *La morphinomanie*, 1885, 69.

102. Rochard, *Questions d'hygiène sociale*, 262.

103. *Dictionnaire populaire de médecine usuelle d'hygiène publique et privée*, s.v. "Morphine," 490.

104. Récamier, *Traitement du cancer*, 172.

105. Warner, *The Therapeutic Perspective*, 248–53.

106. Uterine cancer patients "wake up from time to time, prodded by a pain crisis, beg for their morphine and die relatively calm after months of indescribable suffering." Pozzi, "Le traitement du cancer de l'utérus," 15.

107. Lebert, *Traité pratique des maladies cancéreuses*, 364.

108. Chomel, "De l'importance," 502.

109. Edouard Morel, *La science et la charité en présence des misères humaines. Discours prononcé dans la séance publique du 21 juin 1855 à l'Académie Impériale des Sciences* (Bordeaux: Belles Lettres et Arts de Bordeau, 1855), 7.

110. Quintard, "Forces morales médicatrices," 22.

111. Rochard, *Questions d'hygiène sociale*, 249.

112. Ball, *La morphinomanie*, 1885, 69.

113. Tuffier, "Traitement du cancer inopérable," 2713–14; Récamier, *Traitement du cancer utérin inopérable*, 188.

114. Foxcroft, *The Making of Addiction*, 119, 156–59.

115. Ibid., 43.

116. Yvorel, *Les poisons de l'esprit*, 137–44, 215.

117. Récamier, *Traitement du cancer*, 188.

118. Janet Oppenheim, *"Shattered Nerves": Doctors, Patients, and Depression in Victorian England* (New York: Oxford University Press, 1991), 181–232.

119. Berridge, *Opium*, 153.

120. See also Yvorel, *Les poisons de l'esprit*, 117.

121. Anonymous, *L'éther ou l'art de mourir sans douleur* (Paris: Imprimerie de Lacour, 1847).

122. Rochard, *Questions d'hygiène sociale*, 255.

123. Rochard expressed sympathy for those stricken with painful and lethal diseases and celebrated medicine's ability to make patients' pain "almost completely disappear." Rochard, *Questions d'hygiène sociale*, 237–38.

124. Paul Butel, *L'opium: Histoire d'une fascination* (Paris: Perrin, 1995), 358.

125. Yvorel, *Les poisons de l'esprit*, 20.

126. Roy Porter, "Pain and Suffering," in *Companion Encyclopedia of the History of Medicine*, ed. W. F. Bynum and Roy Porter (London: Rutledge, 1993), 2: 1586.

127. Anne Carol, *Les médecins et la mort XIXe–XXe siècle* (Paris: Aubier, 2004), 56–63

128. Roselyn Rey, "The Church and Pain in France" in *The History of Pain*, trans. Louise Elliot Wallace, J. A. Cadden, and S. W. Cadden (Cambridge, MA: Harvard University Press, 1995), 184–90; quote is from p. 186.

129. Ibid., 184.

130. Porter, "Pain and Suffering," 1585.

131. Simon, *Déontologie médicale*, 23–24, 390 (quote on p. 390).

132. Ibid., 384.

133. Rey, *The History of Pain*, 186.

134. Debreyne, *Thérapeutique appliquée*, 58–60.

135. *Dictionnaire de médecine pratique et des sciences qui lui servent de fondements. Contenant, outre les articles obligés d'anatomie, de physiologie, d'hygiène, d'étiologie, de sémiologie, de pathologie, de thérapeutique, et de matière médicale, la définition des mots qui doivent en rendre le sens intelligible à tous les lecteurs. Ouvrage destiné à MM. les ecclésiastiques, les chefs d'institutions, les membres des sociétés de bienfaisance etc.*, s.v. "Mort," 741.

136. Victor Jean Gourdel, *L'ange consolateur ou méthode pour sanctifier les malades et assister les mourants* (Colmar: C. M. Hoffmann, 1868), 60–62; quote is from p. 61.

137. Lefebvre, *La science de bien mourir, manuel de l'Association de la Bonne Mort*, 218.

138. Lefebvre, *La science de bien mourir, 2e partie*, 3: 40–41.

139. Ibid., 1: 147–48.

140. Martin Pernick, *A Calculus of Suffering: Pain, Professionalism, and Anesthesia in Nineteenth-Century America* (New York: Columbia University Press, 1985), 35.

CHAPTER 8   THE GOOD, THE BAD, AND THE UGLY:
INCURABILITY AND THE QUEST FOR GOODNESS

1. Daremberg, *Les différentes formes*, 99–100.

2. Abel, *Suffering in the Land of Sunshine*, xvi–xvii, 87–88; Kirtsen E. Gardner, *Early Detection: Women, Cancer, and Awareness Campaigns in the Twentieth-Century United States* (Chapel Hill: University of North Carolina Press, 2006), 107; Feudtner, *Bittersweet*, 97, 117, 123, 131, 140, 144, 174–76.

3. Tardieu, "Psychologie du malade," 586–87.

4. "A sick woman readily listens to the suggestive words of her doctor. . . . Women, even the most obstinate and frivolous, let themselves be convinced more easily than men." Daremberg, *Les différentes formes*, 92.

5. "Tuberculosis served as a key vehicle in the nineteenth century through which womanhood was associated with a kind of suffering which was morally and spiritually redeeming." Barnes, *The Making*, 49.

6. Chomel, "De l'importance," 502.

7. Lefebvre, *La science de bien mourir, manuel de l'Association de la Bonne Mort*, 407–8.

8. Drew Gilpin Faust, *This Republic of Suffering: Death and the American Civil War* (New York: Knopf, 2008).

9. Lauvergne claimed that his anthropological/sociological study was based on observations at over a thousand patients' deathbeds. Lauvergne, *De l'agonie et de la mort*, 435. See also Barnes, *The Making*, 48–73.

10. Lauvergne, *De l'agonie et de la mort*, 435–37.

11. Daremberg, *Les différentes formes*, 109–10.

12. Lefebvre, *La science de bien mourir, 2e partie*, 1: 116–17.

13. Ibid., 1: 272–76.

14. Petit, *Essai sur la médecine du cœur*, 190.

15. Lefebvre, *La science de bien mourir, 2e partie*, 3: 258–59.

16. Tardieu, "Psychologie du malade," 590.

17. The rituals included confession, communion, and anointment with holy oils (extreme unction). The idea that one's soul could be lost at the last moment was progressively deemphasized during the eighteenth and nineteenth centuries; one's behavior in the final stage of illness nonetheless remained exceedingly important.

18. McManners, *Death and the Enlightenment*, 231–33; quote is from p. 233.

19. Lefebvre, *La science de bien mourir, manuel de l'Association de la Bonne Mort*, 17 (emphasis in the original).

20. The different lessons were taken up in monthly lectures that were part of a four-year intensive course in the "advanced" science of dying well. Lefebvre, *La science de bien mourir, manuel de l'Association de la Bonne Mort*, 36.

21. Lefebvre, *La science de bien mourir, 2e partie*, 2: 225–26.

22. Ibid., 2: 46–47.

23. Ibid., 1: 226–27, 3: 5, 100.

24. Ibid., 1: 23–26.

25. Ibid., 2: 267–69.

26. Ibid., 1: 103–4.

27. Barnes, *The Making*, 49–50, 63–70.

28. *Dictionnaire de médecine usuelle à l'usage des gens du monde des chefs de famille et de grands établissements, des administrateurs, des magistrats et des officiers de police judiciaire, enfin pouvant servir à tous ceux qui se dévouent au soulagement des malades*, s.v. "Douleur," 536.

29. Lefebvre, *La science de bien mourir, 2e partie*, 1: 184–85. Admiral Henry de Valdailly also "suffered with an admirable patience, and knew how to hide his suffering." Lefebvre, *La science de bien mourir, 2e partie*, 2: 70–71.

30. Ibid., 2: 183–84, 2: 86–87.

31. Ibid., 1: 39–41. These stories may well have been embellished. The fact that stirring displays of self-control were not the norm, however, suggests that it not a simply literary trope or self-congratulatory posturing.

32. Ibid., 1: 154–55.

33. Ibid., 3: 61–63.

34. Ibid., 1: 171–72.

35. Ibid., 1: 169–70.

36. Ibid., 1: 219–20.

37. Ibid., 1: 251–53.

38. Ibid., 1: 249–50.

39. Ibid., 1: 260–61.

40. Ibid., 3: 122.

41. H. Beylard, *Catholicisme: Hier, aujourd'hui, demain*, s.v. "Mort (Congrégation de la Bonne Mort)," 775.

42. Georges Daremberg, *Les grands médecins du XIXe siècle* (Paris: 1907), 161–62.

43. Lefebvre, *La science de bien mourir, 2e partie*, 3: 263.

44. Ibid., 1: 108–14.

45. Weisz, *The Medical Mandarins*, 215, 226–29.

46. Chevreuse, "Influence de l'imagination," 34–35; Simon, *Déontologie médicale*, 128–29.

47. *Dictionnaire de médecine usuelle*, s.v. "Douleur," 536–37.

48. Garoz, "Considérations générales," 20; Chomel, "De l'importance," 502–3.

49. Dechambre, *Le Médecin*, 217–18.

50. Ball, "Phthisie et folie," 174.

51. Pidoux, *Études*, 302–3.

52. Ibid., 536–37.

53. Quintard, "Forces morales," 24–25.

54. Ibid., 14–15.

55. "We die as we are born, according to the *species* of soul which the (hazard) of birth endowed us." Lauvergne, *De l'agonie*, 2: 3, 27.

56. Ibid., I: xi–xii.

57. Ibid., 2: 34.

58. Lefebvre, *La science de bien mourir, manuel de l'Association de la Bonne Mort*, 407–8.

59. One of Mme. Méeary Étard's friends noted that "death frightened her horribly; I have no doubt that she owes to Saint-Joseph the fact that she died quietly almost without seeing it coming, as the doctors had predicted a terrible crisis for her final moments, and nothing of this sort took place." Lefebvre, *La science de bien mourir, 2e partie*, 3: 37.

60. Religiously inspired "moral" fortitude figured prominently in "sociological" analyses of suicide, which stressed that a religious education was a critically important preservative. Dechambre, *Le médecin*, 219.

61. Lauvergne, *De l'agonie*, 2: 144.

62. *Dictionnaire populaire de médecine usuelle d'hygiène publique et privée*, s.v. "Agonie," 59–60.

63. Kselman, *Death*, 95–103.

64. Ibid., 189–99.

65. Patrick Hutton, *The Cult of the Revolutionary Tradition: The Blanquists in French Politics, 1864–1893* (Berkeley: University of California Press, 1981).

66. Jennifer Hecht, "French Scientific Materialism and the Liturgy of Death: The Invention of a Secular Version of Catholic Last Rites 1876–1914," *French Historical Studies*, 20, no. 4 (1997): 714.

67. *The Oxford English Dictionary*, 1989 edition, s.v. "Edify," 71.

68. Lefebvre, *La science de bien mourir, 2e partie*, I: 200–202.

69. Guillaume-Marie-André Ferrus, "Notice historique sur L.-Th. Biett," *Mémoires de l'Académie Royale de Médecine* 8 (1840): 53.

70. Fonssagrives, *Thérapeutique*, 516–17.

71. Daremberg, *Les différentes formes*, 102–3.

72. Ibid., 101.

73. Petit, *Essai sur la médecine du cœur*, 235–36.

74. Jaumes, "Des maladies," 125–26.

## CHAPTER 9    THE FATE OF THE INCURABLY ILL
## BETWEEN THE TWO REVOLUTIONS, 1789–1848

1. Jean-Baptiste Bienvenu-Martin, preface to Edouard Campagnole, *L'assistance obligatoire aux vieillards aux infirmes et aux incurables: Commentaire de la loi du 14 juillet 1905* (Paris: Berger-Levrault, 1908), vii.

2. Gunther Risse, *Mending Bodies, Saving Souls: A History of Hospitals* (New York: Oxford University Press, 1999), 295.

3. Dora Weiner, *The Citizen-Patient in Revolutionary and Imperial Paris* (Baltimore: Johns Hopkins University Press, 1993), 59.

4. Ibid., 59–68.

5. Colin Jones, *The Charitable Imperative: Hospitals and Nursing in Ancien Régime and Revolutionary France* (London: Rutledge, 1989), 9–10.

6. Risse, *Mending Bodies*, 295.

7. Jacques Tenon, *Mémoires sur les hôpitaux de Paris* (Paris: Pierres, 1788), xx, 169.

8. Jones, *The Charitable Imperative*, 10–11, 33, 48–68.

9. Weiner, *The Citizen Patient*, 84.

10. *Procès-verbaux et rapports du comité de mendicité de la Constituante, 1790–1791*, ed. C. Bloch and C. Tuteley (Paris: Imprimerie nationale, 1911), 391, cited in Weiner, *The Citizen Patient*, 87.

11. Weiner, *The Citizen Patient*, 85.

12. Risse, *Mending Bodies*, 301; Weiner, *The Citizen Patient*, 84–87, 321–27.

13. Risse, *Mending Bodies*, 304.

14. Risse, *Mending Bodies*, 302–3; Weiner, *The Citizen Patient*, 26–28.

15. Allan Forrest, *The French Revolution and the Poor* (Oxford: Blackwell, 1981), 174.

16. Risse, *Mending Bodies*, 309.

17. Michael Foucault, *The Birth of the Clinic: An Archaeology of Medical Perceptions* (New York: Vintage, 1994).

18. Foucault's ideas have been taken up by most social scientists. See, for example, Robert Nye, *Crime, Madness, and Politics in Modern France* (Princeton, NJ: Princeton University Press, 1984).

19. Weiner, *The Citizen Patient*, 56.

20. Weiner errs on the side of hyperbole: "health care thus became more efficient, discriminating, diversified and appropriate. Patients now found a number of hospitals equipped to cope with their diseases to the best of contemporary knowledge, while the attending physicians evolved into specialists." Weiner, *The Citizen Patient*, 11–12.

21. Léonard, *La médecine*, 13.

22. The term *selective medicalization* is used in Isabelle von Bueltzingloewen, *Machines à instruire, machines à guérir. Les hôpitaux universitaires et la médicalisation de la société allemande 1730–1850* (Lyon: Presses universitaires de Lyon, 1997), 223–40.

23. Timothy B. Smith, "The Ideology of Charity, the Image of the Poor Law, and Debates over the Right to Assistance in France, 1830–1905," *Historical Journal* 40, no. 4 (1997): 997–1032.

24. William Coleman, *Death Is a Social Disease: Public Health and Political Economy in Early Industrial France* (Madison: University of Wisconsin Press, 1982), 9–11, 32–33, 124–80.

25. Louis-René Villermé, *Tableau de l'état physique et moral des ouvriers employés dans les manufactures de coton, de laine, et de soie*, 2 vols. (Paris: Jules Renouard, 1840).

26. Coleman, *Death*, 219–33.

27. Baron Jean Marie de Gerando, *Le visiteur du pauvre* (Paris: L. Colas, 1820), 26.

28. Epigraph to Théodore Fix, "De l'esprit progressif et de l'esprit de conservation en économie politique," *Journal des économistes* 2 (1842): 222, 237, cited in Coleman, *Death*, 59.

29. The use of Malthus's ideas by French Catholics, socialists, and neo-Malthusians is examined in J. Dupâquier, A. Fauve-Chamoux, E. Grebenik, eds., *Malthus Past and Present* (London: Academic Press, 1983).

30. Yves Charbet, "The Fate of Malthus' Work," in J. Dupâquier, *Malthus*, 25.

31. Smith, "The Ideology of Charity," 1012.

32. Weiner, *The Citizen-Patient*, 154.

33. De Gerando, *Le visiteur*, 91–92.

34. Chevalier, *Laboring Classes*, 137–38, 202–14, 262–67.

35. Timothy B. Smith, *Creating the Welfare State in France, 1880–1940* (Montreal: McGill-Queen's University Press, 2003), 17.

36. Anonymous, "Rapport à Monsieur le Préfet de la Seine et au Conseil général des hospices et des secours à domicile, présenté, au nom de MM. les Maires et adjoints, Présidents des Bureaux de bienfaisance par. M. A. Lefort, Maire du 1er Arrondissement, séance du 4 mai 1836," 8.

37. Smith, "The Ideology of Charity," 999–1000.

38. De Gerando, *Le visiteur*, 68.

39. Anonymous, "Bureau de bienfaisance du 13e arrondissement. Procès-verbal de l'Assemblé Générale du 4 juillet 1837 et compte moral et administratif de l'exercice 1836," Paris, 1837, 6.

40. Gaston Rimlinger, *Welfare Policy and Industrialization in Europe, America, and Russia* (New York: Wiley, 1971).

41. Chevalier, *Laboring Classes*, 224–319.

42. Ibid., 144, 408, 413–16.

43. Louis-René Villermé, "Quelques réflexions sur les établissements de charité publique, à l'occasion d'un ouvrage de M. David Johnson," *Annales d'hygiène publique et de médecine légale* 3 (1830): 99.

44. Coleman, *Death*, xviii–xix, 241–50, 272–73, 277–306.

45. Ibid., 250–61.

46. Anonymous, "Rapport présenté au nom des bureaux de bienfaisance de Paris, à Monsieur le Préfet de la Seine et au Conseil général des hospices et secours à domicile, dans la séance du 6 mai 1835," 25–26.

47. Jacques Orsel, *Essai sur les hôpitaux et sur les secours à domicile distribués aux indigents* (Paris: Le Normant, 1821), 13–14.

48. Anonymous, "Bureau de bienfaisance du 6e arrondissement: Compte moral et administratif pour l'exercice clos 1836. Présenté par M. François, administrateur, rapporteur au nom bu bureau," 7.

49. M. Battelle, "Rapport fait à la société des établissements charitables sur la nécessité de fonder de nouveaux hospices où l'on soit admis en payant (séance du 30 décembre 1834)."

50. Adrien De Gasparin, *Rapport au Roi sur les hôpitaux, les hospices et les services de bienfaisance* (Paris: Imprimerie Royale, 1837), 17.

51. Armand Husson, *Étude sur les hôpitaux considérés sous le rapport de leur construction, de la distribution de leur bâtiments, de l'ameublement, de l'hygiène et du service des asiles des malades* (Paris: P. Dupont, 1862), 277–78.

52. Rachel Ginnis Fuchs, *Abandoned Children: Foundlings and Child Welfare in Nineteenth-Century France* (Albany: State University of New York Press, 1984). See also Weiner, *The Citizen-Patient*, 10, 68–73.

53. Joseph-Henri-Joachim-Holstein Lainé, *Rapport au Roi sur la situation des hospices, des enfants trouvés, des aliénés, de la mendicité et des prisons* (Paris: Imprimerie Royale, 1818), 13, 17 (quote is from p. 17).

54. Ibid., 22–23.

55. Alain Lellouch, "Mortalité, espérance de vie et morbidité dans les hospices parisiens du XIXe," *Histoire des sciences médicales* 23, no. 2 (1989): 96.

56. Weiner, *The Citizen-Patient*, 11.

57. *Lettres patentes du Roy, portant établissement de l'Hôpital des Incurables de Paris* (1634), 2.

58. Jones, *The Charitable Imperative*, 68.

59. Anonymous, "Rapport sur les opérations du bureau central d'admission dans les Hôpitaux, an XII," 18.

60. Anonymous, "Arrêté du Conseil général d'administration des hospices et secours à domicile de Paris. Séance du 11 février 1818."

61. Françoise Huguet, *Les professeurs de la faculté de médecine de Paris, dictionnaire biographique 1794–1939* (Paris: Institut national de recherche pédagogique, editions du CNRS, 1991), 543, 584.

62. Based upon a random sampling of thirty medical and thirty surgical careers in Huguet, *Les professeurs de la faculté.*

63. One example of this universal rule can be found in the statutes of the *Maison nationale de Santé*, a public hospital where patients paid a small daily fee to avoid the stigma of being a charity case. Its admission policy stipulated that "all illnesses are treated there, with the exception of mental illnesses and those that are recognized to be incurable." Meding, *Paris médical*, 2: 76.

64. "Formal criteria in all early voluntary hospitals was similar. None admitted contagious or chronic ills. The former endangered the hospital's staff and the latter undermined its limited ability to provide beds for the potentially curable." Rosenberg, *The Care of Strangers*, 22–23 (quote is from p. 22). Von Buestzingloewen, *Machines à instruire*, 211–16; Olivier Faure, "L'hôpital et les incurables au XIXe siècle: l'exemple de Lyon," *Les cahiers du CTNE-RHI* 50 (1990): 71–78.

65. Anonymous, "Compte moral et administratif du bureau de bienfaisance du 5e arrondissement de Paris, Présenté par M. Vée, adjoint au maire, à l'assemblée générale tenue le 13 juillet 1843," 15.

66. Anonymous, "Rapport sur les opérations du bureau central d'admission dans les hôpitaux, an XII," 6–7.

67. Anonymous, "Mémoire lue à la commission administrative des hospices civiles de Paris, par les médecins du Grand Hospice d'Humanité; ci devant Hôtel Dieu," signé Majault, Danié, Mallet, Duhaume, le Preux, Bosquillon, Thauraux, Defrasne, Montaigu, Asselin, Petit, Bourdier, Médecins du Grand Hospice, Paris An VIII," 7–8.

68. Récamier, *Traitement du cancer*, 210–11.

69. Pierre-Armand Dufau, *Lettres à une dame sur la charité présentant le tableau complet des œuvres, associations et établissements destinés au soulagement des classes pauvres*, 2nd ed. (Paris: Guillaumin, 1847), 148–49.

70. Maxim Du Camp, *Paris: Ses organes, ses fonctions, et sa vie dans le seconde moitié du XIXe siècle*, 6th ed. (Paris: Hachette, 1879), 257–58.

71. Martin-Doisy, "Des hôpitaux et hospices du département de la Somme" *Annales de la charité* (1851): 109.

72. "Institution de Sainte-Périne. Nouveau règlement pour l'admission à l'Institution de Sainte Périne [Arrêté du 26 août 1856 du Conseil Supérieur de l'assistance publique]," 2.

73. Anonymous, "Rapport sur les opérations du bureau central d'admission dans les hôpitaux, an XII," 14.

74. Ibid., 15.

75. "Compte administratif des Hospices Civils de Lyon, 1836: Observations de MM. les médecins et chirurgiens, service de M. Chapleau," 31–32, cited in Faure, *Genèse de l'hôpital moderne*, 174.

76. Anonymous, "Rapport sur les opérations du bureau central d'admissions dans les Hôpitaux, an XII," 18.

77. It included scrofula, pulmonary phthisis, squirrhes, aneurysms, dropsy, gangrene, rickets, concretions [*concrétions*], chlorosis, and scurvy. See Meding, *Paris médical*, I: 155, 157–58.

78. Ariès, *The Hour of Our Death*, 570–71.

79. Referring to an English author who had made the same point, Villermé insisted that "the illnesses that augment the mortality the most in hospitals (in Paris, Berlin, and Vienna) are refused in English ones." Villermé, "Quelques réflexions sur les établissements de charité publique, à l'occasion d'un ouvrage de M. David Johnston," *Annales d'hygiène publique et de médecine légale* 3 (1830): 104–5. This same argument was repeatedly invoked to insulate these institutions from "unfair" comparisons of in-hospital mortality. See Husson, *Étude sur les hôpitaux*, 25–26, 258–59.

80. Anonymous, "Rapport sur les opérations du bureau central d'admissions dans les Hôpitaux, an XII," 5.

81. De Gerando, *Le visiteur*, 93–94.

82. Apollinaire Bouchardat, "Mémoire sur l'hygiène et la statistique des hôpitaux de Paris," *Annales d'hygiène publique et de médecine légale* 18 (1837): 345–46.

83. Charles-Polydore Forget, "Note à consulter pour la statistique médicale de Strasbourg, par M. Forget, professeur de la Faculté de médecine de Strasbourg," *Annales d'hygiène publique et de médecine légale* 23 (1840): 216–24 (quote is from p. 220).

84. Ibid., 221.

85. Orsel, *Essai*, 16.

86. Anonymous, "Rapport du service médicale de l'année 1835 fait par le Docteur Pertus, à L'Assemblée générale du Bureau de bienfaisance du 5e arrondissement de la ville de Paris, dans sa séance du 28 septembre 1836," 6.

87. Anonymous, "Bureau de bienfaisance du 13e arrondissement: Procès-verbale de l'Assemblé Générale du 4 juillet 1837 et compte moral et administratif de l'exercice 1836. Rapport du service médicale par Docteur Lemoine."

88. Both paralytics and the blind were understood to have a limited capacity to earn a living.

89. Orsel, *Essai*, 66.

90. For a worker in 1830, this was defined as age sixty-five or above. See Anonymous, *Manuel des commissaires et dames de charité* (Paris: Mme. Huzard, 1830), 13–14.

91. Ibid., 39–40.

92. "Relief this paltry seems a cruel and atrocious mockery for a poor soul who cannot see to his needs as a result of age, weakness, infirmity, or illness, especially when one imposes formalities, running around, and wasting of time that sometimes aggravate the condition of those requesting it. Assuaging miseries with so little

is not practicing true charity, but pretending to do so." Villermé, "Rapport fait à M. le Préfet de la Seine, président du conseil général des hospices, et à M.M. les membres de ce conseil par les commissaires des douze Bureaux de charité de Pari, dans sa séance du 3 novembre 1830. Notes du conseil général des hospices. Réponse des bureaux de charité à ces notes," *Annales d'hygiène publique et de médecine légale* 6 (1831): 219.

93. Anonymous, "Observations et propositions des douze Bureaux de bienfaisance de la Ville de Paris; présentées au Conseil Général des Hospices, dans la séance du 10 mai 1837," 16.

94. Anonymous, "Bureau de bienfaisance du 12e arrondissement: Procès-verbal de l'Assemblée général du 15 décembre 1838, et compte moral et administratif de l'exercice 1837. Rapport du Dr. Lemoine.," 21.

95. Anonymous, "Observations et propositions présentées au Conseil général des hospices de Paris: Dans la séance du mercredi 10 mai 1843, au nom des douze Bureaux de bienfaisance par M. Vée, Rapporteur," 8.

96. Antoine-Paul-Alphonse Vée, *Considérations sur le décroissement graduel du paupérisme à Paris, depuis le commencement du siècle et les causes des progrès moraux et économiques des classes ouvrières* (Paris: Guillaumin, 1862). This text also appeared in the prestigious *Journal des économistes* in November 1862.

97. Anonymous, "Compte moral et administratif du bureau de bienfaisance du 5e arrondissement de Paris, Présenté par M. Vée, adjoint au maire, à l'assemblée générale tenue le 13 juillet 1843," 15.

98. Interestingly, more was spent on nursing expenses (510 francs) than on medical fees (460 francs) or medications (300 francs). From Anonymous, "Année 1822: Discours de M le Compte de Ségur," *Les Prix de Vertu fondés par M. de Montyon. Discours prononcés à l'Académie Française. Réunis et publiés avec une notice sur M. De Montyon par Frédéric Lock et J. Couly D'Aragon*, vol. 1: 1819–1838 (Paris: Garnier Frères, 1858), 34–36.

99. Anonymous, "Observations et propositions des douze Bureaux de bienfaisance de la Ville de Paris; présentées au Conseil Général des Hospices, dans la séance du 10 mai 1837," 17.

100. Anonymous, "Rapport au Conseil Général des Hospices sur l'admission dans les hospices de Paris des vieillards et infirmes des communes rurales," Paris, 1845, 35–36.

## CHAPTER 10    CAUGHT BETWEEN INITIATIVE AND INERTIA: RESPONSES TO THE INCURABLY ILL FROM 1845 TO 1905

1. Robert Tombs, *France 1814–1914* (London: Longman, 1996), 378.

2. Smith, "The Ideology of Charity," 1010–12.

3. Anonymous, "Rapport au conseil général des hospices sur l'admission dans les hospices de Paris des vieillards et infirmes des communes rurales," 18.

4. Matthew Ramsey, "Public Health in France" in *Doctors, Politics and Society: Historical Essays*, ed. Dorothy Porter and Roy Porter (Amsterdam: Rodopi, 1993), 45–118.

5. Smith, *Creating the Welfare State*, 5–10, 21–23, 29–42.

6. Florence Bourillon, *Les villes en France au XIXe siècle* (Gap, France: Ophrys, 1992), 20–21; Bernard Marchand, *Paris, histoire d'une ville, XIXe–XXe siècle* (Paris: Seuil, 1993), 207, cited in Tombs, *France*, 185.

7. Anonymous, "Rapport au conseil général des hospices sur l'admission dans les hospices de Paris des vieillards et infirmes des communes rurales," Paris, 1845, 42; emphasis in the original.

8. Administration Général de l'Assistance Publique à Paris, "Nouveaux mode d'admission des malades dans les hôpitaux [Arrêté du 29 avril 1854]."

9. Roger Magraw, *France 1815–1914: The Bourgeois Century* (Oxford: Oxford University Press, 1986), 159–205.

10. Tombs, *France*, 397.

11. Magraw, *France*, 169.

12. Philip Nord, *The Republican Moment: Struggles for Democracy in Nineteenth-Century France* (Cambridge, MA: Harvard University Press, 1995).

13. Smith, "The Ideology of Charity," 1013.

14. Gabriel Cros-Mayrevieille, *Traité de l'assistance hospitalière* (Paris: Berger-Levrault, 1912), I: 319.

15. In 1869, the word "charity" was still synonymous with "Catholic." There were an estimated 9,000 nursing sisters working in France's hospitals and hospices, while established charities such as Saint-Vincent-de-Paul and Charité de Nevers societies together had 225 branches scattered account the country. Cros-Mayrevieille, *Traité de l'assistance hospitalière*, I: 319.

16. Magraw, *France 1815–1914*, 169.

17. Harris, *Lourdes*, 361.

18. Pierre Chaffanjon, *Les veuves et la charité. L'œuvre du Calvaire et sa fondatrice* (Lyon: Briday, 1872), 169.

19. Maxim du Camp, "La charité privé à Paris," *Revue des deux mondes* 57 (1883): 285, 299 (quote is from p. 299).

20. Harris, *Lourdes*, 287.

21. Kselman, *Miracles*.

22. Harris, *Lourdes*, 361.

23. Ibid., 287.

24. August Cochin, "Rapport à la Société d'Économie Charitable: Des secours aux indigents atteints d'infirmités incurables," *Annales de la Charité* (1859): 386

25. The census of 1851 indicated that out of a total population of nearly 36 million people, there were 44,970 people classified as insane, over 65,000 who were either blind or deaf-mute, 9,077 paralytics, 44,619 hunchbacks, 75,083 people with one eye, and 22,547 people with clubfeet. Cochin, "Rapport à la Société d'Économie Charitable," 390, 391.

26. Ibid., 392.

27. Ibid., 395.

28. Campagnole, *L'assistance obligatoire*, 10–11.

29. Anonymous, "Procès verbal de l'Assemblée générale du bureau de bienfaisance du cinquième arrondissement et compte moral et administratif de l'exercice 1835, Paris, 1836," 9–10; Anonymous, "Rapport à Monsieur le Préfet de la Seine et au Conseil Général des Hospices et des secours à domicile, présenté, au nom de MM. les Maires et adjoints, Présidents des Bureaux de bienfaisance, par. M. A. Lefort, Maire du 1er Arrondissement, séance du 4 mai 1836," 10.

30. Comtesse Agénor-Étienne de Gasparin, *Il y a des pauvres à Paris . . . et ailleurs, par l'auteur du mariage au point de vue chrétien* (Paris: L.-R. Delay, 1846), 34–37.

31. "Rapport et Projet de loi sur les hôpitaux et les hospices, présentés par M. de Melun (Nord), au nom de la commission d'assistance publique," 11.

32. Eugène Tallon, *Assemblée nationale. Annexe au procès-verbal de la séance du 17 juin 1873: Enquête parlementaire sur l'organisation de l'assistance publique dans les campagnes* (Versailles: Cerf et fils, Eugène Taller, 1873); *Rapport fait au nom de la commission chargée d'examiner les propositions: 1° de M. Lestourgie et plusieurs de ses collègues sur l'organisation de l'assistance dans les campagnes, 2° de M. Eugène Tallon sur l'assistance publique et l'extinction de la mendicité; 3° de MM. Théophile Roussel et Morvan sur l'organisation de l'assistance médicale dans les campagnes, . . . par M. Eugène Tallon, . . . (4 août 1874)* (Versailles: Cerf et fils, n.d.).

33. Du Camp, *Paris*, 152.

34. "Rapport présenté par M. Lafont, au nom de la 4e commission, sur un projet de vœu de M. Dubois et onze de ces collègues: Et tendant à la suppression du Bureau central des hôpitaux Annexe au procès-verbal de la séance du 30 janvier 1877."

35. "Lettre de M. Prieur de l'Hôtel-Dieu à Monsieur le Directeur Général de l'Assistance publique sur le sujet de l'installation à l'Hôtel-Dieu du service du Bureau central d'admission," letter dated 17 November 1875 from *Archives of the Parisian Assistance publique*, folio foss. 32.9–12.

36. It included Drs. Delpech, Cornil, Dujardin-Beaumetz, Rigal, and Duguet.

37. "Rapport présenté par M. Duguet au nom de la commission chargée par la société médicale des hôpitaux d'étudier les questions relatives à la suppression projetée du Bureau central des hôpitaux (Séance du 9 mars 1877)," 14–15.

38. Ibid., 12; emphasis in the original.

39. Ibid., 13.

40. Ibid., 12–13, 14.

41. The surgeons used the word *chronic* to refer to "those patients afflicted with a chronic medical or surgical condition that does not always keep them from working, but who are obliged to rest and often require certain care: these are consumptives, valetudinaries, those with stasis ulcers, etc." Dr. Nicaise, "Le bureau central des hôpitaux: Rapport présenté à la société des chirurgiens des hôpitaux au nom de la commission chargée d'étudier la question de la suppression du bureau central," 13–14, 14–15.

42. Ibid., 15.

43. Maurice Letulle, cited in Louis-Henri Petit, *De l'hospitalisation des tuberculeux d'après l'opinion des médecins des hôpitaux de Paris* (Paris: Masson, 1894), 5.

44. This observation was made during the discussion period of a paper presented at the conference. Petit, *De l'hospitalisation*, 44.

45. Ibid., 5.

46. Grancher, *Maladies*, 362–63.

47. Petit, *De l'hospitalisation*, 15 (emphasis in original).

48. Grancher, *Maladies*, 363.

49. "If the wards of our hospitals were no longer encumbered with consumptives, there would be no need to create new hospitals in Paris." Petit, *De l'hospitalisation des tuberculeux*, 28.

50. Ibid., 7–9.

51. Ibid., 28.

52. Ibid., 16.

53. Grancher, *Maladies*, 363.

54. "Circulaire du Ministère de l'intérieur, Direction de l'assistance et de l'hygiène publiques [3e Bureau]." Reproduced in Édouard Campagnole, *L'assistance médicale gratuite (commentaire de la loi du 15 juillet 1893)* (Paris: Berger-Levrault, 1894), 300.

55. Campagnole, *L'assistance obligatoire*, 9.

56. Ibid., 11.

57. Ellis, *The Physician-Legislators*, 223–25.

58. Campagnole, *L'assistance obligatoire*, 12, 16.

59. Maurice Larkin, *Church and State after the Dreyfuss Affair* (London: Macmillan, 1974), 1–4, 89.

60. Radicals and radical socialists won 233 of 589 seats in the Assembly.

61. Judith Stone, *Sons of the Revolution: Radical Democrats in France 1862–1914* (Baton Rouge: Louisiana State University, 1996), 265–66.

62. France, *Journal des débats* (27 May 1903), 1758–59 (M. Cazeneuve, MNA).

63. Judith Stone, *The Search for Social Peace: Reform Legislation in France, 1890–1914* (Albany: State University of New York Press, 1985), 39.

64. France, *Journal des débats* (27 May 1903), 1712 (Julien Goujon, MNA).

65. France, *Journal des débats* (5 June 1903), 1841 (Government envoy, National Assembly); France, *Journal des débats* (8 June 1905), 979 (Émile Labiche, President of the Senate).

66. In Belgium, for example, workers were entitled to claim their modest pension at age sixty-five. In France's case, essentially everyone accepted that it was better to offer a more generous pension beginning at age seventy as they felt that this would ensure that relief would be more effective while controlling costs by reducing the number of individuals in a position to apply.

67. Stone, *The Search*, 3.

68. Sanford Elwitt, *The Republic Defended: Bourgeois Reform in France, 1880–1914* (Baton Rouge: Louisiana State University Press, 1986), 1.

69. Stone, *The Search*, 30–33, 181–88.

70. Ellis, *The Physician-Legislators*, 175.

71. Smith, "The Ideology of Charity," 1025–26.

72. Barnes, *The Making*, 138–73, 215–46.

73. France, *Journal des débats* (8 June 1905), 974 (M. Guyot, senator).

74. "It is evident that the costs to the country will be more than considerable. We should not regret this, however. We have sought to put in place a reform long awaited by society, that, like Mr. Mirman has asserted, will be the greatest honor to the Republic *(Very good! Very good! On the left)*" France, *Journal des débats* (12 June 1903), 1903 (Emile Rey, MNA).

75. France, *Journal des débats* (9 June 1903), 1896 (Jean Jaurès, MNA).

76. Bienvenu-Martin, from Campagnole, *L'assistance obligatoire*, ix.

77. For but two examples, see France, *Journal des débats* (27 May 1903), 1752 (M. De Gailhard-Bancel, MNA); France, *Journal des débats* (27 May 1903), 1757 (Jules Auffray, MNA).

78. France, *Journal des débats* (29 May 1903), 1793 (Édouard Aynard, MNA).

79. See the exchange between Bienvenu-Martin and M. Jules Contant in the Assembly on June 11, 1903. France, *Journal des débats* (11 June 1903), 1915. The government's allies in the National Assembly repeatedly dared the opposition to vote against the draft legislation. It passed nearly unanimously. France, *Journal des débats* (12 June 1903), 1944–1945 (Charles Monod, Charitable Policy Committee Chair). See also France, *Journal des débats* (12 June 1903), 1975.

80. Bienvenue-Martin in Campagnole, *L'assistance obligatoire*, vii–viii.

81. The government took this matter so seriously that Interior Minister Emile Combes paid a personal visit to the chamber the day of the vote to call for the unanimous passage of the proposed law. See France, *Journal des débats* (15 June 1903), 1973.

82. Radicals had long wanted to abolish the Senate. By the early twentieth century, however, they made up the majority of senators and thus no longer saw the need to do so. Stone, *Sons of the Revolution*, 261.

83. Campagnole, *L'assistance obligatoire*, 42.

84. France, *Journal des débats* (27 May 1903), 1743–1744 (J. Thierry, MNA).

85. Jules Auffray insisted that the plan would likely cost between 60 and 100 million francs. France, *Journal des débats* (27 May 1903), 1757–1758 (Jules Auffray, MNA).

86. France, *Journal des débats* (8 June 1905), 981 (M. Sébline, senator).

87. The finance commissions predicted that the program's total new costs would be 66.7 million francs; the Commerce Ministry came up with the figure of 73 million francs. France, *Journal des débats* (8 June 1905), 981 (Finance committee chair, Senate); France, *Journal des débats* (8 June 1905), 982 (Government envoy, Senate).

88. The exact number was 48,996,000 francs. Bienvenu-Martin in Campagnole, *L'assistance obligatoire*, xii.

89. France, *Journal des débats* (12 June 1903), 1934.

90. Using the formula enshrined in the law on free medical assistance, the finance commission broke down the projected costs of a universal pension plan as follows: communes 31.3 million, departments 18.4 million, and the French state 17 million. France, *Journal des débats* (8 June 1905), 982 (Finance committee chair, Senate).

91. France, *Journal des débats* (9 June 1905), 994 (Milliès-Lacroix, senator).

92. France, *Journal des débats* (15 June 1903), 1976 (M. Borgnet, MNA).

93. France, *Journal des débats* (9 June 1905), 995 (M. Sébline, senator).

94. France, *Journal des débats* (29 May 1903), 1780 (Édouard Vaillant, MNA).

95. France, *Journal des débats* (27 May 1903), 1751 (Édouard Aynard, MNA).

96. France, *Journal des débats* (29 May 1903), 1789, 1791 (François Fournier, MNA); France, *Journal des débats* (29 May 1903), 1792 (M. Féron, MNA).

97. France, *Journal des débats* (4 June 1903), 1836–39.

98. France, *Journal des débats* (4 June 1903), 1838 (M. Defontaine, MNA).

99. France, *Journal des débats* (4 June 1903), 1829 (M. Aynard, MNA); France, *Journal des débats* (4 June 1903), 1830.

100. France, *Journal des débats* (11 June 1903), 1918–21.

101. While the way in which the amount of each pension was calculated was relatively complicated, revenue from personal savings or a worker's pension was to be taxed at a rate of 50 percent. By way of illustration, if the basic pension in a community was 120 francs per year, someone with outside revenue of 40 francs per year would have the amount he received from the state reduced by 20 francs to 100 per year (50 percent of 40 francs). The person of course remained better off than someone receiving a basic pension, earning 140 francs annually instead of 120.

In its original proposal, the government wished to tax private donations at a rate of 75 percent. If one uses the preceding example as a comparison, a "private" donation of 40 francs would trigger a 30-franc decrease in the state pension rather than 20 francs.

102. L. Larrivé, *L'assistance publique en France* (Paris: Alcan, 1899), 53–54.

103. Larkin, *Church and State*, 90–92, 102–16.

104. M. le commissaire du gouvernement, "Chambre des députées. Séance du 4 juin 1903," *Journal des débats*, 1903, 1843.

105. France, *Journal des débats* (16 June 1905), 1023.

106. Larkin, *Church and State*, 24.

107. Maxim du Camp, "La charité privée à Paris. I. Les petites-sœurs des pauvres," *Revue des deux mondes* 56 (1883): 519.

108. Ibid., 523.

## CONCLUSION

1. Récamier, "Traitement des malades inopérables et questions d'assistance," 191.

2. Ernest P. Boas and Nicholas Michelson, *The Challenge of Chronic Diseases* (New York: Macmillan, 1929), 8–9.

3. Gerald Grob, *The Deadly Truth: A History of Disease in America* (Cambridge, MA: Harvard University Press, 2002), 217–42.

4. Anonymous, "Announcement," *Journal of Chronic Disease* 1, no. 1 (January 1955): 1.

5. The term appeared in the Magnuson report and was reprinted in Anonymous, "Announcement," 4.

6. In preparing these concluding arguments, I've benefited from various discussions with George Weisz, who is currently preparing a transnational comparative history of chronic disease.

7. In each instance, the process by which they were legitimized was nearly as challenging professionally as it was scientifically. See John V. Pickstone, "Contested Cumulations: Configurations of Cancer Treatments through the Twentieth Century," *Bulletin of the History of Medicine* 81, no. 1 (2007): 164–96.

8. J. C. Gavey, *The Management of the Hopeless Case* (London: Lewis, 1952).

9. In 1939, Robert Le Bret noted, "Here's what happens with cancer patients: physicians declare themselves disarmed in most cases. They declare them 'incurable,' they are refused in the clinics. Hospitals, even specialized cancer hospitals, push them away." Quoted in Patrice Pinel, *Naissance d'un fléau: Histoire de la lutte contre le cancer en France, 1890–1940* (Paris: Métaillié, 1992), 239.

10. Cantor, "Cancer, Quackery, and the Vernacular Meanings of Hope in 1950s America," 333; 337–40.

11. Cicely Saunders, "Care of the Dying 1. The Problem of Euthanasia," *Nursing Times*, 9 October 1959, 960–61; "Care of the Dying 2. Should a Patient Know . . . ?," *Nursing Times*, 16 October 1959, 994–95; "Care of the Dying 3. Control of Pain in Terminal Cancer," *Nursing Times*, 23 October 1959, 1031–32; "Care of the Dying 4. Mental Distress in the Dying," *Nursing Times*, 30 October 1959, 1067–69; "Care of the Dying 5. The Nursing of Patients Dying of Cancer," *Nursing Times*, 6 November 1959, 1091–92. "Care of the Dying 6. When a Patient Is Dying," *Nursing Times*, 19 November 1959, 1129–30.

12. Barron H. Lerner, *The Breast Cancer Wars: Hope, Fear, and the Pursuit of a Cure in Twentieth-Century America* (Oxford: Oxford University Press, 2001).

13. For a compelling account of present-day end-of-life practices and decision making, see Sharon R. Kaufman, *And a Time to Die: How American Hospitals Shape the End of Life* (New York: Scribner, 2005).

# SELECT BIBLIOGRAPHY

Abel, Emily K. *Suffering in the Land of Sunshine: A Los Angeles Illness Narrative*. New Brunswick, NJ: Rutgers University Press, 2006.

Ackerknecht, Erwin. "Diathesis: The Word and the Concept in Medical History." *Bulletin of the History of Medicine* 56 (1982): 317–25.

———. *La médecine hospitalière à Paris*. Translated from English by Françoise Blateau. Paris: Payot, 1986.

Adams, Mark B., ed. *The Wellborn Science: Eugenics in Germany, France, Brazil, and Russia*. New York: Oxford University Press, 1990.

Anonymous. "Announcement." *Journal of Chronic Disease* I, no. I (1955): I–II.

Appel, Toby. *The Cuvier-Geoffroy Debate: French Biology in the Decades before Darwin*. Oxford: Oxford University Press, 1987.

Ariès, Philippe. *The Hour of Our Death*. Translated by Helen Weaver. New York: Oxford University Press, 1991.

Aronowitz, Robert A. *Unnatural History: Breast Cancer and American Society*. Cambridge: Cambridge University Press, 2007.

Bardet, Jean-Pierre, P. Bourdelais, P. Guillaume, and F. Lebrun. *Peurs et terreurs face à la contagion: Cholera, tuberculose, syphilis, xix$^e$–xx$^e$ siècles*. Paris: Fayard, 1988.

Barnes, David S. *The Making of a Social Disease: Tuberculosis in Nineteenth-Century France*. Berkeley: University of California Press, 1995.

Barthélemy-Maudale, Maurice. *Lamarck, the Mythical Precursor: A Study of the Relations between Science and Ideology*. Translated by M. H. Shank. Cambridge, MA: MIT Press, 1982.

Bataille, Georges. *Eroticism: Death and Sensuality*. Translated by M. Dalwood. San Francisco: City Light Books, 1986.

Bates, Barbara. *Bargaining for Life: A Social History of Tuberculosis, 1876–1938*. Philadelphia: University of Pennsylvania Press, 1992.

Becker, Ernest. *The Denial of Death*. New York: Free Press, 1973.

Becker, Howard Saul. *Outsiders: Studies on the Sociology of Deviance*. New York: Free Press, 1963.

Berridge, Virginia. *Opium and the People: Opiate Use and Drug Control Policy in Nineteenth and Early Twentieth Century England*, 2nd ed. London: Free Association Books, 1999.

Berlin, Isaiah. *The Roots of Romanticism*. Edited by H. Hardy. Princeton, NJ: Princeton University Press, 1999.

Beylard, H. "Mort (Congrégation de la Bonne Mort)." *Catholicisme: Hier, aujourd'hui, demain*. vol. 9. Paris: Letouzey et Ané, 1982.

Bogdan, Robert. *Freak Shows: Presenting Human Oddities for Amusement and Profit.* Chicago: University of Chicago Press, 1990.

Bosk, Charles L. *Forgive and Remember: Managing Medical Failure.* Chicago: University of Chicago Press, 1979.

Bourillon, Florence. *Les villes en France au XIXe siècle.* Gap: Ophrys, 1992.

Bowe, Frank G. *Handicapping America: Barriers to Disabled People.* New York: Harper and Row, 1978.

Bowler, Peter J. *Evolution: The History of an Idea.* Berkeley: University of California Press, 1989.

Brandt, Allen M. *No Magic Bullet: A Social History of Venereal Disease in the United States since 1880.* New York: Oxford University Press, 1985.

Braunstein, Jean-François. *Broussais et le matérialisme: Médecine et philosophie au XIXe siècle.* Paris: Méridiens Klincksieck, 1986.

Bryder, Linda. *Below the Magic Mountain: A Social History of Tuberculosis in Twentieth-Century Britain.* Oxford: Oxford University Press, 1988.

Bury, Michel. "Chronic Illness as Disruption." *Sociology of Health and Illness* 4, no. 2 (1982): 167–82.

———. "The Sociology of Chronic Illness: A Review of Research and Prospects." *Sociology of Health and Illness* 13, no. 4 (1991): 451–68.

Butel, Paul. *L'opium: Histoire d'une fascination.* Paris: Perrin, 1995.

Cantor, David. "Cancer, Quackery, and the Vernacular Meanings of Hope in 1950s America." *Journal of the History of Medicine and Allied Sciences* 61, no. 3 (2006): 324–68.

Chamberlin, J. Edward, and S. L. Gilman. *Degeneration: The Dark Side of Progress.* New York: Columbia University Press, 1985.

Charbit, Y. "The Fate of Malthus' Work." In J. Dupâquier, A. Fauve-Chamoux, and E. Grebenik, eds., *Malthus Past and Present,* 17–30. London: Academic Press, 1983.

Charmaz, Kathy. "Experiencing Chronic Illness." In G. Albrecht, R. Fitzpatrick, and S. Scrimshaw, eds., *Handbook of Social Studies in Health and Medicine.* London: Sage, 2000.

———. *Good Days, Bad Days: The Self in Chronic Illness and Time.* New Brunswick, NJ: Rutgers University Press, 1991.

———. "Identity Dilemmas of Chronically Ill Men." *Sociological Quarterly* 35, no. 2 (1994): 269–88.

Chevalier, Louis. *Laboring Classes and Dangerous Classes in Paris during the First Half of the Nineteenth Century.* Translated by F. Jellinek. New York: Howard Fertig, 1973.

Christakis, Nicholas A. *Death Foretold: Prophecy and Prognosis in Medical Care.* Chicago: University of Chicago Press, 1999.

Clow, Barbara. *Negotiating Disease: Power and Cancer Care, 1900–1950.* Montreal: McGill-Queen's University Press, 2001.

Coleman, William. *Death Is a Social Disease: Public Health and Political Economy in Early Industrial France.* Madison: University of Wisconsin Press, 1982.

Corbin, Alain. *The Foul and the Fragrant: Odor and the French Imagination.* Cambridge, MA: Harvard University Press, 1986.

———. "Hereditary Syphilis or the Impossible Redemption: A Contribution to the History of Morbid Heredity." *Time, Desire, and Horror: Towards a History of the Senses.* Translated by J. Birrell. Oxford: Polity Press, 1995.

———. *Women for Hire: Prostitution and Sexuality in France after 1850.* Cambridge, MA: Harvard University Press, 1990.

Corsi, Pietro. *The Age of Lamarck: Evolutionary Theories in France, 1790–1830.* Translated by J. Mandelbaum. Berkeley: University of California Press, 1988.

Courtwright, David T. *Dark Paradise: A History of Opiate Addiction in America.* Cambridge, MA: Harvard University Press, 2001.

Couser, G. Thomas. *Recovering Bodies: Illness, Disability, and Life Writing.* Madison: University of Wisconsin Press, 1997.

Cunningham, Andrew. "Transforming Plague: The Laboratory and the Identity of Infectious Disease." In A. Cunningham and P. Williams, eds., *The Laboratory Revolution in Medicine,* 209–44. Cambridge: Cambridge University Press, 1992.

Daniel, Thomas M. *Captain of Death: The Story of Tuberculosis.* Rochester, NY: University of Rochester Press, 1997.

Davidson, Iain, G. Woodhill, and E. Bredberg. "Images of Disability in Nineteenth-Century British Children's Literature." *Disability and Society* 9, no. 1 (1994): 33–46.

Davis, Fred. *Passage through Crisis: Polio Victims and Their Families.* Indianapolis: Bobbs-Merrill, 1963.

Davis, Lennard J. *Enforcing Normalcy: Disability, Deafness, and the Body.* New York: Verso, 1995.

Delvecchio Good, Mary-Jo, and B. J. Good. "Clinical Narratives and the Study of Contemporary Doctor-Patient Relationships." In G. L. Albrecht, R. Fitzpatrick, and S. C. Scrimshaw, eds., *Handbook of Social Studies in Health and Medicine.* London: Sage, 2000.

Delvecchio Good, Mary-Jo, et al. "American Oncology and the Discourse of Hope." *Culture, Medicine, and Society* 14 (1990): 59–79.

Duffin, Jacalyn. *To See with a Better Eye: A Life of R.T.H. Laënnec.* Princeton: Princeton University Press, 1998.

Duprat, Catherine. *Pour l'amour de l'humanité: Le temps des philanthropes. La philanthropie parrisienne des Lumières à la monarchie de Juillet.* Paris: Ed. du CTHS, 1993.

Ehrenreich, Barbara, and Deirdre English. *For Her Own Good: 150 Years of the Experts' Advice to Women.* Garden City, NY: Anchor Press, 1978.

Ellis, Jack D. *The Physician-Legislators of France: Medicine and Politics in the Early Third Republic.* Cambridge: Cambridge University Press, 1990.

Elwitt, Sanford. *The Third Republic Defended: Bourgeois Reform in France, 1880–1914.* Baton Rouge: Louisiana State University Press, 1986.

Evans, Martha Noel. *Fits and Starts: A Genealogy of Hysteria in Modern France.* Ithaca, NY: Cornell University Press, 1991.

Farmer, Paul. "Social Scientists and the New Tuberculosis." *Social Sciences of Medicine* 44, no. 3 (1997): 347–58.

Faure, Olivier. *Genèse de l'hôpital moderne: Les Hospices Civils de Lyon de 1802 à 1845.* Lyon: Presses Universitaire de Lyon, 1982.

———. "L'hôpital et les incurables au XIXe siècle: L'exemple de Lyon." *Les cahiers du CTNE-RHI* 50 (1990).

Feifel, Herman. "Epilogue." In H. Feifel, ed. *New Meanings of Death.* New York: McGraw-Hill, 1977.

Feldberg, Georgina D. *Disease and Class: Tuberculosis and the Shaping of Modern North American Society.* New Brunswick, NJ: Rutgers University Press, 1995.

Feudtner, John C. *Bittersweet: Diabetes, Insulin, and the Transformation of Illness.* Chapel Hill: University of North Carolina Press, 2003.

Forrest, Alan. *The French Revolution and the Poor.* Oxford: Blackwell, 1981.

Foucault, Michel. *The Birth of the Clinic: An Archaeology of Medical Perceptions.* New York: Vintage, 1994.

Fox, Renée-Claire. *Experiment Perilous: Physicians and Patients Facing the Unknown.* Glencoe, IL: Free Press, 1959.

Fox, Renée C., and Judith P. Swazey. *The Courage to Fail: A Social View of Organ Transplants and Dialysis.* Chicago: University of Chicago Press, 1974.

———. *The Courage to Fail: A Social View of Organ Transplants and Dialysis,* 2nd ed. Chicago: University of Chicago Press, 1978.

Foxcroft, Louise. *The Making of Addiction: The "Use and Abuse" of Opium in Nineteenth-Century Britain.* Aldershot, UK: Ashgate, 2007.

Frank, Arthur. *At the Will of the Body: Reflections on Illness.* Boston: Houghton Mifflin, 2002.

Freidson, Eliot. "Disability as Social Deviance." In M. B. Sussman, ed., *Sociology and Rehabilitation.* Washington, DC: American Sociological Association, 1965.

———. *Profession of Medicine: A Study of the Sociology of Applied Knowledge.* New York: Dodd, Mead, 1974.

Fuchs, Rachel Ginnis. *Abandoned Children: Foundlings and Child Welfare in Nineteenth-Century France.* Albany: State University of New York Press, 1984.

Fulton, Robert Lester. *Death, Grief, and Bereavement: A Bibliography, 1845–1975.* New York: Arno, 1977.

Gardner, Kirsten Elizabeth. *Early Detection: Women, Cancer, and Awareness Campaigns in the Twentieth-Century United States.* Chapel Hill: University of North Carolina Press, 2006.

Garfinkel, Susan. "'This Trial Was Sent in Love and Mercy for My Refinement': A Quaker Woman's Experience of Breast Cancer Surgery in 1814." In J. W. Leavitt, ed., *Women and Health in America,* 2nd ed. Madison: University of Wisconsin Press, 1999.

Garland-Thomson, Rosemarie, ed. *Freakery: Cultural Spectacles of the Extraordinary Body.* New York: New York University Press, 1997.

Gartner, Alan, and T. Joe, eds. *Images of the Disabled, Disabling Images.* New York: Praeger, 1987.

Gaudillière, Jean-Paul, and I. Löwy, eds. *Heredity and Infection: The History of Disease Transmission.* London: Routledge, 2001.

Gavey, C. J. *The Management of the Hopeless Case.* London: Lewis, 1952.

Geison, Gerald L. *The Private Science of Louis Pasteur.* Princeton, NJ: Princeton University Press, 1995.

Gilman, Sander L. *Disease and Representation: Images of Illness from Madness to AIDS.* Ithaca, NY: Cornell University Press, 1988.

Gilpin-Faust, Drew. *The Republic of Suffering: Death and the American Civil War.* New York: Knopf, 2008.

Glaser, Barney G., and Anselm L. Strauss. *Anguish: A Case History of a Dying Trajectory.* Mill Valley, CA: Sociology Press, 1970.

———. *Awareness of Dying.* Chicago: Aldine, 1965.

Glenn, Evelyn. "Citizenship and Inequality: Historical and Global Perspectives." *Social Forces* 47 (2000): 1–20.

Goetz, Christopher G., M. Bonduelle, and T. Gelfand. *Charcot: Constructing Neurology.* New York: Oxford University Press, 1995.

Goffman, Erving. *Asylums: Essays on the Social Situation of Mental Patients and Other Inmates.* Chicago: Aldine, 1961.

———. *The Presentation of Self in Everyday Life.* Garden City, NY: Doubleday, 1959.

————. *Stigma: Notes on the Management of Spoiled Identity*. Englewood Cliffs, NJ: Prentice-Hall, 1963.

Golden, Richard L. "Sir William Osler: Humanist and Thanatologist." *OMEGA: Journal of Death and Dying* 36 (1997–98): 241–58.

Good, Byron. *Medicine, Rationality, and Experience*. Cambridge: Cambridge University Press, 1994.

Grabar, Sophie, et al. "Factors Associated with Clinical and Virological Failure in Patients Receiving a Triple Therapy Including a Protease Inhibitor." *AIDS* 14, no. 2 (2000): 141–49.

Greene, Jeremy A. *Prescribing by Numbers: Drugs and the Definition of Disease*. Baltimore: Johns Hopkins University Press, 2007.

Grob, Gerald *The Deadly Truth: A History of Disease in America*. Cambridge, MA: Harvard University Press, 2002.

Guillaume, Pierre. *Du désespoir au salut: Les tuberculeux aux XIXe et XXe siècles*. Paris: Aubier, 1986.

————. *Médecins, église et foi XIXe–XXe siècles*. Paris: Aubier, 1990.

Guillaumin, Émile. *The Life of a Simple Man*. Hanover, NH: University Press of New England, 1983.

Harrington, Anne. *The Cure Within: A History of Mind-Body Medicine*. New York: Norton, 2008.

Harris, Ruth. *Lourdes: Body and Spirit in the Secular Age*. London: Allen Lane, 1999.

————. *Murders and Madness: Medicine, Law, and Society in the Fin de Siècle*. Oxford: Clarendon Press, 1989.

Hecht, Jennifer Michael. "French Scientific Materialism and the Liturgy of Death: The Invention of a Secular Version of Catholic Last Rites, 1876–1914." *French Historical Studies* 20, no. 4 (1997): 703–35.

Herzlich, Claudine, and Janine Pierret. *Illness and Self in Society*. Translated by E. Forster. Baltimore: Johns Hopkins University Press, 1987.

Hodgson, Barbara. *In the Arms of Morpheus: The Tragic History of Laudanum, Morphine, and Patent Medicine*. Vancouver: Greystone Books, 2001.

Hughes, Everett C. "Dilemmas and Contradictions of Status." *American Journal of Sociology* 50 (1945): 353–59.

Huguet, Françoise. *Les professeurs de la faculté de médecine de Paris, dictionnaire biographique, 1794–1939*. Paris: Institut national de recherche pédagogique, editions du CNRS, 1991.

Hunter, Tera W. *To Joy My Freedom: Southern Black Women's Lives and Labors after the Civil War*. Cambridge, MA: Harvard University Press, 1997.

Hutton, Patrick. *The Cult of the Revolutionary Tradition: The Blanquists in French Politics, 1864–1893*. Berkeley: University of California Press, 1981.

Huxley, Thomas Henry. "On the Reception of the Origin of Species." In F. Darwin, ed., *Life and Letters of Charles Darwin*, vol. 1. New York: D. Appleton, 1925.

Jones, Colin. *The Charitable Imperative: Hospitals and Nursing in Ancien Régime and Revolutionary France*. London: Routledge, 1989.

————. "Plague and Its Metaphors in Early Modern France." *Representations* 53 (Winter 1996): 97–127.

Kaufman, Suzanne. "Miracles, Medicine, and the Spectacle of Lourdes." Ph.D. dissertation, Rutgers University, 1996.

Kaufman, Sharon. R. *And a Time to Die: How American Hospitals Shape the End of Life*. New York: Scribner, 2005.

Kearney, Michael. *A Place of Healing: Working with Suffering in Living and Dying.* Oxford: Oxford University Press, 2000.

Kelly, Michael. "Self, Identity, and Radical Surgery." *Sociology of Health and Illness* 14, no. 3 (1992): 390–415.

Kelly, Michael, and D. Field. "Medical Sociology, Chronic Illness, and the Body." *Sociology of Health and Illness* 18 (1996): 241–57.

Kevles, Daniel J. *In the Name of Eugenics: Genetics and the Uses of Human Heredity.* New York: Knopf, 1985.

Kleinman, Arthur. *The Illness Narratives: Suffering, Healing, and the Human Condition.* New York: Basic Books, 1988.

Kleinman, Arthur, V. Das, and M. Locke, eds. *Social Suffering.* Berkeley: University of California Press, 1997.

Kraut, Alan M. *Silent Travelers: Germs, Genes, and the Immigrant Menace.* Baltimore: Johns Hopkins University Press, 1994.

Kristeva, Julia. "Holbein's Dead Christ." In M. Fehr, ed., *Fragments of a Human Body,* part I. New York: Zone, 1989.

Kselman, Thomas A. *Death and the Afterlife in Modern France.* Princeton, NJ: Princeton University Press, 1993.

———. *Miracles and Prophecies in Nineteenth-Century France.* New Brunswick, NJ: Rutgers University Press, 1983.

Kudlick, Catherine J. "Disability History: Why We Need Another 'Other.'" *American Historical Review* 108, no. 3 (2003): 763–93.

Kushner, Howard I. "Taking Biology Seriously: The Next Task for Historians of Addiction?" *Bulletin of the History of Medicine* 80, no. 2 (2006): 115–43.

Kusow, Abdi M. "Contesting Stigma: On Goffman's Assumptions of Normative Order." *Symbolic Interaction* 27, no. 2 (2004): 179–97.

Larkin, Maurice. *Church and State after the Dreyfus Affair.* London: Macmillan, 1974.

Latour, Bruno. *The Pasteurization of France.* Translated by A. Sheridan and J. Law. Cambridge, MA: Harvard University Press, 1988.

Lawlor, Clark, and Akihoto Suzuki. "The Disease of the Self: Representing Consumption, 1700–1830." *Bulletin of the History of Medicine* 74, no. 3 (2000): 458–94.

Lederer, Susan E. "Dark Victory: Cancer and Popular Hollywood Film." *Bulletin of the History of Medicine* 81, no. 1 (2007): 94–115.

Lellouch, A. "Mortalité, espérance de vie et morbidité dans les hospices parisiens du XIXe." *Histoire des sciences médicales* 23, no. 2 (1989).

Léonard, Jacques. "Les guérisseurs en France au XIXe siècle." *Revue d'histoire moderne et contemporaine* 27 (1980): 501–16.

———. *La médecine entre les savoirs et les pouvoirs: Histoire intellectuelle et politique de la médecine française au XIXe siècle.* Paris: Aubier Montaigne, 1982.

———. *Médecins, malades, et société dans la France du XIXe siècle.* Paris: Sciences en situation, 1992.

———. *La vie quotidienne du médecin de province au XIXe siècle.* Paris: Hachette, 1977.

Lerner, Barron. *The Breast Cancer Wars: Hope, Fear, and the Pursuit of a Cure in Twentieth-Century America.* Oxford: Oxford University Press, 2001.

Link, Bruce G., and J. C. Phelan. "Conceptualizing Stigma." *Annual Review of Sociology* 27 (2001): 363–85.

Mackaman, Douglas Peter. *Leisure Settings: Bourgeois Culture, Medicine, and the Spa in Modern France.* Chicago: University of Chicago Press, 1998.

Magraw, Roger. *France 1815–1914: The Bourgeois Century.* Oxford: Oxford University Press, 1986.

Mann, Thomas. *The Magic Mountain: A Novel.* New York: Knopf, 1996.

Marchand, Bernard. *Paris: Histoire d'une ville, XIXe–XXe siècle.* Paris: Seuil, 1993.

Martin, Emily. *The Woman in the Body: A Cultural Analysis of Reproduction.* Boston: Beacon Press, 1987.

Matthews, J. Rosser. *Quantification and the Quest for Medical Certainty.* Princeton, NJ: Princeton University Press, 1995.

McGann, Jerome J. *The Romantic Ideology: A Critical Investigation.* Chicago: University of Chicago Press, 1983.

McKeown, Thomas. *The Modern Rise of Population.* London: Edward Arnold, 1976.

McManners, John. *Death and the Enlightenment: Changing Attitudes to Death among Christians and Unbelievers in Eighteenth-Century France.* Oxford: Oxford University Press, 1981.

Mendelsohn, J. Andrew. "Medicine and the Making of Bodily Inequality in Twentieth-Century Europe." In J.-P. Gaudrillière and I. Löwy, eds., *Heredity and Infection: The History of Disease Transmission,* 21–79. London: Routledge, 2001.

Micale, Mark S. "On the 'Disappearance' of Hysteria: A Study in the Clinical Deconstruction of a Diagnosis." *Isis* 84, no. 3 (1993): 496–526.

Micale, Mark S., and P. Lerner, eds. *Traumatic Pasts: History, Psychiatry, and Trauma in the Modern Age, 1870–1930.* Cambridge: Cambridge University Press, 2001.

Mitchinson, Wendy. "Gynecological Operations on Insane Women: London, Ontario, 1895–1901." *Journal of Social History* 15 (2001): 467–84.

Mitchell, David T., and S. L. Snyder, eds. *The Body and Physical Difference: Discourses of Disability.* Ann Arbor: University of Michigan Press, 1997.

Morantz-Sanchez, Regina Markell. *Conduct Unbecoming a Woman: Medicine on Trial in Turn-of-the-Century Brooklyn.* New York: Oxford University Press, 1999.

Moscucci, O. *The Science of Woman: Gynaecology and Gender in England, 1800–1929.* Cambridge: Cambridge University Press, 1990.

Mueller, Paul S. "William Osler's Study of the Act of Dying: An Analysis of the Original Data." *Journal of Medical Biography* 15, supplement 1 (2007): 55–63.

Murard, Lion, and Patrick Zylberman. *L'hygiène dans la République: La santé publique en France ou l'utopie contrariée 1870–1918.* Paris: Fayard, 1996.

Murphy, Terence D. "Medical Knowledge and Statistical Methods in Early Nineteenth-Century France." *Medical History* 25 (1981): 301–19.

Musto, David F. *The American Disease: Origins of Narcotic Control.* New Haven: Yale University Press, 1973.

Nagi, Saad Zaghloub. *Disability and Rehabilitation: Legal, Clinical, and Self-Concepts and Measurements.* Columbus: Ohio State University Press, 1970.

Nord, Philip. *The Republican Moment: Struggles for Democracy in Nineteenth-Century France.* Cambridge, MA: Harvard University Press, 1995.

Nye, Robert A. *Crime, Madness, and Politics in Modern France: The Medical Concept of National Decline.* Princeton, NJ: Princeton University Press, 1984.

———. *Masculinity and Male Codes of Honour in Modern France.* Oxford: Oxford University Press, 1993.

Oliver, Michael. *Disabled People and Social Policy: From Exclusion to Inclusion.* London: Longman, 1998.

Oppenheim, Janet. *Shattered Nerves: Doctors, Patients, and Depression in Victorian England.* New York: Oxford University Press, 1991.

Ott, Katherine. *Fevered Lives: Tuberculosis in American Culture since 1870*. Cambridge, MA: Harvard University Press, 1996.

Patterson, James T. *The Dread Disease: Cancer and Modern American Culture*. Cambridge, MA: Harvard University Press, 1987.

Paul, Harry W. *The Edge of Contingency: French Catholic Reaction to Scientific Change from Darwin to Duhem*. Gainesville: University Presses of Florida, 1979.

Pelling, Marageret. *Cholera, Fever, and English Medicine, 1825–1865*. Oxford: Oxford University Press, 1978.

Pernick, Martin S. *A Calculus of Suffering: Pain, Professionalism, and Anesthesia in Nineteenth-Century America*. New York: Columbia University Press, 1985.

Persell, Stuart Michael. *Neo-Lamarckism and the Evolution Controversy in France, 1870–1920*. Lewiston, ME: Edwin Mellen Press, 1999.

Peyre, Henri. *Qu'est-ce que le Romantisme?* Paris: Presses universitaires de France, 1971.

Pick, Daniel. *Faces of Degeneration: A European Disorder, circa 1848–1918*. Cambridge: Cambridge University Press, 1993.

Pickstone, John. "Bureaucracy, Liberalism, and the Body in Post-Revolutionary France: Bichat's Physiology and the Paris School of Medicine." *History of Science* 19 (1981): 115–42.

———. "Contested Cumulations: Configurations of Cancer Treatments through the Twentieth Century." *Bulletin of the History of Medicine* 81, no. 1 (2007): 164–96.

Pinell, Patrice. *Naissance d'un fléau histoire de la lutte contre le cancer en France (1890–1940)*. Paris: Métaillé, 1992.

Porter, R. "Pain and Suffering." In W. F. Bynum and R. Porter, eds., *Companion Encyclopedia of the History of Medicine*, vol. 2. London: Rutledge, 1993.

Porter, Roy, and G. S. Rousseau. *Gout: The Patrician Malady*. New Haven: Yale University Press, 1998.

Proctor, Robert N. *Cancer Wars: How Politics Shapes What We Know and Don't Know about Cancer*. New York: Basic Books, 1995.

———. *The Nazi War on Cancer*. Princeton, NJ: Princeton University Press, 1999.

———. *Racial Hygiene: Medicine Under the Nazis*. Cambridge, MA: Harvard University Press, 1988.

Ramsey, M. "Academic Medicine and Medical Industrialism: The Regulation of Secret Remedies in Nineteenth-Century France." In A. La Berge and M. Feingold, eds., *French Medical Culture in the Nineteenth Century*, 25–78. Amsterdam: Rodopi, 1994.

———. "Alternative Medicine in Modern France." *Medical History* 43, no. 3 (1999): 286–322.

———. *Professional and Popular Medicine in France, 1770–1830: The Social World of Medical Practice*. Cambridge: Cambridge University Press, 1988.

Rey, Roselyne. *The History of Pain*. Translated by L. E. Wallace, J. A. Cadden, and S. W. Cadden. Cambridge, MA: Harvard University Press, 1995.

Richey, W. "Boycott Groups: Klein Ads Carry Scent of Heroin Chic." *Christian Science Monitor*. October 25, 1996.

Riessman, Catherine. "Stigma and Everyday Resistance Practices: Childless Women in South India." *Gender and Society* 14 (2000): 111–35.

Rimlinger, Gaston V. *Welfare Policy and Industrialization in Europe, America, and Russia*. New York: Wiley, 1971.

Risse, Guenther B. *Mending Bodies, Saving Souls: A History of Hospitals*. New York: Oxford University Press, 1999.

Rosenberg, Charles E. "Banishing Risk: Continuity and Change in the Moral Management of Disease." In A. M. Brandt and P. Rozin, eds., *Morality and Health*. London: Routledge, 1997.

———. "The Bitter Fruit: Heredity, Disease, and Social Thought." In *No Other Gods: On Science and American Social Thought*, 2nd ed. Baltimore: Johns Hopkins University Press, 1987.

———. *The Care of Strangers: The Rise of America's Hospital System*. Baltimore: Johns Hopkins University Press, 1987.

———. *The Cholera Years: The United States in 1832, 1849, and 1866*. Chicago: University of Chicago Press, 1962.

———. "Pathologies of Progress: The Idea of Civilization at Risk." *Bulletin of the History of Medicine* 72 (1998): 714–30.

———. "The Therapeutic Revolution: Medicine, Meaning, and Social Change in Nineteenth-Century America." *Perspectives in Biology and Medicine* 20 (1977): 485–506.

Roth, Julius A. *Timetables*. New York: Bobbs-Merrill, 1963.

Rothman, Sheila. *Living in the Shadow of Death: Tuberculosis and the Social Experience of Illness in American History*. New York: Basic Books, 1994.

Saunders, Ciecly. "Care of the Dying 1: The Problem of Euthanasia." *Nursing Times* (October 9, 1959): 960–61.

———. "Care of the Dying 2: Should a Patient Know . . . ?" *Nursing Times* (October 16, 1959): 994–95.

———. "Care of the Dying 3: Control of Pain in Terminal Cancer." *Nursing Times* (October 23, 1959): 1031–32.

———. "Care of the Dying 4: Mental Distress in the Dying." *Nursing Times* (October 30, 1959): 1067–69.

———. "Care of the Dying 5: The Nursing of Patients Dying of Cancer." *Nursing Times* (November 6, 1959): 1091–92.

———. "Care of the Dying 6: When a Patient Is Dying." *Nursing Times* (November 19, 1959): 1129–30.

Scambler, Graham, and A. Hopkins. "Being Epileptic: Coming to Terms with Stigma." *Sociology of Health and Illness* 8, no. 1 (1986): 26–43.

Schiller, Francis. *Paul Broca: Founder of French Anthropology, Explorer of the Brain*. Berkeley: University of California Press, 1979.

Schneider, William H. "The Eugenics Movement in France 1890–1940." In M. B. Adams, ed., *The Wellborn Science: Eugenics in Germany, France, Brazil, and Russia*. New York: Oxford University Press, 1990.

Shakespeare, Tom. "Cultural Representations of Disabled People: Dustbins for Disavowal." *Disability and Society* 9, no. 3 (1994): 283–99.

Smith, Timothy B. *Creating the Welfare State in France, 1880–1940*. Montreal: McGill-Queens University Press, 2003.

———. "The Ideology of Charity, the Image of the English Poor Law, and Debates over the Right to Assistance in France, 1830–1905." *Historical Journal* 40, no. 4 (1997): 997–1032.

Sontag, Susan. *Illness as Metaphor*. New York: Random House, 1979.

Stebbins, Robert E. "France." In T. F. Glick, ed., *The Comparative Reception of Darwinism*. Austin: University of Texas Press, 1972.

Stiker, Henri-Jacques. *A History of Disability*. Translated by W. Sayers. Ann Arbor: University of Michigan Press, 1993.

Stone, Judith. *The Search for Social Peace: Reform Legislation in France, 1890–1914.* Albany: State University of New York Press, 1985.

———. *Sons of the Revolution. Radical Democrats in France 1862–1914.* Baton Rouge: Louisiana State University, 1996.

Strauss, Anselm L. *Chronic Illness and the Quality of Life.* St. Louis: Mosby, 1975.

Strauss, Anselm L., and J. Corbin, et al. *Chronic Illness and the Quality of Life,* 2nd ed. St. Louis: Mosby, 1984.

Szreter, Simon. "The Importance of Social Intervention in Britain's Mortality Decline, c. 1850–1914: A Reinterpretation of the Role of Public Health." *Social History of Medicine* 1 (1988): 1–37.

Thomas, Keith. *Religion and the Decline of Magic.* New York: Scribner, 1971.

Tombs, Robert. *France 1814–1914.* London: Longman, 1996.

Tomes, Nancy. *The Gospel of Germs: Men, Women, and the Microbe in American Life.* Cambridge, MA: Harvard University Press, 1998.

Tone, Andrea. *Devices and Desires: A History of Contraceptives in America.* New York: Hill and Wang, 2001.

Turner, Bryan S. *The Body and Society.* Oxford: Blackwell, 1984.

Twitchell, James B. *The Living Dead: A Study of the Vampire in Romantic Literature.* Durham, NC: Duke University Press, 1981.

Von Bueltzingloewen, Isabelle. *Machines à instruire, machines à guérir: Les hôpitaux universitaires et la médicalisation de la société allemande 1730–1850.* Lyon: Presses universitaires de Lyon, 1997.

Vovelle, Michel. *La mort et l'occident: De 1300 à nos jours.* Paris: Gallimard, 1983.

Waddington, Ivan. "The Role of the Hospital in the Development of Modern Medicine: A Sociological Analysis." *Sociology* 72 (1973): 211–24.

Wainwright, L. "Profound Lesson for the Living." *Life,* November 21, 1969, 36–43.

Waksman, Selman A. *The Conquest of Tuberculosis.* Berkeley: University of California Press, 1964.

Warner, John H. *Against the Spirit of System: The French Impulse in Nineteenth-Century American Medicine.* Princeton, NJ: Princeton University Press, 1998.

———. *The Therapeutic Perspective: Medical Practice, Knowledge, and Identity in America, 1820–1885.* Cambridge, MA: Harvard University Press, 1986.

Weiner, Dora B. *The Citizen-Patient in Revolutionary and Imperial Paris.* Baltimore: Johns Hopkins University Press, 1993.

Weisz, George. *The Medical Mandarins: The French Academy of Medicine in the Nineteenth and Early Twentieth Centuries.* New York: Oxford University Press, 1995.

Williams, Elizabeth A. *A Cultural History of Medical Vitalism in Enlightenment Montpellier.* Aldershot, UK: Ashgate, 2003.

Williams, G. "Theorizing Disability." In G. L. Albrecht, K. D. Seelman and M. Bury, eds., *Handbook of Disability Studies.* Thousand Oaks, Calif.: Sage, 2000.

Williams, Simon J. "Chronic Illness as Biographical Disruption or Biological Disruption as Chronic Illness? Reflections on a Core Concept." *Sociology of Health and Illness* 22, no. 1 (2000): 40–67.

Wohl, Anthony S. *Endangered Lives: Public Health in Victorian Britain.* Cambridge, MA: Harvard University Press, 1983.

Wood, Ann D. "The Fashionable Diseases: Women's Complaints and Their Treatment in Nineteenth-Century America." *Journal of Interdisciplinary History* 4, no. 1 (1973): 25–52.

Worboys, Michael. *Spreading Germs: Disease Theories and Medical Practice in Britain 1865–1900*. New York: Cambridge University Press, 2000.

Yvorel, Jean-Jacques. *Les poisons de l'esprit. Drogues et drogués au XIXe siècle*. Paris: Quai Voltaire, 1992.

Zeldin, Theodore. *France 1848–1945*, vol. I. Oxford: Clarendon Press, 1973.

Zola, Irving K. "Bringing Our Bodies and Ourselves Back In: Reflections on the Past, Present, and Future Medical Sociology." *Journal of Health and Social Behaviour* 32 (1991): 1–16.

———. *Ordinary Lives: Voices of Disability and Disease*. Cambridge, MA: Applewood, 1982.

Zweig, Stefan. *The World of Yesterday*. Lincoln: University of Nebraska Press, 1964.

# INDEX

abandonment, 11, 80, 91, 107–12, 120, 130–31, 134, 152, 157; of the pope by France, 170, 201
Académie Française: *Prix de vertu*, 81
Academy of Medicine: French/Paris/Royal, 20, 21, 30–33, 35, 41, 44, 51, 68, 81, 92, 96, 103, 114, 121, 127, 129, 171; of Lyon, 21
Academy of Sciences, 66; of Bordeaux, 151
acute illnesses, 1–3, 5, 9, 17–18, 27, 92, 97, 191, 207
acquired immunodeficiency syndrome (AIDS), 1, 55, 216; iconography of, 77–78
addiction, 12, 40, 69, 77, 136–40, 143–48, 151, 153–55, 172; among doctors, 145, 152; among literati, 144
*Adélaïde Perrin et les jeunes filles incurables*, 70
AIDS. *See* acquired immunodeficiency syndrome
Albutt, Clifford, 140
alcoholism, 40, 58, 60–61, 64, 67, 69, 143–45, 154, 183, 205, 212
Alibert, Jean, 59, 62
alternative medicine, 8, 11, 16, 34–35, 62, 93–94, 98, 107, 125–31, 141
ambiguity, 10, 84, 115–16, 120, 156. *See also* prognosis
Amussat, Jean-Zuléma, 31
anatomico-pathology/pathologists, 19–23, 36, 38, 40, 46, 54, 96, 192; Catholicism and, 24–25
ancien régime, 176–77, 187–88, 200
Andral, Gabriel, 27, 92
anesthesia, 33, 49, 121, 155, 158
Anthropological Society of Paris, 60
antibiotics, 2, 4, 42, 48, 83, 116, 216
anticlericalism, 24, 118–19, 133, 158, 168–70, 183, 202, 213–15
Ariès, Philippe, 5, 89, 191
Association de la Bonne Mort, 157, 163–67, 170
Auber, Edouard, 97
Aubergier, Hector, 139–40

Audin-Rouvière, Dr., 93, 100
Aurelianus, Coelius, 92
autopsy/dissection, 17, 19–20, 22, 28, 43–44, 47, 87, 97, 170, 179, 192

bacillus, tubercle, 5–6, 43, 45, 69, 84–85, 96, 205
bacteriology, 43, 83–85, 118
Balzac, Honoré de, 76–77
Ball, Benjamin, 68, 110, 144, 148, 153, 168
Barrier, Jean, 96
Bashkirtseff, Marie, 73
Bataille, Georges, 89
Bayle, Gaspard, 19–23, 27, 31, 36, 128
Beard, George, 153
Becker, Howard, 78
Béhier, Louis-Jules, 138, 167
Benoit, Dr., 34
Berlioz, Hector, 129
Bertrand, Dr. Amédée, 117–18
Bichat, Xavier, 24
Bernard, Claude, 29
Bourchardat, Apollinaire, 41, 192
Bouvart, Michel Philip, 35
Brouardel, Paul, 148
Brierre de Boismont, Alexandre, 80, 106
Broca, Paul, 25, 33, 60, 130
Broussais, François-Joseph-Victor, 2, 3, 24–28, 30, 35, 38–40, 60, 65, 103, 117; *Histoire des phlegmasies chroniques*, 103; "Napoleon of medicine," 24; therapeutic system, 23–28, 40
Broussaisism, 23–27, 30, 38
Buchez, Philippe, 64

cancer, 3–4, 55–56; breast, 6, 30–33, 53, 96, 106, 116; causes of, 21–23, 25, 40, 42, 49, 58–61, 63; cervical/uterine, 21, 49–53, 63, 77, 84, 105, 121, 146, 150, 194; contagion and, 84–85; degeneration and, 65, 67–68; demographic importance of, 3, 61, 63; Hollywood and, 89; incurability of, 15–22, 26, 30–32, 36–37, 41, 53, 56, 96, 108;

# ABOUT THE AUTHOR

**DR. JASON SZABO** has been involved in AIDS care and clinical research at McGill University since 1991. He also received a Ph.D. in history from McGill followed by postdoctoral training at Harvard University. His research focuses on the history of chronic disease and other complex illness experiences. He recently received a multiyear research fellowship from the Canadian Institutes of Health Research to write a history of the AIDS epidemic. He lives in Montreal with his two children.